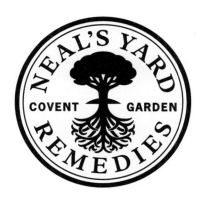

COMPLETE
WELLNESS

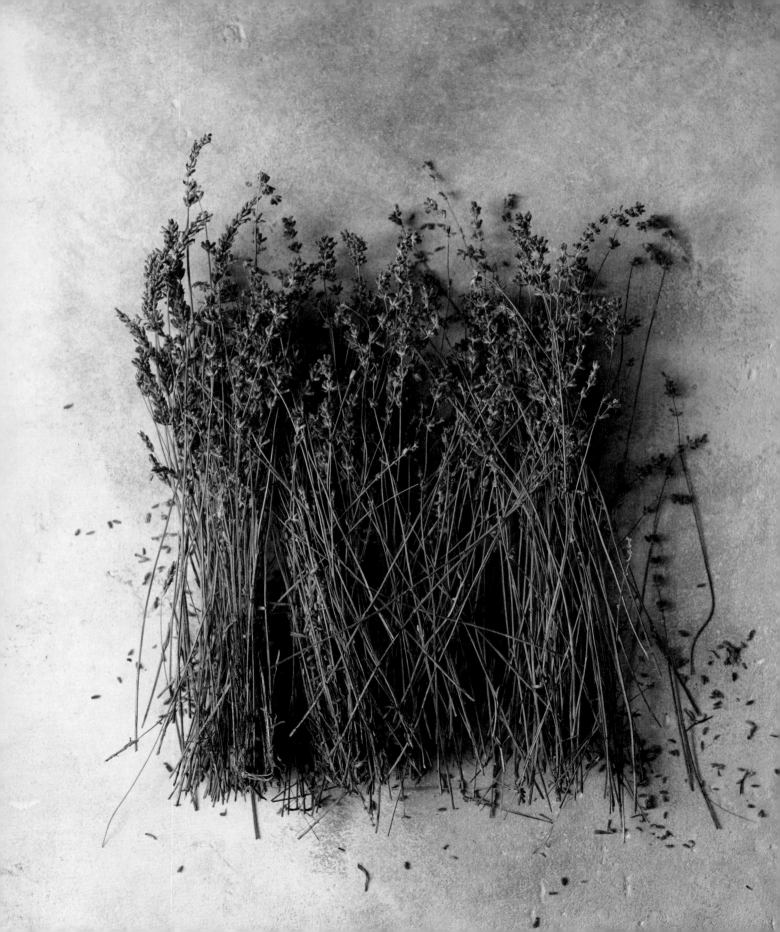

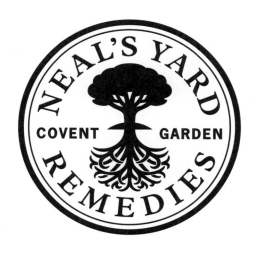

COMPLETE
WELLNESS

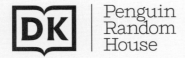

Senior Editor Claire Cross
Senior Designer Collette Sadler
Designers Mandy Earey, Louise Brigenshaw,
and Jade Wheaton
Editorial Assistant Megan Lea
Managing Editor Dawn Henderson
Managing Art Editor Marianne Markham
Senior Jacket Creative Nicola Powling
Jackets Co-ordinator Lucy Philpott
Senior Producer, Pre-Production Tony Phipps
Producer Luca Bazzoli
Art Director Maxine Pedliham
Publisher Mary-Clare Jerram

First published in Great Britain in 2018
by Dorling Kindersley Limited
One Embassy Gardens, 8 Viaduct Gardens, London,
SW11 7BW

A Penguin Random House Company

6 8 10 9 7
016–305966–Sept/2018

Copyright © 2018 Dorling Kindersley Limited

DISCLAIMER See page 304

A CIP catalogue record for this book
is available from the British Library.

ISBN 978-0-2413-0213-2

Printed and bound in China

All images © Dorling Kindersley Limited. For further
information see: www.dkimages.com

**A WORLD OF IDEAS:
SEE ALL THERE IS TO KNOW**
www.dk.com

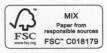

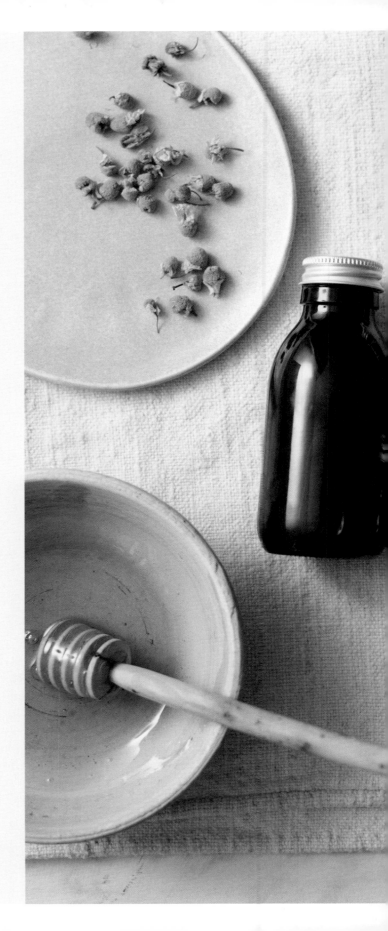

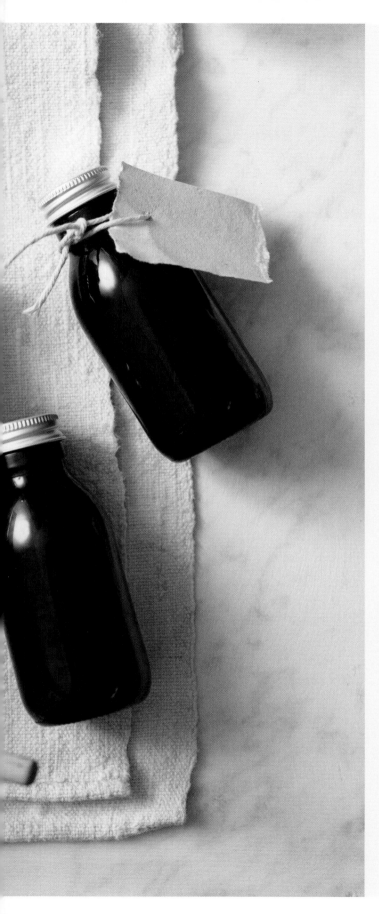

THE AUTHORS

Susan Curtis is an experienced natural health practitioner, having originally qualified as a homeopath and naturopath and then going on to study and work with herbs and essential oils. She has written numerous books and articles on helping people to improve their health and wellbeing by using natural remedies and adopting a natural lifestyle. Susan has worked for the ethical natural health and beauty company Neal's Yard Remedies since the 1980s. She is their Director of Natural Health, helping to champion awareness of natural and organic ingredients and products.

Pat Thomas is a journalist, author, and advocate for natural health, sustainable living, and a clean environment. She is editor of the Natural Health News website and, in addition to her own books such as the guide to alternative healthcare: *What Works, What Doesn't*, she has contributed to several Neal's Yard Remedies' titles including *Healing Foods*, *Essential Oils*, and *The Beauty Book*.

Julie Wood, MNIMH, is a herbal practitioner who has worked for Neal's Yard Remedies since 2003, making tinctures, working on the customer advice line, and teaching on the Introduction to Herbal Remedies' course. Julie's interest in the roots of plant medicine also helped to develop the Anglo-Saxon herb garden at Shaftesbury Abbey along with their guided herb walks and talks, which have been taking place for over 15 years.

Fran Johnson is a passionate cosmetic scientist and aromatherapist and has been part of the Product Development team at Neal's Yard Remedies since 2006, formulating therapeutic products for healing and wellbeing. She has written for and teaches a number of Neal's Yard Remedies' courses, which cover aromatherapy, natural perfumery, and making cosmetic products.

Fiona Waring is a qualified nutritional therapist with 27 years' experience in the health and fitness industry. Fiona is passionate about nutrition; she has just completed an MSc, and her main priority is keeping current and up to date with nutritional research. Using her extensive knowledge, Fiona runs a busy consultancy service, clinic, and workshops.

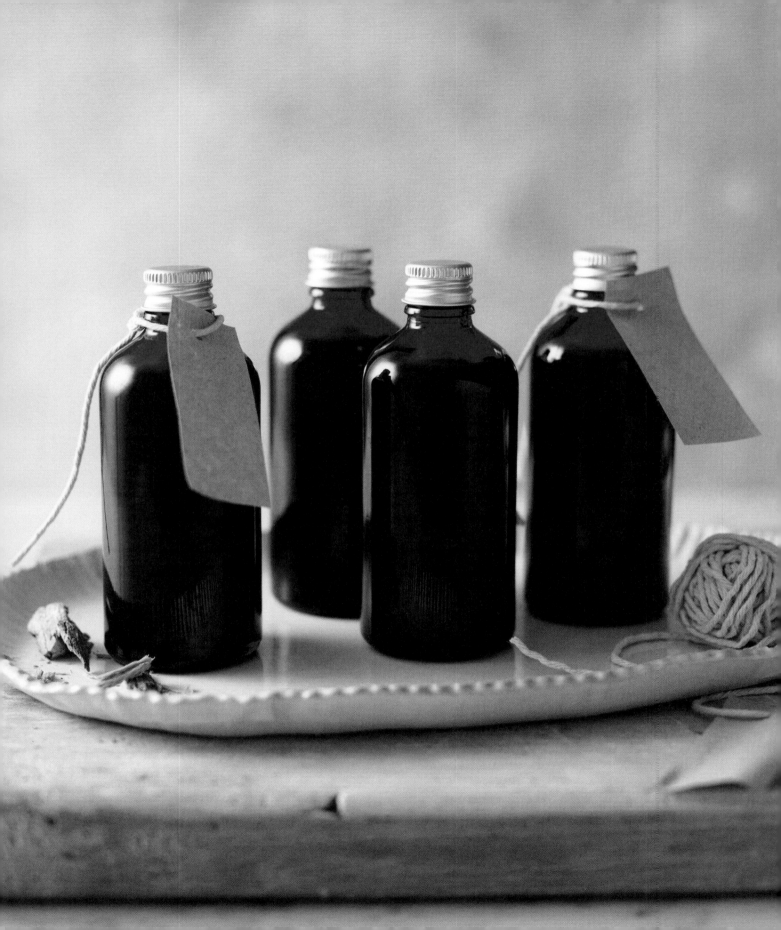

CONTENTS

INTRODUCTION

Natural remedies are an increasingly important part of many people's approach to wellness. As we live longer and become more concerned about the side effects of pharmaceutical drugs, many more of us are seeking a natural solution for the troublesome and distressing ailments that we can fall prey to.

Conditions such as stress, insomnia, low vitality, digestive problems, eczema, and poor immunity are the classic areas where a herbal or essential oil remedy, a change of diet or lifestyle, or a well-chosen supplement can be of great benefit. Natural remedies and healthy diet and lifestyle choices support a person's overall health and wellbeing, rather than undermine it with potentially addictive medications or with treatments that simply suppress the symptoms of a condition rather than address its root causes.

Our expertise

Neal's Yard Remedies first opened its doors in 1981 and since that time we have sold a wide range of herbal remedies and essential oils. The customers who come into our stores are seeking solutions to the many everyday problems that can undermine our health and wellbeing. We like to think of ourselves as "the herbalist on the high street".

Our staff are trained in how to use the herbs, tinctures, and essential oils that make up our natural remedies and are skilled in helping customers find out more about which remedy might be most helpful for their health concern. The aim always is to help the customer choose a herb, oil, or other solution themselves, rather than simply prescribe a remedy for them. In this way, the customer has an opportunity to find out more about the wonderful plant remedies that are available and also learns something about how natural remedies can be used to support a healthy lifestyle.

New discoveries

One thing that has changed considerably over the past few decades is the number of studies and clinical trials that have been carried out on natural remedies and foods. There is now a mass of evidence on the medicinal and health benefits of so many herbs and foods; most often reinforcing their traditional

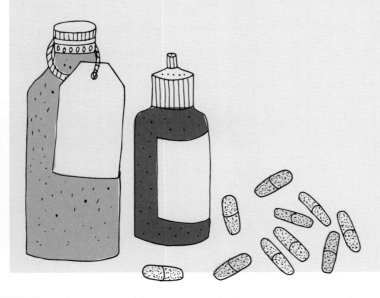

> *"Natural remedies support overall health and wellbeing."*

use, but sometimes revealing new and even surprising outcomes. Lemon balm, for example, is a herb that has long been used for relieving stress and anxiety, but modern research has shown that it is also specifically active against the virus that causes herpes. Several studies have also shown how pine bark extract, originally developed to improve blood circulation and help lower high blood pressure, is also very effective for improving symptoms and sex drive in menopausal women.

REMEDIES FOR ALL

This book is divided into the body systems with separate sections on the health issues particularly relevant to women, men, and children, as well as a first aid section. So if you have an area of health that is of particular concern, you can read around the remedies and suggestions that are likely to be of benefit. Some more minor ailments should respond quite quickly to a timely taken herb or essential oil. For more serious health concerns,

or for problems that have continued over a long period of time, the suggestions and remedies are often supportive, to help you manage symptoms while taking a prescribed medication or while making necessary lifestyle changes.

We have been able to draw on a wide range of expertise in writing this book, with input from well-qualified and experienced practitioners of herbalism, aromatherapy, nutrition, homeopathy, and naturopathy. We very much hope that you find it inspiring, helpful, and also enjoyable as you learn to prepare and use the wonderful array of herbal and aromatherapy remedies and try out some of the delicious recipes.

Susan Curtis
Director of Natural Health, Neal's Yard Remedies

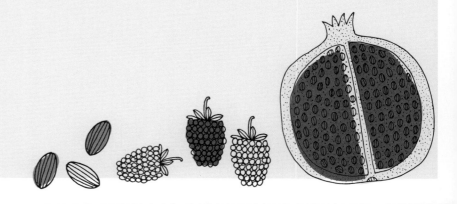

THE HOLISTIC APPROACH

Holistic health and healing work on the premise that the mind, body, and spirit are interconnected, so imbalances in one area can impact elsewhere. By treating the whole person, rather than an illness or symptom, a deeper level of healing is reached and complete wellness enjoyed. In this chapter we explore how herbal and essential oil remedies, dietary choices, and complementary therapies, all used throughout the book, work holistically. Naturally, lifestyle choices that keep you physically and mentally active, provide a supportive network, and avoid harmful habits support this holistic approach.

HERBS

Herbs are aromatic plants with medicinal and culinary uses whose chemical constituents have healing actions. In herbal medicine, the whole plant or a part, such as the root, leaf, flower, or seed, is used. Knowledge of how herbs work and safe usage, explored over millennia, is increasingly supported by scientific research.

HOW HERBS HEAL

Herbs offer safe, effective holistic healing that focuses on the root cause of a problem and herbalists tailor remedies to work on the body, mind, and emotions. A range of actions, listed below, strengthen the body and support wellness. Many herbs "multi-task" to combine several actions. Cautions on specific herbs are given in the book and page 295 gives general guidance on safe usage.

Tonic herbs, traditionally taken in the spring, refresh, strengthen, and rebuild health. They work either on the whole body or on specific areas such as the circulation, boosting energy, or the mind, for example St John's wort is a nerve tonic with antidepressant effects. Tonic herbs also help to rebalance dysfunctional and stressed body systems. Popular tonic herbs include ashwagandha, skullcap, nettle, and hawthorn.

Bitter herbs, such as dandelion root and mugwort, stimulate bitter taste receptors on the tongue and gastric juices to boost digestion. They promote appetite, for example during convalescence; support a healthy gut "microbiome", balancing good and bad bacteria; aid nutrient absorption; and help the elimination of waste.

A large proportion of immune cells are located in the digestive tract and many neurotransmitters originate in the gut, so a healthy gut flora boosts immunity and mental health.

Mucilaginous herbs, also called demulcents, have a protective effect in the gut. They make a gel-like substance that forms a coating to soothe irritation and inflammation and they are used for a range of digestive complaints as well as for respiratory problems. Emollient herbs, used externally to soften skin, are also mucilaginous. Mucilaginous herbs include marshmallow, plantain, fenugreek, mullein, and chia seed.

Adaptogens, such as Siberian ginseng, astragalus, and liquorice, are a type of powerful tonic that help the body adapt to physical and emotional stress, restoring balance and building resilience.

Sedative herbs, such as valerian, passionflower, wild lettuce, and ashwagandha calm the nerves, reducing the effects of stress on the body and mind. Sedative herbs are also referred to as nervines, relaxants, or hypnotics.

Carminative herbs, such as cardamom and fennel, are often aromatic and rich in essential oils. They relieve gastrointestinal spasms and expel excess gas to ease griping pains.

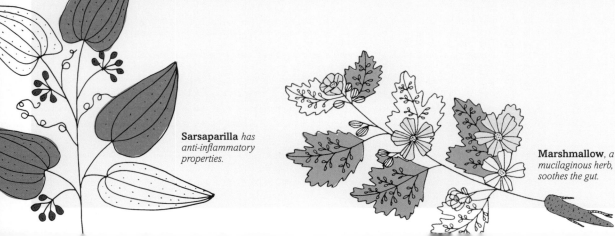

Sarsaparilla *has anti-inflammatory properties.*

Marshmallow, *a mucilaginous herb, soothes the gut.*

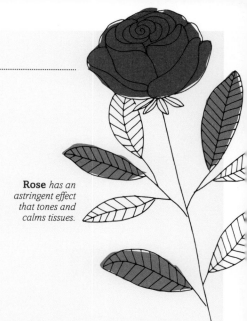

Rose has an astringent effect that tones and calms tissues.

Antioxidants inhibit cell oxidation to stop free radicals forming. Rosemary and milk thistle are powerful antioxidant herbs.

Astringent, or toning, herbs, such as witch hazel, rose, or sage tighten tissues, helping to protect against fluid loss and inflammation. They can be applied internally to calm inflamed mucous membranes and reduce excess mucus; or externally to tone skin, treat sores, and help stem bleeding.

Expectorants, such as elecampane and mullein, loosen mucus, ease spasms, and make coughs productive to expel catarrh. Anticatarrhal herbs, which remove mucus, and antitussive herbs, which soothe coughs, are related to expectorants.

Diuretic herbs increase the production and flow of urine, making them beneficial for problems such as fluid retention and for flushing the urinary tract when an infection is present. Diuretic herbs include dandelion, cleavers, buchu, and corn silk.

Antimicrobial herbs, such as calendula and garlic, have a range of protective properties, including being antibacterial, antiviral, antifungal, and anti-infective. They increase resistance to – and inhibit the action of – pathogenic microorganisms, strengthening the body's resilience and limiting infection.

Anti-inflammatory herbs, such as sarsaparilla and cayenne, help reduce excessive inflammation, in turn relieving pain.

Antispasmodic herbs, such as wild yam, relax muscles and reduce spasms. They can work on smooth muscle, such as in the stomach, as well as relieve general muscle tension.

Styptic herbs, such as lady's mantle, have a "haemostatic" action to help stem bleeding when applied topically.

MAKING HERBAL REMEDIES

In this book, herbal remedies are given for each ailment and area of health, and step-by-step features, listed below, show how to prepare these. The remedies use dried herbs, but fresh can be used where available, with quantities for fresh herbs given on the features.

- **30–31 How to make a herbal infusion**
- **66–7 How to make a tincture**
- **78–9 How to make a macerated oil**
- **100–101 How to make a decoction**
- **136–7 How to make a syrup**
- **146–7 How to make herbal capsules**
- **180–81 How to make a poultice**

ESSENTIAL OILS

Essential oils are aromatic, volatile components derived from plants. These highly concentrated essences are extracted from a variety of plant parts, including the bark, stems, seeds, roots, and flowers. A single oil can contain more than 100 different chemical components, each of which has a specific therapeutic property.

HOW ESSENTIAL OILS HEAL

Essential oils are inhaled or absorbed, for example in a massage. Each oil has a unique chemistry with therapeutic psychological and physiological effects. Aromatherapy treats the whole person and promotes the body's ability to balance itself. The oils' wide-ranging properties have numerous benefits, explored below, which in turn enhance immunity and wellbeing. Cautions on specific oils are given in the book and page 295 gives general guidance on safe usage.

Mood-enhancing essential oils, such as bergamot, lavender, chamomile, and ylang ylang, can be used as antidepressants to revive the spirits and promote wellbeing; to sedate and relax, easing anxiety and assisting meditation; and as aphrodisiacs.

Focusing essential oils clear the mind, ground emotions, and enhance concentration. Studies show that rosemary stimulates neurotransmitters to improve memory function. Cardamom, peppermint, and thyme also refresh and focus the mind.

Strengthening essential oils have a stimulating effect, similar to tonic herbs. Geranium, myrrh, and clary sage are examples of stimulating oils that help to strengthen body systems.

Adaptogenic essential oils, such as lavender and geranium, help the body adapt to stress by supporting the adrenal glands, which release the stress hormone cortisol. They stimulate or calm, as required, to restore balance, and by helping the body to cope with stress also help to boost immunity. Oils such as basil and clary sage help to balance female hormones to control mood swings caused by fluctuating hormone levels.

Anti-inflammatory essential oils, such as frankincense, thyme, and eucalyptus, have pain-relieving properties. In massage blends, they ease muscle and joint problems and soothe localized pain, relieving problems such as tension headaches.

Antimicrobial essential oils act against a range of pathogens and can be antiseptic, antibacterial, antiviral, and antifungal. Tea tree is a poweful antimicrobial used as an essential oil to help fight and prevent infection. Other antimicrobial oils include thyme and clove, which are applied topically or inhaled to fight germs in the respiratory tract.

Cleansing essential oils support waste elimination to prevent a buildup of toxins. Some oils are mildly diuretic, aiding the kidneys and helping to remove excess fluid to relieve fluid retention. Dill, grapefruit, and juniper are all used as diuretics.

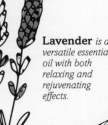

Lavender *is a versatile essential oil with both relaxing and rejuvenating effects.*

Lemon *stimulates and cleanses and has a toning action on the skin.*

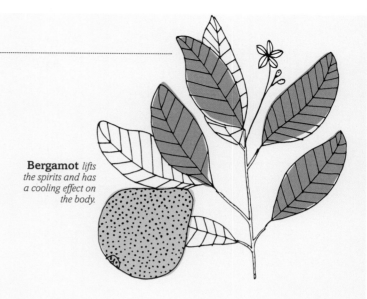

Bergamot *lifts the spirits and has a cooling effect on the body.*

These oils also stimulate the blood and lymphatic system, boosting circulation to help remove waste. Citrus oils, such as lemon and orange, support liver and kidney function.

Digestion-boosting essential oils support digestion and provide relief from bloating, gas, and constipation. Oils such as fennel and chamomile are calming, soothing indigestion caused by emotional upset or rushed eating; and citrus oils such as sweet orange calm unsettled digestion and help release trapped wind.

Antispasmodic essential oils relieve spasms in voluntary and involuntary muscles. Warming oils such as rosemary used in a massage relieve cramps and sore muscles and joints.

Toning essential oils, such as geranium, sandalwood, cypress, rose, lemon, and bergamot, are astringent, reviving and rejuvenating skin. Used in a well-diluted massage blend, they can help to even out blotchy, irregular skin tone.

Decongestant essential oils help to reduce the swelling of blood vessels in the nasal passages, in turn opening up the airways to make breathing easier. Essential oils such as helichrysum and eucalyptus have effective decongestant properties to help boost respiratory function during colds and coughs.

Expectorant essential oils, such as cedarwood, fennel, bay laurel, and niaouli, can be inhaled to thin secretions, breaking up catarrh and increasing mucus flow to help expel excess mucus.

Deodorizing essential oils, such as lemongrass, bergamot, and peppermint, cool and refresh, neutralizing strong odours.

Rubefacient essential oils, such as sweet marjoram and ginger, stimulate local blood flow in the skin and muscle tissues; their warming effect can help back pain, cramps, and osteoarthritis.

USING ESSENTIAL OILS

Essential oil remedies are suggested for each ailment and area of health in the book, and step-by-step features, listed below, show how to prepare and use essential oils. These features explain how to make essential oil blends and how to incorporate oils into different preparations and bases.

- **192–3 How to make an essential oil blend**
- **232–3 How to make a balm**
- **262–3 How to make a cream**
- **292–3 How to make an essential oil compress**

FOOD

Nutritious food is the foundation of good health. As well as supplying calories to fuel daily activities, a balanced, nutrient-dense diet also provides a complete package of vitamins, minerals, antioxidants, enzymes, and a variety of fats and fibre, all of which are necessary to optimize health in the mind and body.

HOW FOODS HEAL

Today it is recognized that many chronic diseases are related to poor diet. What we eat plays a vital role in preventing disease and supporting healing. Here we explore the ways in which nutrients benefit physical and mental health. Within the book you will find recipes for wellness that incorporate these healing nutrients.

Anti-inflammatory foods promote good health. Inflammation is the body's natural protective response, but if it is chronic it can affect areas such as the digestive tract and the muscles, joints, and bones. Nutrients help to control inflammation. Essential fatty acids, such as omega-3, antioxidants, especially flavonoids (see below), and minerals are the basis of an anti-inflammatory diet. Oily fish, such as salmon and mackerel; walnuts; and chia and flaxseeds provide omega-3, while bright-coloured produce, leafy greens, and clear broths have minerals and antioxidants.

Antioxidants are key to a healthy diet. These powerful substances help to fight the effects of free radicals, which, if left unchecked, lead to oxidative stress and disease. A range of antioxidants provides a variety of benefits. For example, flavonoids reduce the risk of diseases such as heart disease and cancer, while

carotenoids such as beta-carotene and lycopene support eye health. Brightly coloured fruit and vegetables, such as mangoes, peppers, squash, tomatoes, and berries, including blueberries and goji berries, and pulses and beans, are high in antioxidants.

Energy-providing foods ensure that cells have fuel to function. Basing the diet around unprocessed, whole foods with complex carbohydrates, which release energy slowly; healthy proteins; and fibre, sustains energy over time, reducing the temptation to resort to unhealthy snacks and avoiding spikes in blood sugar levels. Wholegrain breads and pasta, pulses, beans, fish, poultry, and fresh fruit and vegetables all help to fuel the body.

Calming foods promote restful sleep, vital for health and wellbeing. Foods with natural sources of melatonin, the substance that prepares us for sleep, and tryptophan, an amino acid that converts to melatonin, help the body to relax. Tart cherries, rice, turkey, yogurt, tomatoes, and seafood are good sources.

Immune-boosting foods support the immune response. A healthy gut flora with good bacteria boosts immunity. Probiotic foods, such as kefir and natural yogurt, contain good bacteria, and prebiotic foods, such as garlic and onions, feed these bacteria. Some foods, such as mushrooms, garlic, ginger, coconut oil,

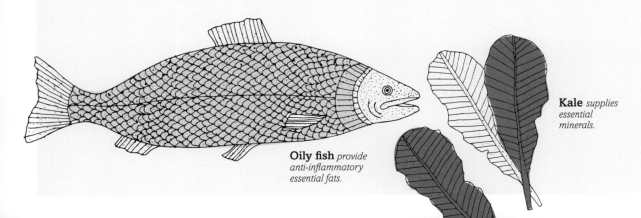

Oily fish *provide anti-inflammatory essential fats.*

Kale *supplies essential minerals.*

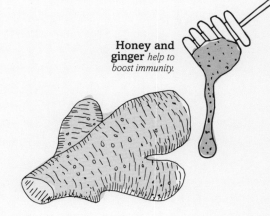

Honey and ginger *help to boost immunity.*

honey, and oats, are antimicrobial, fighting bacteria, viruses, and fungal infections. Antioxidant vitamins A and C, found in citrus, kiwi, broccoli, carrots, and squash also boost immunity.

Cleansing foods support the removal of waste. Fibre-rich foods such as wholegrains, vegetables and fruit, and pulses bulk up waste to help it through the gut. Chlorophyll-containing foods, such as cruciferous vegetables, support the liver and kidneys.

Mood-enhancing foods support wellbeing. Omega-3 in oily fish boosts brain function and helps balance mood, while vitamin D, in foods such as mushrooms and eggs, boosts levels of the mood-enhancing neurotransmitter serotonin.

Cholesterol-lowering foods help to control levels of bad cholesterol. Oats contain a soluble fibre called beta-glucan, which aids the removal of cholesterol from the body.

Hydrating foods such as watermelon, cucumber, and celery help to maintain fluid levels and prevent dehydration.

Alkalizing foods, such as green leafy vegetable, almonds, and ginger, contain minerals such as sodium and potassium, which help to balance the body and support health.

TAKING SUPPLEMENTS

Ideally, our nutrients should come from food, but stress, poor diet, declining soil quality with fewer nutrients, and medications all affect nutrient intake and absorption. Also, some ailments mean the body needs more of specific nutrients. Supplements can therefore be beneficial. Guidance on doses is given on pages 294–95 and throughout the book. If in doubt, consult a nutritional therapist.

- High-quality supplements have greater nutritional benefits, so buy the best you can afford, ideally free from additives.
- Choose wholefood supplements derived from food such as rice bran and alfalfa, which aid the absorption of vitamins.
- A daily multi-vitamin and mineral supplement ensures at least the minimum recommended intake of key nutrients.
- The fat-soluble vitamins, A, D, E, and K, need to be taken with sources of fat to aid their absorption and utilization.

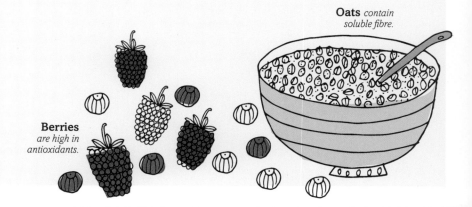

Oats *contain soluble fibre.*

Berries *are high in antioxidants.*

THERAPIES

Complementary therapies carried out by qualified practitioners offer a variety of holistic benefits that can support natural remedies managed at home as well as conventional treatments. The aim of therapies is to heal, restore balance, and strengthen the body to prevent illness.

HOW THERAPIES HEAL

Holistic complementary treatments work on a variety of levels, supporting the mind and emotions as well as the physical body, and sometimes offering support for the spirit, too. Here we explore some of the most common therapies, how these work, and their particular benefits.

Acupressure and acupuncture are ancient techniques used in Chinese medicine. Both therapies work on key points along the body's "meridians", or energy channels, to help balance Chi – the body's energy force. The theory is that blockages in these energy channels can lead to disease, and so removing blockages restores health.

Acupressure applies gentle pressure to specific points along the meridians, while acupuncture inserts very fine needles at these points, to stimulate and balance Chi. With acupuncture, the needles are left in place for a certain amount of time and may be gently turned or stimulated with heat or a small electrical charge to increase the effects. The therapies are used for pain relief, circulatory problems, fatigue, digestive disorders, arthritis, fertility problems, menstrual concerns, migraines, and stress disorders.

Massage involves a variety of techniques to relax muscles, increase oxygen in the blood, and release toxins. Types of massage include deep tissue, holistic, shiatsu, aromatherapy, manual lymph drainage, remedial, sports, Indian head, and hot stone. As well as the medical benefits, massage induces relaxation and wellbeing by stimulating nerve endings. There is also evidence that physical touch can help boost immunity and decrease heart rate and blood pressure.

Reflexology works on the premise that all parts of the body are connected by energy pathways that end in the hands, feet, and head. Pressure on specific areas of the feet or hands stimulate healing in corresponding organs and glands. It is useful for migraine, sinus problems, hormone imbalances, breathing disorders, digestive and circulatory problems, and stress.

Chiropractic and osteopathy treat musculoskeletal problems, including sports injuries, and some circulatory and digestive problems. Chiropractic believes that illness arises from spinal misalignment and the disruption this causes to nerves, and also looks at restricted joint movement. Osteopathy diagnoses and treats problems to correct imbalances in muscles, bones, and ligaments. Practitioners manually manipulate and gently adjust the spine, joints, and muscles to restore alignment.

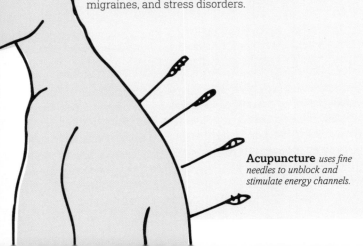

Acupuncture *uses fine needles to unblock and stimulate energy channels.*

Massage has multiple benefits, helping to stimulate, relax, and boost immunity.

The Alexander technique addresses postural bad habits such as slouching, damaging patterns of movement, muscular tension, and breathing problems. All of these can hinder full recovery from injury and make it hard to eliminate aches and pains. The technique teaches self-awareness of our responses to stressful situations. By paying attention to how we hold ourselves, breathe, and work, unhelpful habits can be undone and balance restored. The technique is especially helpful for back pain, low energy, respiratory problems, anxiety, and stress.

Hydrotherapy uses water to support healing, whether in a mineral salt bath, a high-pressure shower, a mud bath, or a high-temperature bath in natural thermal mineral waters. It can be combined with physiotherapy to help problems such as arthritis. Warm water relaxes and soothes muscles. Water also supports weight to release tension and is a resistant force to strengthen muscles. Hydrotherapy supports rheumatological conditions, osteoarthritis, fibromyalgia, ankylosing spondylitis, rheumatoid arthritis, chronic low back pain, and psoriasis.

Flower essence therapy, which includes Bach Flower Remedies and Australian Bush Flower Remedies, uses tinctures selected to match a person's emotional "type" to help balance and harmonize emotions and enhance health.

Homeopathy works on the premise that "like cures like". Symptoms are treated with tiny amounts of potentized remedies that cause similar symptoms in healthy people. The aim is to stimulate the body's ability to heal itself. This gentle therapy strengthens the whole body, in turn offering support for specific symptoms.

Counselling and psychotherapy identify difficult feelings and negative ways of coping, and aim to change entrenched beliefs or behaviours that affect health, self-esteem, and relationships. Counselling helps to find coping mechanisms and change behaviour patterns. Psychotherapy involves a deeper exploration of long-standing issues to enhance understanding of emotions.

Hypnotherapy and biofeedback retrain the body's and mind's processes and responses to cope with problems such as pain and anxiety, and to break harmful habits. Hypnotherapy reaches to the subconscious to get to the root of a problem or change a behaviour and can involve visualization, a technique that focuses the mind on a desired outcome. It is often used to deal with emotional and psychological problems and to manage pain.

Biofeedback uses electronic monitoring to measure processes such as heart rates, brain waves, and perspiration. The aim is to increase awareness of how emotional responses affect us physiologically and then to control and change behaviour.

MIND AND EMOTIONS

Looking after our mental health helps us to enjoy healthy relationships, feel productive, cope with stress, and muster resilience in the face of setbacks. Discover how key nutrients and natural remedies can nourish the mind and balance emotions, optimizing mental health and ensuring we are well-equipped to cope under pressure. When stress does take its toll, find out which herbs, essential oils, and mind-nourishing nutrients can help to restore vitality and wellbeing.

STAYING WELL
MIND AND EMOTIONS

Our mental and emotional wellbeing is influenced by the health of the whole body and by factors such as anxiety levels and relationship dynamics. A holistic approach to wellness can help to ensure mental clarity and balanced emotions. Here we explore how nutrients nourish the mind and how herbs and essential oils strengthen mental health and lift spirits to optimize wellbeing.

FOOD

A varied, nutrient-dense diet is a key component to robust mental health and wellbeing, helping to maintain energy levels, balance moods, and promote mental and emotional resilience.

SLEEP-PROMOTING NUTRIENTS

Regular sleep is one of the cornerstones of mental health. A lack of restful sleep can increase anxiety and impact on mental wellbeing, while getting adequate rest bolsters energy and resilience. Certain nutrients actively help to promote good-quality, restful sleep. Some foods are a natural source of melatonin, the hormone that helps prepare our bodies for rest and sleep. Melatonin-rich foods include tart cherries, or cherry juice, tomatoes, chillies, white and black mustard seeds, fenugreek, corn, rice, sprouted seeds, and lupin, a legume that is ground down and used in some flours and pasta. In addition, some foods, including turkey, dairy, and seafood, supply the amino acid tryptophan, which converts to melatonin in the body, so incorporate these into an evening meal to promote sleep.

BALANCING ANTIOXIDANTS

Anti-inflammatory and antioxidant-rich foods, such as green tea, turmeric, brightly coloured fruit and vegetables, and dark chocolate, help to support healthy blood pressure, which in turn provides support during times of stress and mental endurance, and so reduces the negative impact of stress on mental health and emotional wellbeing.

MOOD-BOOSTING HEALTHY FATS

The brain requires a steady supply of healthy fats to keep it working optimally and help balance our moods and emotions. Oily fish contain essential fatty acids such as omega-3, low levels of which have been linked to depression, while olive oil and

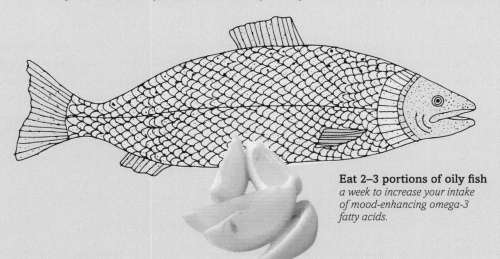

Eat 2–3 portions of oily fish
a week to increase your intake of mood-enhancing omega-3 fatty acids.

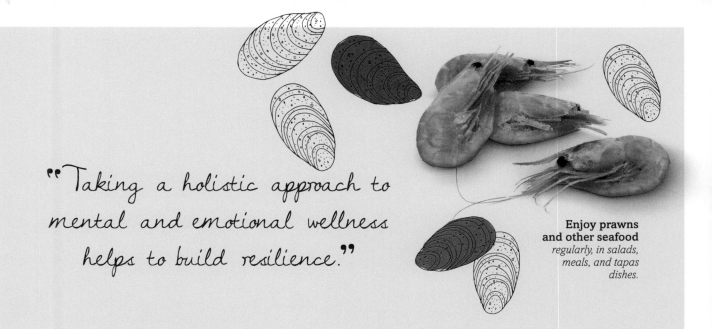

"*Taking a holistic approach to mental and emotional wellness helps to build resilience.*"

Enjoy prawns and other seafood *regularly, in salads, meals, and tapas dishes.*

coconut oil are thought to boost the body's levels of serotonin, a neurotransmitter that is linked to mood and wellbeing. Enjoy oily fish, such as salmon, trout, mackerel, and sardines, up to three times a week and incorporate olive and coconut oils into dressings and meals daily.

NERVE-CALMING AMINO ACIDS
Magnesium-rich foods, such as almonds and cashews, contain the amino acids gamma-aminobutyric acid (GABA), tryptophan, and l-theanine, which help to calm the nerves.

THE SUNSHINE VITAMIN
Vitamin D, which our bodies make from sunlight, is important for many bodily functions and low levels of vitamin D3 in particular are thought to affect mood. It can be hard to get enough vitamin D from our diets alone, but eating foods such as organic eggs helps to top up supplies in the winter months, energizing the mind and promoting feelings of positivity.

HERBS
Herbal remedies can help to strengthen us mentally and emotionally, restoring energy levels and vitality when these are depleted by stress and anxiety, and helping to restore a sense of calm and equilibrium.

HERBS TO REVIVE THE MIND
Strengthening tonic herbs support mental robustness, helping to reduce the impact of stress and fatigue on our ability to think and focus, while gently stimulating brain function. Some tonic herbs have relaxing properties, too; for example, lemon balm, oats, and bacopa strengthen and nourish the mind and are calming for the nervous system. Another herb, damiana, a traditional tonic herb that boosts motivation, also has aphrodisiacal properties to support healthy sexual function, beneficial when a lack of libido is linked to low mood and lack of motivation.

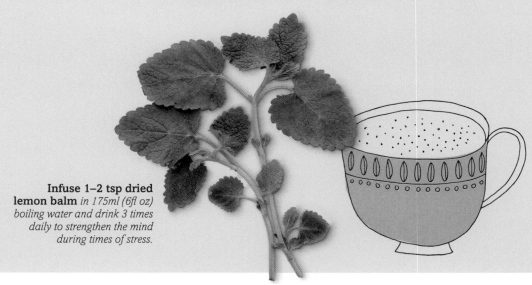

Infuse 1–2 tsp dried lemon balm *in 175ml (6fl oz) boiling water and drink 3 times daily to strengthen the mind during times of stress.*

Herbs to rest the mind

Certain herbs have a relaxing and sedative action on the body. Passionflower and valerian, for example, encourage deep, restful sleep, ensuring that the body is able to rest, repair, rebalance, and refocus, all of which help to boost mental resilience and support emotional health.

Balancing herbs

Herbs known as adaptogens help the body to adapt to varying circumstances, most notably during periods of stress. These herbs support the health of the adrenal system, helping it to regulate the release of the stress hormone cortisol to manage the body's response to stress. The adaptogenic herbs ashwagandha and liquorice are both physically strengthening and promote emotional resilience so are used to support the body, mind, and emotions through challenging times.

Uplifting herbs

Uplifting herbs can help when mental resilience is low and depression sets in. St John's wort, recommended in the following treatment pages, helps to lift depression gently, and has fewer side effects than many conventional medications.

Essential oils

Both stimulating and calming essential oils can be used alongside other therapies as a supportive treatment to help improve mental clarity and even out moods.

Oils for focus

Rosemary is renowned for its ability to improve concentration and focus, and studies have conclusively demonstrated its capacity to enhance memory and mental clarity. Rosemary also has uplifting properties that can help to raise vitality in the body and mind and encourage a positive outlook overall.

Grounding and uplifting oils

Essential oils can be uplifting and physically grounding, helping you reconnect to your body if the mind is distracted. Grounding and uplifting oils are especially beneficial if there is a tendency to depression and anxiety that can lead to feelings of wishing to escape reality. Uplifting oils such as bergamot, lemongrass, neroli, and grapefruit have compounds to boost wellbeing and mood, while rosewood and carrot seed help to ground emotions.

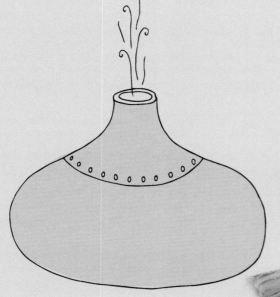

Add 4 drops lemongrass essential oil *to a diffuser, or sprinkle on a tissue, and inhale to lift the spirits.*

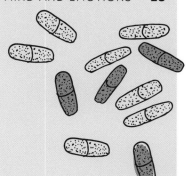

Relaxing oils

Soothing oils promote relaxation, calming breathing and moderating the stress response to prevent anxiety building up.

Stimulating oils

Oils such as basil and ginger boost circulation to the brain, enhancing mental sharpness and focus. Aphrodisiacal oils, such as ylang ylang and clary sage, also stimulate the mind, relieving stress and energizing the body to reignite and stimulate passion.

Supplements

Supplementing a healthy diet can provide sustained energy to support mental health and wellbeing.

Stress-fighting vitamins

Stress can deplete the body of B vitamins, which help balance neurotransmitters, leaving you vulnerable to fatigue, depression, and anxiety. B vitamins also support energy and circulation, boosting libido. Take a B-complex supplement with the vitamin-like substance coenzyme Q10 (CoQ10), for the range of B vitamins.

Nerve-supporting nutrients

Regular probiotic supplements help to optimize gut health and support the production of neurotransmitters in both the gut and the brain. Neurotransmitters are involved in balancing moods and work as a buffer against the effects of shock and trauma.

Vitamin C aids the production of the neurotransmitter norepinephrine, which increases alertness to help the body and mind cope during stressful situations. Omega-3 fatty acid supplements can help to normalize neurotransmitter activity in the brain to lift and balance moods and promote concentration.

Adrenal-boosting minerals

Zinc and magnesium support the action of the adrenal system, which regulates stress hormones, to help calm the nerves. Low levels of these minerals are linked to anxiety and depression.

Mood-lifting vitamin D

Vitamin D is another important vitamin for regulating mood and enhancing wellbeing. Our levels of vitamin D, synthesized mainly from sunlight, are often low in the winter and in places with little sunshine, making us vulnerable to low mood and depression, so a supplement is advised to top up levels when sunlight is scarce.

"Essential oils can be used to stimulate the mind and enhance focus."

TREATMENTS
MIND AND EMOTIONS

Modern-day living can affect our mental health and wellbeing, with busy lives, social pressures, and multiple demands all taking their toll on how we think and feel. Holistic treatments using herbs and essential oils can have profound effects on our mental states, helping to calm, stimulate, and rejuvenate emotions, and a healthy diet that provides essential nutrients is vital for a healthy mind and the ability to cope.

ANXIETY

Anxiety is a general feeling of unease, often without a specific cause. Left to become a chronic problem, anxiety can affect both mental and physical health and wellbeing. Exercise and activities such as yoga can help relieve tension and stress.

HERBS

Relaxing and strengthening tonic herbs can be used to nourish the mind and can also help to release irrational fears. These actions are supported by antispasmodic herbs, to help calm the nerves.

Lemon balm induces a relaxed state of mind, easing tension and lifting the spirits. Avoid with hypothyroidism.
➡*Infuse 1–2 tsp dried lemon balm in 175ml (6fl oz) boiling water and drink 3 times daily.*

Skullcap is powerfully relaxing and nourishes the central nervous system, helping to ease feelings of anxiety and allay fears. Lemon balm and skullcap partner well in a calming infusion.
➡*Infuse 1–2 tsp dried skullcap in 175ml (6fl oz) boiling water and drink 3 times daily, or see remedy, right.*

Wood betony soothes, restores, and strengthens nerves, releasing tension.
➡*Add 1–2ml tincture to a lemon balm or skullcap infusion 3 times daily.*

ESSENTIAL OILS

Essential oils can be used to help steady breathing and calm the stress response, relieving anxiety.

Frankincense calms the mind and deepens breathing.
➡*Add 3 drops to a diffuser.*

Lemon balm reduces anxiety and panic.
➡*Add 5 drops to 10ml almond oil for a soothing massage oil.*

Mandarin is relaxing and calming.
➡*Add 5 drops to 10ml apricot oil for a massage, or add 1 tsp to a bath dispersant for a bedtime bath.*

FOOD

Magnesium-rich foods and those containing the amino acids gamma-aminobutyric acid (GABA), tryptophan, and l-theanine calm nerves. Neurotransmitters are made in the gut so fermented foods support the nervous system by promoting gut health.

Natural yogurt feeds good gut bacteria to restore balance to the gut.
➡*Add to fruits, cereals, and meals.*

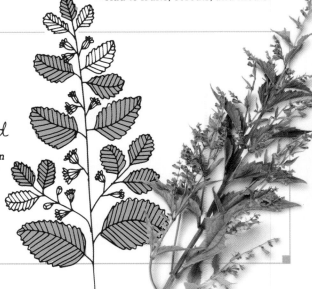

REMEDY

Relaxing infusion blend

*Add 1 tsp each of dried **lemon balm** and **skullcap** herbs to 175ml (6fl oz) boiling water. Drink 3 times daily.*

Kimchi, a traditionally fermented spicy side dish, contains probiotics that produce the nerve-calming neurotransmitter, GABA.
➡*Enjoy as a side dish or use as a condiment.*

Oolong tea has high levels of GABA.
➡*Swap coffee for a daily cup of this.*

Almonds and cashews have calming magnesium and the amino acid tryptophan, which is converted to mood-regulating serotonin in the body.
➡*Eat as nut butters or add to salads and stir-fries.*

WHAT TO AVOID
Caffeine and alcohol.

SUPPLEMENTS

Supplements that are aimed at strengthening a healthy connection between the gut and the brain, both of which produce essential neurotransmitters, help relieve anxiety, while antioxidants and trace elements support the nervous system.

Probiotic supplements populate the gut with beneficial bacteria.
➡*Look for ones with up to 10 billion live organisms per dose.*

Vitamin C aids in the production of the neurotransmitter norepinephrine, promoting a sense of calm.
➡*Take 1g daily.*

Vitamin B5 has antioxidant properties and aids in the production of calming brain chemicals serotonin, dopamine, and norepinephrine.
➡*Take as part of a B complex.*

Zinc, calcium, magnesium, potassium, and selenium help regulate the stress hormone cortisol.
➡*Take a multi-mineral supplement.*

OTHER THERAPIES

Hypnotherapy and biofeedback, a technique that helps to control the heart rate, can help to relieve anxiety.

"Herbs that are balancing and restorative work on the central nervous system to help ease the symptoms of depression and lift mood."

DEPRESSION

Depression affects quality of life and can raise the risk of stroke, diabetes, heart disease, and early death.

HERBS

Restorative, balancing herbs act on the nervous system, while tonic digestive herbs support gut neurotransmitters, helping lift mood and increase vitality.

St John's wort is a proven antidepressant for mild to moderate depression. Avoid internally in pregnancy and high doses in strong sunlight. Taken internally, interacts with many prescription medicines.
➡*Take 2–5ml tincture in a little water daily for a minimum of 4 weeks.*

Oats are a restorative, nutritious nerve tonic that strengthen the mind and lift the spirits. Avoid with gluten sensitivity.
➡*Infuse 1–2 tsp dried oats in 175ml (6fl oz) boiling water and drink 3 times daily.*

Rhodiola is a strengthening tonic that helps lift depression and balance mood. Avoid if bipolar or suffering paranoia; rarely, may trigger insomnia.
➡*Take 2–4 480mg capsules daily.*

Damiana is stimulating and restorative, enhancing vitality in mind and body.
➡*Take 1–5ml tincture in a little water 3 times daily.*

ESSENTIAL OILS

Oils act on the part of the brain that controls mood. Some are proven antidepressants.

Jasmine is a powerful antidepressant, relieving a low mood and revitalizing. Avoid on hypersensitive skin.
➡*Add 4 drops to 10ml unfragranced base cream and apply to the skin.*

Neroli eases depression and stress.
➡*Use neat as a fragrance, or add 3 drops to a diffuser.*

Clary sage lifts mind and emotions.
➡*Add 5 drops to a bath dispersant.*

FOOD

The risk of depression drops with higher intakes of folate, monounsaturated fats, omega-3 fatty acids, and selenium.

Oily fish is high in omega-3 fatty acids, which have brain-boosting chemicals linked to lower depression rates and may increase the effectiveness of conventional antidepressants.
➡*Eat 2–3 portions a week.*

Wholegrain bread is rich in gut-boosting fibre and other essential nutrients.
➡*One slice provides more than half the daily selenium requirements.*

Spinach, asparagus, Brussels sprouts, and dried legumes are high in folate.
➡*Eat several portions a week.*

WHAT TO AVOID
Sugar, refined cereals, fried and fast foods, processed meats, and alcohol.

➤ CONTINUED...

SUPPLEMENTS

Deficiencies in B vitamins, magnesium, potassium, and selenium are all linked to an increased incidence of depression, while vitamins C and D can also help to lift mood and balance emotions. It is hard to obtain sufficient amounts of vitamin D from diet alone; our bodies synthesize the vitamin from sunlight so supplements are beneficial in the darker months.

B vitamins, especially B12 and folic acid, boost mood-affecting brain chemicals.
➡ *Take a B complex supplement.*
Vitamin D promotes uplifting serotonin.
➡ *Take 600–800iu vitamin D3 daily.*
Vitamin C supports norepinephrine, a mood-lifting brain chemical.
➡ *Take 1g daily with food.*

LIFESTYLE

Exercise and time outdoors is restorative and boosts vitamin D.
Yoga and meditation help lift mood.

OTHER THERAPIES

Counselling and psychotherapy can be highly effective.

> **"** *Deficiencies in B vitamins, magnesium, potassium, and selenium are linked to depression.* **"**

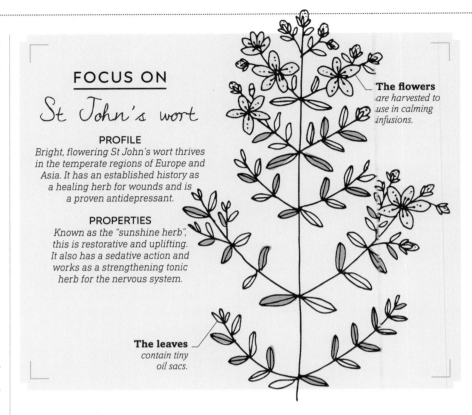

FOCUS ON

St John's wort

PROFILE
Bright, flowering St John's wort thrives in the temperate regions of Europe and Asia. It has an established history as a healing herb for wounds and is a proven antidepressant.

PROPERTIES
Known as the "sunshine herb", this is restorative and uplifting. It also has a sedative action and works as a strengthening tonic herb for the nervous system.

The flowers *are harvested to use in calming infusions.*

The leaves *contain tiny oil sacs.*

SEASONAL AFFECTIVE DISORDER (SAD)

SAD is a form of depression linked to the darker, shorter days of winter. Symptoms include insomnia, loss of libido, fatigue, overeating, and a general feeling of depression.

HERBS

Herbs refresh the spirit and lift mood. Some act directly on the nervous system, while others support the liver, helping it to regulate hormones to avoid mood swings.

St John's wort. See box, above. Avoid in pregnancy and high doses in strong sunlight. Taken internally, interacts with many prescription drugs.
➡ *Take 2–5ml tincture in water daily.*

Lemon balm activates the nerves to lift spirits, and improves digestion to revitalize. Avoid with hypothyroidism.
➡ *Infuse 1–2 tsp dried lemon balm in 175ml (6fl oz) boiling water and drink 3 times daily.*
Rosemary boosts vitality by improving sluggish digestion. Avoid therapeutic doses in pregnancy.
➡ *Take 1–2ml tincture 3 times daily.*
Rhodiola is a traditional remedy for winter sadness. It has a tonic action that lifts mood. Avoid with bipolar or paranoia; rarely, may trigger insomnia.
➡ *Take 2–4 500mg capsules daily.*

ESSENTIAL OILS

Energizing and uplifting oils boost vitality, and calming oils promote restful sleep.

Orange imparts a sense of optimism.
➡ *Add 5 drops to a bath dispersant.*
Cinnamon rekindles enthusiasm in life.
➡ *Add 1–2 drops to a diffuser.*

Petitgrain is an antidepressant oil with refreshing and uplifting properties.
➥*Add 3 drops to 5ml wheatgerm oil for a restorative massage blend.*

Lavender promotes relaxation and a good night's sleep. Avoid with epilepsy.
➥*Put 1–2 drops on the pillow before bed.*

FOOD

Eat foods with vitamin D to increase levels of this mood-boosting vitamin in the winter.

Oily fish, such as salmon, mackerel, and trout, provide vitamin D.
➥ *Aim for 2–3 servings a week.*

Free range and organic eggs have been shown to contain more vitamin D in the yolks than other eggs.
➥*Snack on hard-boiled eggs.*

WHAT TO AVOID
Sugar and stimulants such as caffeine.

SUPPLEMENTS

Food may not deliver all the vitamin D you need, so supplements are advised. They can also support neurotransmitter activity.

Vitamin D supports the mood-boosting chemical serotonin.
➥*Take 600–800iu vitamin D3 daily.*

5-HTP (5-hydroxytryptophan) is a precursor to serotonin.
➥*Take 100mg 3 times daily.*

Probiotic supplements containing L reuteri NCIMB 30242 can significantly increase vitamin D levels in the blood.
➥*Look for ones with at least 10 billion live organisms per dose.*

LIFESTYLE

Use a full-spectrum light box.

OTHER THERAPIES

Acupuncture, visualization, massage, counselling, and psychotherapy can all help to ease symptoms.

STRESS
Chronic stress can lower immunity and cause insomnia, anxiety, and general aches and pains.

HERBS

"Adaptogenic" herbs, which help regulate adrenal hormones, promote resilience.

Ashwagandha is restorative. Avoid in pregnancy or with hyperthyroidism.
➥*Take 1–2ml tincture in water 3 times daily, or add the powder to smoothies.*

Astragalus boosts immunity. Avoid with acute infections and with immune-suppressant and blood-thinning drugs.
➥*Take 2–4ml tincture in a little water 3 times daily.*

Liquorice balances stress hormones. Avoid in pregnancy, with hypertension, and large doses over prolonged periods.
➥*Add ½ tsp dried shredded root to 250ml (9fl oz) boiling water, and drink 2–3 times daily.*

Lavender relaxes nerves to ease tension.
➥ *Add 1–2 cups lavender and limeflower infusion to a foot bath.*

ESSENTIAL OILS

These are highly effective in treating stress and stress-related symptoms.

Rose is both calming and uplifting.
➥*Add 5 drops to 10ml almond oil for a massage blend.*

Ylang ylang calms and soothes.
➥*Add up to 3 drops to a diffuser.*

Basil strengthens resistance to stress. Avoid in pregnancy.
➥*Add 3 drops to a diffuser.*

FOOD

Our bodies use up B vitamins, which boost the nervous system, faster under stress.

Spinach contains multiple B vitamins.
➥*Top with a hard-boiled egg and sunflower seeds for all the B vitamins.*

Lean beef, pork, lamb, calf's liver, and salmon, supply multiple B vitamins.
➥*Have 1–2 servings a week.*

Mushrooms have beta-glucans, naturally occurring polysaccharides, which support mood and immune function.
➥*Lightly steam to up the beta-glucans.*

Fermented foods boost nerve pathways from gut to brain: the "brain-gut axis".
➥*Enjoy sauerkraut or kimchi.*

WHAT TO AVOID
High-fat, high-sugar foods.

SUPPLEMENTS

Use supplements to help replenish depleted B vitamins.

B vitamins work synergistically.
➥*Take a high-dose B complex.*

Pro- and prebiotic supplements support nerve pathways to the gut.
➥*Look for ones with at least 10 billion live organisms per dose.*

Magnesium – low levels are linked to symptoms such as depression, psychosis, irritability, or confusion.
➥*Take 350–400mg a day.*

OTHER THERAPIES

Homeopathy and Bach Flower Remedies support emotional balance.

HEADY SCENT
Ylang ylang has a very strong aroma, which some can find overpowering. Start with just 1–2 drops in a diffuser to see if this is enough for you, then add another drop if desired.

HOW TO MAKE
A HERBAL INFUSION

Infusions, made using the softer parts of a herb such as the leaves and flowers, are simple and quick to make and effective. Depending on the herb, infusions are used either as medicinal remedies or therapeutic teas. The method below uses a standard ratio of herbs to water, but instructions may vary depending on the herb. For convenience you can use a tea-ball infuser instead of a teapot.

Makes 1 cup, or multiply ingredients for a bigger batch

YOU WILL NEED

1–2 tsp dried herbs, or
2–4 tsp fresh herbs (or
recommended dosage): either
a single herb or a blend

175ml (6fl oz) freshly
boiled water

teapot, or tea-ball infuser

tea cosy (optional)

strainer

teacup

honey (optional)

jug if storing in the fridge

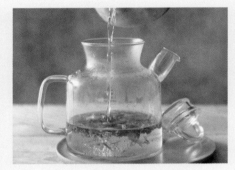

1 Warm the teapot. Place the herbs in the teapot and add the freshly boiled water. If you wish, treble the ingredients to make enough for a day's dosage.

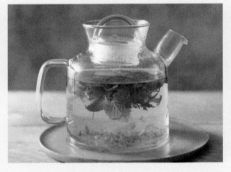

2 Place the lid on the teapot to prevent the volatile oils from escaping. This is especially beneficial for aromatic herbs such as lemon balm and chamomile. Leave the herbs to infuse in the teapot for 10–15 minutes, using a tea cosy to keep the teapot warm if you wish.

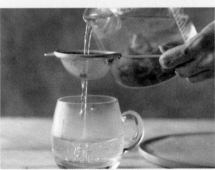

3 Strain the liquid, pouring it into a teacup, then drink warm or leave to cool, as required. Add half a teaspoon of honey for sweetness, if desired.

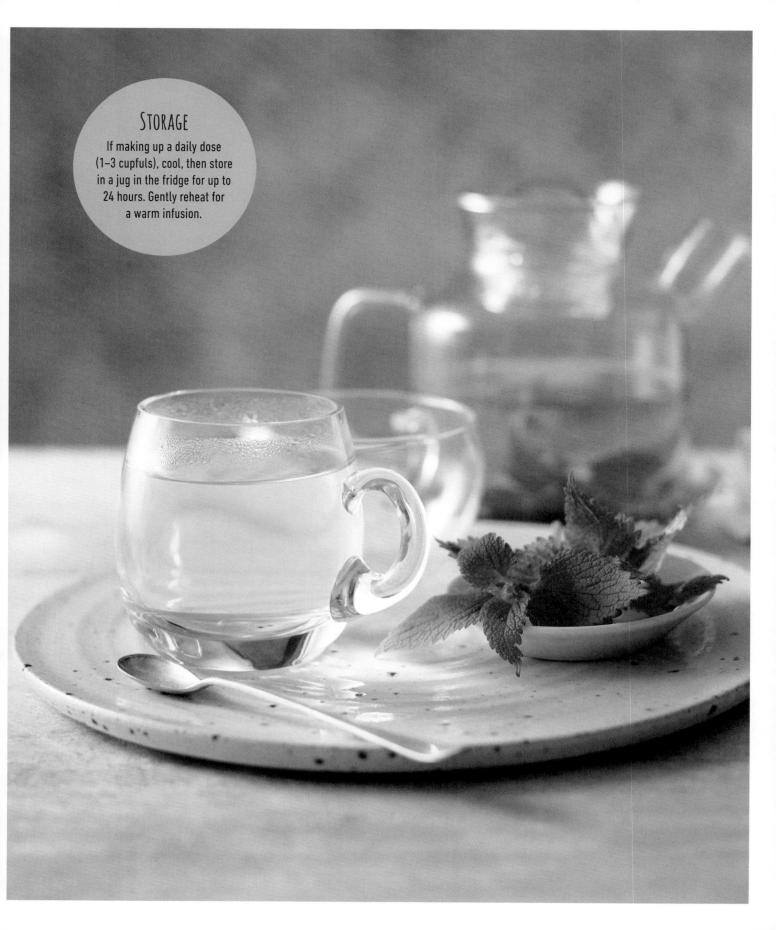

STORAGE

If making up a daily dose
(1–3 cupfuls), cool, then store
in a jug in the fridge for up to
24 hours. Gently reheat for
a warm infusion.

CONCENTRATION AND FOCUS

Our ability to focus is affected by levels of stress, quality and amount of sleep, nutrition, and age. A loss of focus can also be related to conditions such as depression, diabetes, or thyroid problems.

HERBS

Herbs can improve concentration when this is compromised by other mental health conditions. Tonic herbs, which strengthen vitality, reduce the impact of stress and fatigue on cognitive ability and gently stimulate brain function.

Ashwagandha, a tonic herb, relaxes and gently stimulates the mind to enhance mental clarity. Avoid in pregnancy or with hyperthyroidism.
➡ *Take 1–2ml tincture in a little water 3 times a day, or add the powder to smoothies or sprinkle over cereals.*

Holy basil has antioxidant properties and enhances cerebral circulation, boosting memory and concentration. Avoid in pregnancy.
➡ *Infuse 1–2 tsp dried holy basil in 175ml (6fl oz) boiling water. Drink 2–3 times a day.*

Bacopa has an antioxidant action and helps to strengthen nerves, in turn improving focus.
➡ *Take 1–3ml tincture in a little water 3 times daily.*

ESSENTIAL OILS

Essential oils can both refresh and stimulate brain circulation, boosting mental sharpness.

Rosemary is known for improving concentration and focus. Avoid with epilepsy.
➡ *Add 3 drops to a diffuser or 2 drops to a tissue and inhale as needed.*

Frankincense is a traditional aid to meditation, helping to enhance focus and concentration.
➡ *See remedy with sunflower oil, left.*

Clove is a profoundly stimulating oil that can help to focus the mind.
➡ *Add 3 drops to a diffuser, or 5 drops to 10ml vodka and 40ml (1⅓fl oz) water to make a focus-enhancing room spray.*

FOOD

Sub-optimal levels of essential nutrients and beneficial fats in the diet can affect the brain's ability to function properly. A varied, nutrient-dense diet with 1.5–2 litres (2¾–3½ pints) water daily optimizes blood flow and protects the brain from free radical damage and inflammation. Staying well hydrated is especially beneficial for improving focus and reaction times.

Dark chocolate, green tea, and curcumin – a component of turmeric – have antioxidant and anti-inflammatory properties that support a healthy brain function.
➡ *Treat yourself to an occasional square of minimum 70 per cent cocoa chocolate, drink a cup of green tea daily, and add turmeric to dishes.*

Blueberries and blackcurrants are high in the antioxidants anthocyanin and gallic acid, which help to protect the brain from degeneration and the effects of stress.
➡ *Add a handful to yogurts or scatter over porridge or cereals.*

Coconut and olive oils are rich in medium-chain fatty acids, which are natural anti-inflammatories.
➡ *Use in salads and for cooking in place of other oils.*

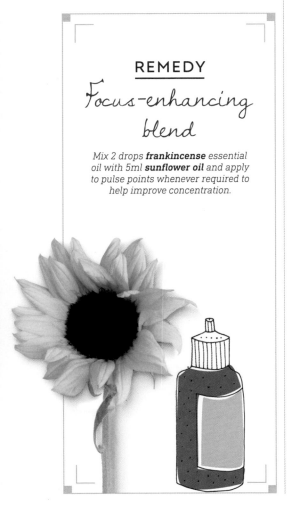

REMEDY
Focus-enhancing blend

*Mix 2 drops **frankincense** essential oil with 5ml **sunflower oil** and apply to pulse points whenever required to help improve concentration.*

> "Essential oils can have a refreshing effect, stimulating circulation to the brain and boosting mental sharpness."

Seaweed and oily fish contain polyunsaturated fatty acids such as docosahexaenoic acid (DHA), which boost brain cell connections.
➡️*Aim for at least 2 servings a week.*

Maca is high in antioxidants, B vitamins, and magnesium, all of which can help to enhance focus.
➡️*Add the powder to smoothies, yogurts, and dressings.*

WHAT TO AVOID
High-fat, high-sugar diets, which can cause blood sugar levels to spike and affect mental focus and energy.

SUPPLEMENTS

B vitamin supplements and those with the vitamin-like substance CoQ10 help to improve focus. In addition, supplements with unsaturated fatty acids support the production and functioning of neurotransmitters that aid concentration.

Iodine supports a healthy nervous system to keep the mind sharp.
➡️*Take as part of a multi-vitamin and mineral supplement.*

Folate, vitamins B6 and B12, and CoQ10 increase alertness by aiding cellular energy production and regulating nerve transmissions in the brain.
➡️*Take a B complex with added CoQ10.*

Omega-3 helps to increase the speed of neural connections and plays a role in repairing damaged neural connections.
➡️*Take a daily 500mg to 1g EPA/DHA supplement from fish or plant sources.*

Vitamin C is important in the synthesis of the neurotransmitter dopamine and it also protects the brain against oxidative stress.
➡️*Take 1g daily.*

LIFESTYLE

Meditation and yoga help train the mind to focus.

Reading, crosswords, and puzzles keep the mind active and engaged.

FATIGUE

Occasional tiredness is normal and our bodies are equipped to recover quickly. But long-term fatigue can be debilitating, robbing you of physical energy, mental sharpness, and the "get up and go" to enjoy life.

HERBS

Herbs can strengthen physically, mentally, and emotionally, restoring energy levels and vitality depleted by stress and anxiety.

Ashwagandha restores physical strength and vitality and enhances relaxation to promote restful sleep. Avoid in pregnancy or with hyperthyroidism.
➡️*Take 1–2ml tincture 3 times a day, or add the powder to smoothies or cereals.*

Oatstraw is deeply restorative for nervous exhaustion. Try using with lavender. Avoid with gluten sensitivity.
➡️*See remedy, below.*

Siberian ginseng (Eleuthero) is a tonic herb, which boosts stamina, alertness, and energy. Avoid with acute infections.
➡️*Take 3–5ml tincture in a little water 3 times daily.*

Nettle is rich in iron, acting as a strengthening, revitalizing blood tonic.
➡️*Infuse 1–2 tsp dried nettle in 175ml (6fl oz) boiling water and drink 3 times daily*

ESSENTIAL OILS

Oils that have a stimulating effect on the body and mind help to relieve feelings of fatigue and boost energy levels.

Bergamot is refreshing and uplifting.
➡️*Add 3 drops to a diffuser or add 5 drops to a bath dispersant.*

Juniper stimulates and strengthens both body and mind.
➡️*Add 5 drops to 10ml sunflower oil for a massage blend.*

Ginger boosts energy and vitality.
➡️*Add 1–2 drops to a diffuser or 5 drops to 10ml almond oil for a massage blend.*

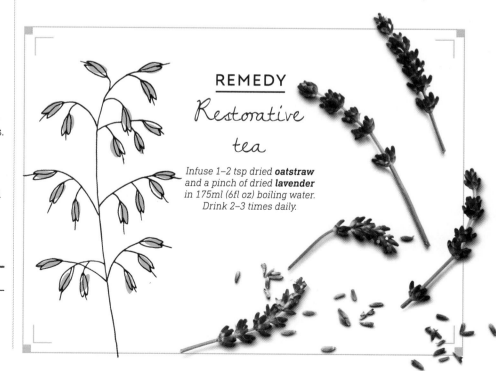

REMEDY
Restorative tea

*Infuse 1–2 tsp dried **oatstraw** and a pinch of dried **lavender** in 175ml (6fl oz) boiling water. Drink 2–3 times daily.*

➤ CONTINUED...

FOOD

Staying well hydrated with water and herbal teas and eating a nutritious, wholefood diet helps to stabilize blood sugar levels to avoid dips in energy throughout the day.

Chia seeds contain protein, fats, and fibre to provide sustained energy.
➡ *Grind and add to smoothies, porridge, and salads.*
Mushrooms have gut-friendly prebiotic inulin and energy-boosting chromium.
➡ *Grill or microwave to preserve and enhance the nutrient content.*
Bananas are high in potassium and are as effective as sports drinks for keeping energy levels up.
➡ *Snack on a banana daily.*
Pulses provide plant-based protein, slow-release carbohydrates, and fibre.
➡ *Enjoy chickpeas in a hummus dip or add pulses to stews and soups.*

SUPPLEMENTS

Additional antioxidants and essential fatty acids help to stabilize energy levels.

Magnesium is crucial for energy production and insulin metabolism.
➡ *Take 350–400mg daily.*
CoQ10 supports the adrenal glands, which influence energy levels, and improves symptoms of chronic fatigue.
➡ *Take 20mg daily.*
Chromium aids cellular energy and helps digest fats, sugars, and proteins.
➡ *Take 50–500mcg daily.*
WHAT TO AVOID
Caffeine energy supplements such as guarana and yerba mate.

LIFESTYLE

Time in nature relieves fatigue and improves mental health and wellbeing.
Regular exercise, 3–4 times a week, boosts energy levels.

INSOMNIA

If you have frequent sleepless nights this can create anxiety and cause a chronic problem. Keeping your bedroom dark and at around 18.5°C (65°F) promotes restful sleep, as will taking regular exercise.

HERBS

Herbs that relax the mind help to induce sleep and reduce disturbed sleep patterns. Anti-anxiety herbs can also be helpful.

Valerian is strongly sedative on the central nervous system and relaxes the internal organs. Avoid with sleep-inducing medication.
➡ *Take 2.5–5ml tincture twice in a little water between 6pm and bedtime.*
Hops is a sedative and aromatic herb that helps to ease tension and feelings of restlessness that accompany insomnia. Avoid with depression.
➡ *Infuse 1 tsp dried flowers in 175ml (6fl oz) boiling water for a bedtime tea.*

Passionflower is deeply relaxing for mind and body. Try using with chamomile. May cause drowsiness.
➡ *See remedy, below.*
Wild lettuce is an extremely relaxing sedative and an antispasmodic herb, which can help induce sleep.
➡ *Add 1ml tincture to a cup of passionflower tea.*

ESSENTIAL OILS

Some essential oils, such as lavender, have been proven to both induce sleep and promote a restful night's sleep.

Lavender has been shown in trials to be a safe, effective insomnia remedy.
➡ *Add 5 drops to 10ml vodka and 40ml (1⅓fl oz) water for a room spray.*
Roman chamomile is a calming and sedative oil to aid sleep.
➡ *Add 2 drops to 5ml almond oil for a pre-bedtime massage.*
Vetiver is helpful for relieving stress and tension when these block restful sleep.
➡ *Add 2–3 drops to a diffuser, or add 5 drops to a bath dispersant for a pre-bedtime bath.*

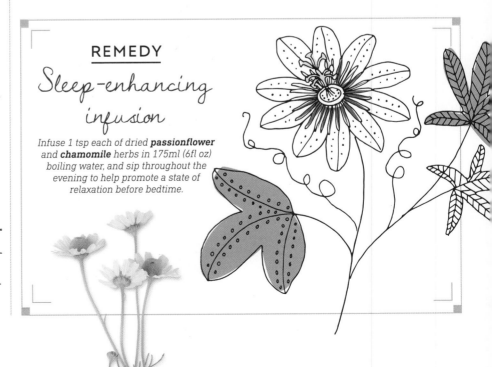

REMEDY

Sleep-enhancing infusion

*Infuse 1 tsp each of dried **passionflower** and **chamomile** herbs in 175ml (6fl oz) boiling water, and sip throughout the evening to help promote a state of relaxation before bedtime.*

FOOD

Choose foods that contain the amino acid tryptophan, which boosts levels of sleep-inducing melatonin, or ones with naturally high levels of melatonin.

Sour cherries, cherries, goji berries, tomatoes, chillies, fenugreek, white or black mustard seeds, sprouted seeds, corn, rice, and lupin provide melatonin.
➡ *Include sources regularly in your diet. A bedtime glass of sour cherry juice has been shown to aid sleep.*
Yogurt, poultry, nuts, and seeds are all good sources of tryptophan.
➡ *Include sources in your daily diet.*
WHAT TO AVOID
Junk food, which studies have shown can disrupt restorative sleep.

SUPPLEMENTS

We need a broad spectrum of nutrients to remain healthy and therefore sleep better. There are also certain nutrients that have been specifically linked to improvements in relaxation and a reduction in insomnia.

Omega-3 has been shown to promote restful sleep in children.
➡ *Take 500mg to 1g daily for adults and 300–500mg daily for children, from marine or plant sources.*
Magnesium is a trace mineral that helps the body to release tension and in turn relax.
➡ *Take 350–400mg daily.*
Vitamin D – low levels are associated with daytime sleepiness and musculoskeletal pain.
➡ *Take 600–800iu vitamin D3 daily.*

OTHER THERAPIES

Regular massage, such as shiatsu, is effective in promoting sleep.
Counselling and psychotherapy can help to address early morning waking that is linked to depression.

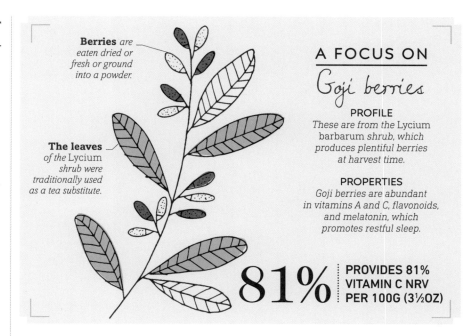

Berries *are eaten dried or fresh or ground into a powder.*

The leaves *of the* Lycium *shrub were traditionally used as a tea substitute.*

A FOCUS ON
Goji berries

PROFILE
These are from the Lycium barbarum shrub, which produces plentiful berries at harvest time.

PROPERTIES
Goji berries are abundant in vitamins A and C, flavonoids, and melatonin, which promotes restful sleep.

81%
PROVIDES 81% VITAMIN C NRV PER 100G (3½OZ)

LIBIDO

It's common to experience periods when desire is low, which may be linked to tiredness, stress, or recovery. However, if these periods become chronic – and your relationship is otherwise happy – natural remedies can help to restore desire and renew your energy levels.

HERBS

Strengthening tonic herbs support the health of the nervous system and sexual organs and boost general motivation, helping to raise libido and restore essential vitality.

Damiana is a well-known traditional aphrodisiac used for its energizing and uplifting tonic actions that help to reignite desire.
➡ *Infuse 1–2 tsp dried damiana in 175ml (6fl oz) boiling water and drink 3 times daily.*

Saw palmetto is a restorative and stimulating herb. It is also used to help balance hormone levels and can boost sexual function for both men and women.
➡ *Take 1–3ml tincture in a little water 3 times daily.*
Lycium is a traditional Chinese remedy used as a strengthening tonic, which can help to increase testosterone levels and in turn restore a flagging libido. Avoid with digestive irritability.
➡ *Take 1–3ml tincture in a little water 3 times daily.*

BEST BEFORE

Cherries don't fare well when kept at room temperature, quickly losing quality and nutrients. Store cherries in the fridge for up to 5 days, or freeze fresh cherries.

➤ CONTINUED...

ESSENTIAL OILS

Essential oils act therapeutically on the mind and body to help stimulate passion and reawaken sexual arousal by gently working to relieve stress and anxiety and energize the body.

Sandalwood has restorative properties and a subtle earthy aroma that can help to strengthen sex drive, particularly in men.
➡️*Add 1–2 drops to a diffuser, or add 10 drops to 20ml (¾fl oz) coconut oil for a sensual massage blend.*
Coriander is a warming, toning oil that can be used to relieve held-in tension, which can dampen libido, and to help clear the mind.
➡️*Add 5 drops to 10ml almond oil for a relaxing massage blend.*
Jasmine is a classic aphrodisiacal oil. It has a sensual, heady, and exotic aroma that is both extremely relaxing and powerfully uplifting.
➡️*Add 2–3 drops to a diffuser, or add 5 drops to 10ml jojoba oil for a massage blend.*

FOOD

Include foods in your diet that support sustained energy release and ones that are high in important trace elements such as zinc, which are necessary for maintaining healthy circulation.

LOCKING IN OILS

A high oil content means that walnuts can turn rancid quickly. Buy just a few at a time, in their shells, and store in the fridge in an airtight container.

"Therapeutic essential oils stimulate arousal by working gently to relieve stress and anxiety and re-energize."

Oysters, clams, and scallops, as well as crab and lobster are all excellent sources of zinc, which helps to boost blood flow around the body, in turn promoting desire.
➡️*Eat a serving a week. Try oysters raw, or, if you prefer, smoked.*
Walnuts are rich in zinc and the amino acid l-arginine, both of which improve circulation. They are also a good source of omega-3 fats, which can heighten sexual arousal by raising dopamine levels in the brain.
➡️*Snack on a handful of walnuts.*
Goji berries contain beneficial polysaccharides, which can help protect testosterone levels from the effects of stress.
➡️*Eat up to 30g (1oz) goji berries daily, on cereals, in salads, and as a snack.*
Eggs contain energy-sustaining protein and amino acids, one of which, tyrosine, helps produce the feel-good hormones norepinephrine and dopamine to boost levels of desire.
➡️*Feel free to eat eggs daily.*
Beetroot juice contains significant levels of dietary nitrate, which the body metabolizes into nitric oxide, a gas that widens blood vessels. It is also high in boron, the mineral that stimulates the production of sexual hormones.
➡️*Enjoy a glass daily.*

SUPPLEMENTS

Boosting the diet with supplements that support circulation and both aid the production of sex hormones and help to balance hormones can be helpful for restoring libido.

Vitamin E enhances mood and desire, aids in the production of sex hormones, and protects these hormones from the damaging effects of oxidation.
➡️*Take 400iu daily.*
Pine bark extract increases micro-circulation and is well researched to improve libido and sexual enjoyment, especially in women.
➡️*Take a 100mg capsule daily.*
Amino acids, especially l-arginine and l-carnitine, support a healthy blood flow to help boost sexual function.
➡️*Amino acids work synergistically, meaning their effects tend to be enhanced when combined, so take a broad-spectrum supplement that includes all 20 amino acids.*
Zinc helps improve sperm count, supports prostate health, and boosts testosterone to increase sex drive.
➡️*Take up to 40mg daily.*

LIFESTYLE

Losing weight and taking regular exercise will improve fitness and stamina, relieve tension, and help to boost confidence.

OTHER THERAPIES

Counselling and psychotherapy can be helpful when loss of libido is linked to emotional problems such as depression.
Massage therapy is an effective way to promote feelings of relaxation, relieve stress, and help you to get back in touch with your body.

EMOTIONAL SHOCK

Emotional pain, which can be caused by factors such as bereavement, illness, or an upsetting event, can be as real to the brain as physical pain. If unaddressed, it can cause the same damage to the body as chronic stress.

HERBS

Relaxing herbs that calm the mind and body are beneficial. In addition, herbs that support the heart and central nervous system can be strengthening during times of trauma and stress.

Valerian, a natural tranquillizer, acts on the central nervous system to calm the mind. It also has an antispasmodic action that releases held-in tension. Avoid with sleep-inducing medication.
➡*Take 2.5–5ml tincture in a little water 3 times daily.*
Passionflower is deeply relaxing. It has a sedative action that relaxes the body and mind in difficult times. The herb may cause feelings of drowsiness.
➡*Infuse 1–2 tsp dried passionflower in 175ml (6fl oz) boiling water and drink 3 times daily.*

Rose is emotionally uplifting and strengthening, and has a mildly sedative action.
➡*Combine equal parts rose, valerian, and passionflower in a tincture. Take 1ml in a little water when needed.*

ESSENTIAL OILS

Calming and relaxing essential oils that help to balance the emotions and impart a sense of wellbeing can be extremely supportive after experiencing emotional shock, grief, or trauma.

Lavender is the "go-to" essential oil remedy for treating emotional shock and trauma. It has a gently relaxing action and is deeply soothing.
➡*Add 3 drops to a diffuser or 5 drops to a bath dispersant for a warm, relaxing bedtime bath.*
Helichrysum is a profoundly healing oil that can help to relieve acute anxiety and the symptoms of stress.
➡*Add 5 drops to 10ml wheatgerm oil for a massage blend.*
Rose is both calming and uplifting, helping to relieve the stress of emotional shock.
➡*Add 1–2 drops to a diffuser or 5 drops to 10ml jojoba oil for a soothing massage blend.*

FOOD

Shock causes a spike in cortisol levels, which in turn can lead to food cravings and the release of enzymes that cause the body to hang on to its fat stores. Include satiating foods in your diet, which release energy slowly and contain nutrients with calming and steadying properties.

Asparagus is high in the folate – vitamin B12 – which helps to balance emotions.
➡*Grill or steam to preserve nutrients; add to salads or eat as a side dish.*
Summer berries, such as strawberries, raspberries, blackberries, and blueberries are high in the stress-busting vitamin C.
➡*See recipe suggestion, below.*
Cashews are an especially good source of zinc, low levels of which have been linked to both anxiety and depression.
➡*Snack on a handful of cashews, or add to salads and stir-fries.*
Dark chocolate, with at least 70 per cent cocoa content, contains flavonoids that can help lower blood pressure, helping induce a feeling of calm.
➡*A square of chocolate once or twice a week is a healthy indulgence.*
WHAT TO AVOID
Stimulants such as caffeine, which can make you feel more jittery.

RECIPE

Vitamin C stress buster

*Add 150g (5½oz) mixed organic berries, such as **blackberries**, **strawberries**, and **raspberries**, to 100ml (3½fl oz) natural or coconut **yogurt**. Place in a blender and blitz until smooth, then drink immediately.*

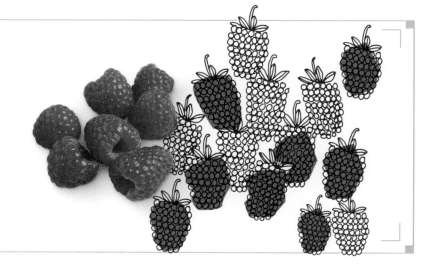

➤ CONTINUED...

SUPPLEMENTS

Certain nutrients act as buffers against shock and trauma so supporting the diet with supplements during difficult emotional periods can help to boost recovery. Probiotics support gut health, which in turn supports emotional health by boosting neurotransmitters between the brain and gut. In addition, calcium, magnesium, and zinc are important for combating the effects of stress.

Calcium helps to transmit impulses through neural pathways and has a calming effect on nerves.
➺*Take up to 1g daily.*

Magnesium levels can be depleted in those suffering from chronic shock or long-term stress, so a regular supplement can help to ensure that there are sufficient levels of magnesium circulating in the body.
➺*Take 350–400mg daily.*

Probiotic supplements help to rebalance gut flora, which in turn supports emotional balance.
➺*Look for a probiotic that has at least 10 billion live organisms per dose and that can resist stomach acid.*

LIFESTYLE

Relaxation techniques, such as yoga and meditation, when practised regularly, help to reduce levels of stress hormones, which in turn helps to balance the emotions, calm the mind, and leads to a sense of enhanced wellbeing.

Absorbing hobbies and activities can be extremely beneficial for lowering stress levels.

OTHER THERAPIES

Counselling and psychotherapy can provide a safe space in which to express emotions.

Massage helps to ground the body.

POST-TRAUMATIC STRESS DISORDER

Post-traumatic stress disorder (PTSD) can follow a life-threatening, terrifying, and/or horrific event. Sufferers may experience flashbacks and have feelings of guilt and anxiety. Women are more susceptible than men and multiple trauma increases risk.

HERBS

Herbs can support emotional healing gently and powerfully. They can be used to ease the associated numbness and pain that accompanies PTSD and to restore strength, helping to calm the nerves and lift the spirits.

Rose is emotionally uplifting, strengthening, and has a mildly sedative action.
➺*Infuse 2–6 tsp rose petals in 400–600ml (14fl oz to 1 pint) boiling water. Add to a warm bath, with some rosebuds floating on the water.*

Oatstraw is a nutritious and restorative nerve tonic, ideal for long-term convalescence. Avoid taking with gluten sensitivity.
➺*See remedy, below.*

Hawthorn is a potent heart tonic. See box, opposite, and remedy below for use. Avoid with heart medication unless under medical supervision.
➺*Take 2–5ml tincture in a little water 3 times daily.*

ESSENTIAL OILS

Aromatherapy essential oils can be used as a supportive treatment for PTSD, working alongside other therapies to help balance emotions.

Cedarwood is a deep-acting oil that helps to steady the mind and strengthen the nerves.
➺*Add 5 drops to 10ml almond oil for a massage blend, or 5 drops to 10ml bath dispersant for a warm bath.*

Lemon balm is one of the most effective oils for treating post-trauma anxiety and depression.
➺*Add 1–2 drops to a diffuser or a tissue and inhale as needed.*

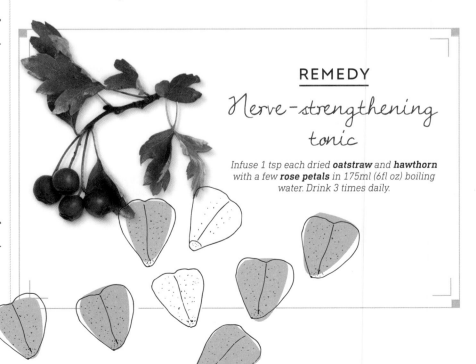

REMEDY

Nerve-strengthening tonic

Infuse 1 tsp each dried **oatstraw** and **hawthorn** with a few **rose petals** in 175ml (6fl oz) boiling water. Drink 3 times daily.

PALATE SWEETENER

Try soaking sour-tasting goji berries in hot water for a few minutes until softened to sweeten the flavour.

Ylang ylang has a sedative effect and can calm symptoms of anxiety such as palpitations and hyperventilation.
➥*Add 1–2 drops to a diffuser.*

FOOD

Staying hydrated with 1.5–2 litres (2¾–3½ pints) water daily and eating plenty of fresh fruit and vegetables, high-quality protein, and healthy fats, in particular, omega-3 fatty acids, provides essential nutrients and helps to balance blood sugar levels to support coping mechanisms after trauma.

Cherries, goji berries, fenugreek, corn, rice, sprouted seeds, and lupin are all rich in melatonin, the hormone that helps to regulate sleep–wake cycles, allowing you to rest and in turn speed recovery and maintain equilibrium.
➥*Include at least 2–3 servings in your diet each week.*

Citrus fruits, summer berries, guava, red peppers, tomatoes, and kale are high in vitamin C, which supports and restores the release of stress hormones from the adrenal glands.
➥*Try juicing to obtain nutrients in an easily absorbed form.*

Spinach, kale, tomatoes, broccoli, cauliflower, cucumber, onions, and asparagus have slow-release carbohydrates that stabilize the energy supply to the muscles and brain.
➥*Eat raw or lightly steamed.*

Oily fish contain omega-3 fatty acids that support nerve and brain function.
➥*Serve with mixed steamed vegetables for a calming, sustaining meal.*
WHAT TO AVOID
Processed and "white" foods made with refined flours and sugars; caffeine and alcohol.

SUPPLEMENTS

Trauma and stress deplete the body of nutrients and can exacerbate the symptoms of PTSD. A regular supplement regime may help to speed recovery.

Vitamin C is an antioxidant and an adrenal enhancer, helping to control the release of stress hormones.
➥*Take 1g with added bioflavonoids daily.*
Omega-3 fatty acids improve immunity and protect nerve transmission.
➥*Aim for 500mg to 1g daily.*
Vitamins B12, B6, and B5 play a role in producing the chemicals involved in regulating mood and cellular metabolism and help reduce fatigue.
➥*Take as part of a daily B complex.*
Melatonin aids restful sleep. Supplements should be taken for a short period of time only and should be a low dosage.
➥*Take up to 5mg 2 hours before bedtime. Use for no longer than 2 months.*

LIFESTYLE

Practise stress management with regular exercise and yoga.

OTHER THERAPIES

Counselling and psychotherapy are essential to provide support and help work through issues surrounding traumatic events.
Homeopathy helps to support and promote emotional wellness.

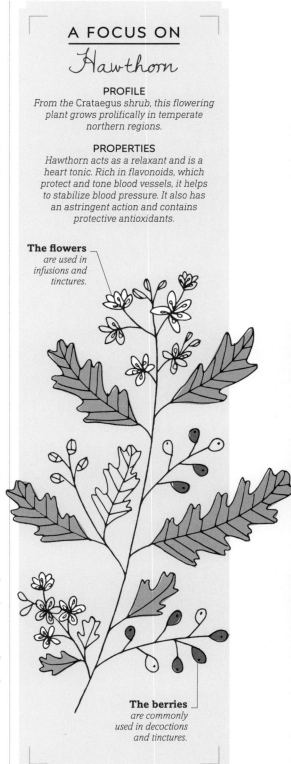

A FOCUS ON
Hawthorn

PROFILE
From the Crataegus shrub, this flowering plant grows prolifically in temperate northern regions.

PROPERTIES
Hawthorn acts as a relaxant and is a heart tonic. Rich in flavonoids, which protect and tone blood vessels, it helps to stabilize blood pressure. It also has an astringent action and contains protective antioxidants.

The flowers *are used in infusions and tinctures.*

The berries *are commonly used in decoctions and tinctures.*

SKIN, HAIR, AND NAILS

Our skin, hair, and nails have several important roles, including helping to regulate temperature, providing a protective barrier, and supplying sensory information. Find out how nourishing foods and cleansing, toning, and antimicrobial herbs and essential oils strengthen and protect the fabric of the skin, hair, and nails, leaving them looking healthy and conditioned. If the health of these areas is compromised, discover how healing nutrients and holistic remedies can soothe, balance, and repair.

STAYING WELL

SKIN, HAIR, AND NAILS

For healthy skin and well-conditioned hair and nails, it's important to get the right balance of nourishing nutrients and to stay well hydrated to prevent the dryness that can make skin and hair more vulnerable to damage. In addition, herbs and essential oils provide all-natural-ingredient treatments that can help to keep the skin, hair, and nails looking and feeling their very best.

FOOD

A broad range of nutrients promotes a healthy skin barrier and helps to condition the hair and nails. Aim for more than half of your diet to consist of fresh, raw, organic produce, and eat more vegetables than fruit.

CLEANSING FOODS

Your skin is a major detoxification pathway, and if it is working hard to remove toxins this can lead to flare-ups. High-fibre pulses and wholegrains support the removal of waste through the digestive system, taking pressure off the skin.

SKIN-STRENGTHENING NUTRIENTS

Certain foods help to strengthen the skin barrier and boost immunity to protect the skin. Garlic, onions, leeks, and chives are excellent immune-boosting foods, and cruciferous vegetables, such as spinach, collard greens, and kale, are rich in skin-loving sulphur compounds, which support immunity and promote healthy connective tissue to strengthen the hair, nails, and skin and ensure that these are in optimum condition.

SKIN-HEALTHY FATS

Healthy fats are key for skin, hair, and nails. Polyunsaturated fats have omega-3 fatty acids, which are part of the building blocks for cell membranes, supporting the skin's natural oil barrier to keep skin supple. Omega-3 fats also aid the absorption of vitamins A and E, vital for skin, hair, and nail health. Use olive and coconut oils daily and eat oily fish, chia and flaxseeds, eggs, and nuts.

SKIN-TONING NUTRIENTS

As we age, or if we put on excess weight, skin on the body can lose its smooth appearance and appear dimpled, known as cellulite. Eating a low-carbohydrate diet alongside healthy fats helps to maintain weight to keep skin toned and reduce the

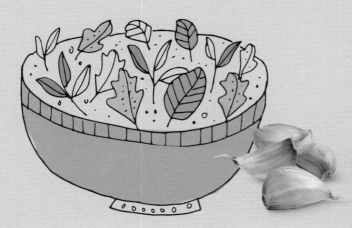

Add 1–2 cloves of crushed garlic *to a vinaigrette dressing made with extra virgin olive oil and toss over a salad or add to lightly steamed green vegetables.*

> *"Herbal preparations can help the skin to retain moisture."*

Enjoy a daily egg, *boiled or poached, on wholemeal toast, to provide nail-boosting amino acids.*

appearance of cellulite. Another skin-toning nutrient is magnesium, found in foods such as seaweed, nuts, and yogurt, which has a diuretic effect that helps to eliminate excess water and reduce fluid retention. In addition, antioxidant-rich green tea boosts metabolism to help control weight gain and reduce the risk of cellulite forming.

NUTRIENTS FOR HEALTHY HAIR

Support hair health by including sources of zinc and vitamin B6 in your diet. Zinc plays a role in cell metabolism, helping to keep the scalp clean and flake free, and vitamin B6 is thought to aid hair growth. Nuts, wholegrains, turkey, chicken, and fish provide vitamin B6, while chickpeas, cashews, and seeds supply zinc.

NAIL-CONDITIONING NUTRIENTS

Nails are made from the protein keratin so need protein to stay strong. Eggs provide complete protein, with all the essential amino acids; the amino acid cysteine in particular supports nail growth.

HERBS

Medicinal plants and herbal preparations can help the skin to retain moisture, support immunity to prevent infections, and boost the condition of hair and nails.

HERBAL SKIN TONERS

Astringent herbs help to tone skin and reduce the likelihood of spider veins. Horse chestnut, used traditionally to tone capillaries and stimulate circulation, helps to nourish and hydrate skin.

CLEARING HERBS

Mahonia, blue flag, and thyme are effective herbs for supporting the liver, lymph, and urinary systems, helping to cleanse the body and promote cleaner- and clearer-looking skin. Herbs that have a diuretic effect, such as parsley, promote the effective elimination of waste and support skin and hair health.

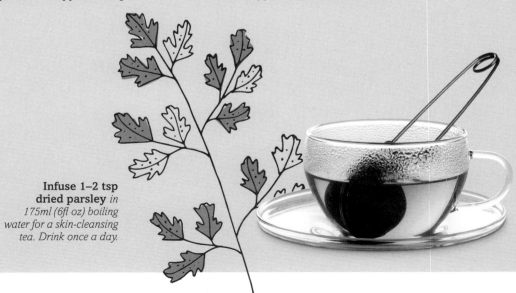

Infuse 1–2 tsp dried parsley *in 175ml (6fl oz) boiling water for a skin-cleansing tea. Drink once a day.*

Infection-fighting herbs

Herbs with antifungal properties boost the skin's resistance to infection. Calendula, a popular healing remedy, promotes cell regeneration, while exotic myrrh is antifungal and antibacterial.

Skin-calming and protective herbs

Chickweed cools and calms skin prone to breakouts and itching. Comfrey, used externally only, has a gel-like mucilage to protect skin from toxins, and a healing compound allantoin; while anti-inflammatory St John's wort conditions the skin and scalp.

Nutrient boost

Some herbs, eaten as foods, provide nutrients that help to optimize skin, hair, and nail health. Nettles supply both calcium and silica for healthy nails, and dandelion leaves are also high in calcium.

Balancing herbs

Our skin can reflect our emotional state. Used holistically, herbs balance the body, allowing healing in one area to boost health elsewhere. Calming infusions, such as chamomile and lemon balm, balance mood and create a feeling of wellbeing, promoting health and vitality across the body.

Essential oils

Cleansing, toning, and rejuvenating diluted aromatherapy oils support skin, hair, and nail health.

Oils to cleanse and stimulate

Detoxifying oils help to cleanse skin, lymphatic-stimulating oils ward off infection, and diuretic oils help reduce water retention to promote smooth skin. Refreshing grapefruit, uplifting cypress, and astringent and earthy juniper berry cleanse and stimulate, while mandarin, neroli, and frankincense revitalize the complexion. Massage with oils to stimulate cell growth and rejuvenate skin.

Toning oils

Oils can help to brighten skin tone. Rose, a time-honoured choice for skin, is emollient and hydrating for smooth, radiant skin.

Oils to refresh

Refreshing oils help to calm the mind and body and reduce flushing and sweating in warm weather. Petitgrain refreshes skin, lemon cools and dries, and cypress is a strong deodorizer.

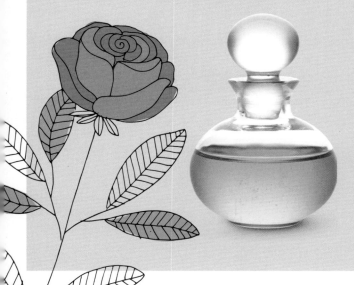

Add 2 drops rose essential oil *to 10ml almond oil and gently massage into the face, avoiding the area around the eyes, to brighten the complexion.*

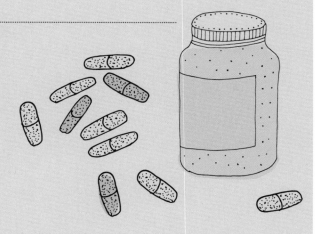

HAIR-CONDITIONING OILS

Massaging an oil blend into the scalp stimulates follicles to boost scalp health and give hair a sheen. Antimicrobial rosemary protects the scalp and boosts circulation to follicles. Cedarwood also stimulates the follicles, and antifungal sage wards off dandruff and helps balance sebum to condition the hair and scalp.

SUPPLEMENTS

A range of nutrients helps optimize skin, hair, and nail health; a supplement regime supports a varied diet.

NUTRIENT BASICS

Base a supplement regime around a good-quality multi-vitamin and mineral supplement as well as an omega-3 fatty acid supplement to support healthy skin cells and moisture balance.

FAT-BURNING NUTRIENTS

If cellulite is a concern, a brown seaweed supplement derived from kelp and wakame could help to burn fat more efficiently. It has a carotenoid, fucoxanthin, which helps burn fat over time.

NUTRIENTS FOR SUPPLE SKIN

Stretch marks can be hard to prevent, with some skin types more prone. A nutrient-dense diet boosts skin elasticity, and zinc and vitamin E in particular strengthen the skin's structure to minimize the appearance of stretch marks. A supplement ensures adequate levels of these skin-supporting nutrients.

INFECTION-FIGHTING SUPPLEMENTS

Supplements that support immunity improve resistance to skin and nail infections when these strike. Vitamin C boosts immunity, while zinc helps sustain levels of vitamin E and aids in the absorption of vitamin A – both vital for immunity and skin health. Probiotic supplements help to populate the gut with beneficial bacteria to fight infections. Look for a supplement that contains at least 10 billion live organisms to colonize the gut and promote a healthy gut flora.

NAIL STRENGTHENERS

Two supplements specifically target nail health. Biotin, a B vitamin, helps to thicken weak nails and reduces splitting, while colloidal silica, also known as orthosilicic acid, strengthens nails – and also boosts hair and skin health.

"Essential oil blends can be massaged into the scalp to help give hair a glossy sheen."

TREATMENTS

SKIN, HAIR, AND NAILS

The condition of our skin, hair, and nails can reflect our inner health, and these visible parts of us are also vulnerable to damage and infection. Healing treatments and nutritional therapy can help to combat complaints and boost appearance.

DRY, CRACKED, CHAPPED SKIN

Dry skin can be delicate, flaky, and prone to fine lines and/or itchiness. Overuse of soaps and detergents is a major cause of dry skin.

HERBS

Soothing, anti-inflammatory, and healing herbs help to protect and moisturize and accelerate healing.

Comfrey is high in moisturizing mucilage and allantoin, which promotes healing. Avoid on infected or deep lesions as it heals rapidly so could trap bacteria. Take advice before internal use.
➡ *Apply a comfrey-based cream or ointment to affected areas as needed.*
Elderflower can be used topically as an emollient to soften dry, chapped skin.
➡ *Apply an elderflower hand cream with other protective ingredients such as shea butter or almond oil daily.*
Calendula is an anti-inflammatory with skin moistening, healing properties. Avoid internal use in pregnancy.
➡ *Infuse 1–2 tsp dried calendula in 175ml (6fl oz) boiling water and drink 3 times daily.*

> "Soothing, anti-inflammatory herbs can be used to help protect and moisturize dry skin."

ESSENTIAL OILS

Regular massage increases circulation and improves skin health.

Sandalwood soothes and moisturizes.
➡ *Add 2 drops to 5ml almond oil and massage into the skin.*
Rose is both emollient and hydrating.
➡ *Add 2 drops to 5ml avocado oil and massage into the skin.*
Geranium helps to balance the production of sebum.
➡ *Add 2 drops to 5ml jojoba oil and massage into the skin.*
Sweet orange has healing properties and is antibacterial.
➡ *Add 2 drops to a balm for chapped lips.*

FOOD

Healthy fats aid the absorption of skin-loving nutrients such as vitamins A and E. Hydration is essential, too. Drink 1.5–2 litres (2¾–3½ pints) of water, herbal teas, or coconut water daily.

Olive oil is a good source of skin-healing vitamin E and omega-9 (oleic acid).
➡ *Use up to 2 tbsp cold-pressed extra-virgin olive oil in dressings or meals daily.*
Coconut oil has skin-nourishing medium-chain fatty acids. Coconut water has hydrating trace elements, such as zinc and manganese, to boost skin elasticity.
➡ *Use 2 tbsp of the oil daily or drink 300ml (10fl oz) of coconut water.*
Berries are high in vitamin C, which boosts circulation and collagen.
➡ *Add to smoothies or porridge.*

SUPPLEMENTS

Supplementing the diet with healthy fats helps support very dry skin.

Flaxseed oil contains both omega-3 and omega-6 polyunsaturated fatty acids.
➡ *Take 500mg twice daily with food.*
Borage oil has anti-inflammatory gamma-linolenic acid (GLA).
➡ *Take 500mg 3 times daily.*

ABSCESSES AND BOILS

These painful sacs of pus are infected sebaceous cysts. Medical treatment is needed to release pus.

HERBS

Herbs cleanse, heal, and boost immunity.

Burdock root is deeply cleansing.
➥ *Make a decoction to wash the area or infuse 1–2 tsp dried burdock in 175ml (6fl oz) boiling water. Drink 3 times daily.*
Echinacea aids immunity and used externally cleanses skin. See box, below. Avoid with immunosuppressants.
➥ *Apply a poultice made with slippery elm powder and echinacea tincture.*

ESSENTIAL OILS

Anti-inflammatory, antibacterial oils ease discomfort and support healing.

Thyme has thymol, a powerful antiseptic.

Tea tree is a broad antimicrobial, fighting bacteria, viruses, and fungi.
Oregano is antibacterial and calming.
➥ *Use 6 drops of any of the above oils, or 2 drops of each, in a warm compress.*

FOOD

Eat immune-supporting, detoxifying foods.

Pulses and wholegrains are high in fibre to remove waste and toxins.
➥ *Eat wholewheat bread and pasta.*
Garlic, onions, and cruciferous vegetables have immune-boosting sulphur.
➥ *Use liberally in meals and eat raw.*

SUPPLEMENTS

These support immunity and aid healing.

Vitamin C boosts collagen production to help heal wounds and prevent scarring.
➥ *Take 1g with meals daily.*
Vitamin B6 supports efficient immunity.
➥ *Take 25–50mg of a B complex daily.*
Zinc supports vitamin E levels and aids vitamin A absorption for skin health.
➥ *Take at least 11mg daily.*

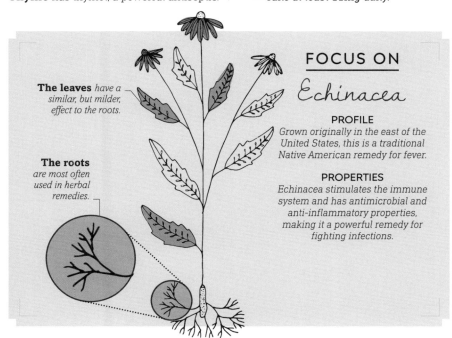

The leaves *have a similar, but milder, effect to the roots.*

The roots *are most often used in herbal remedies.*

FOCUS ON
Echinacea

PROFILE
Grown originally in the east of the United States, this is a traditional Native American remedy for fever.

PROPERTIES
Echinacea stimulates the immune system and has antimicrobial and anti-inflammatory properties, making it a powerful remedy for fighting infections.

ACNE

Caused by chronic inflammation of hair follicles and sebaceous glands, acne usually occurs in the early to mid teens and may last until the mid-20s.

HERBS

Use herbs that help to cleanse the liver, lymphatic, and urinary systems and which reduce inflammation.

Thyme has an antibacterial action against the acne-linked bacterium *Propionibacterium acnes* and is also a tonic for the immune system. Avoid internal use in pregnancy.
➥ *Infuse 1–2 tsp dried thyme in 175ml (6fl oz) boiling water and apply as a skin wash twice daily, or drink as a tea twice daily.*
Calendula is anti-inflammatory and promotes skin healing. It also helps fight *Propionibacterium acnes* bacteria.
➥ *Add 10 drops tincture to the thyme infusion, above, and apply directly to the affected skin.*
Mahonia (Oregon grape), a liver tonic, boosts skin health. Avoid in pregnancy.
➥ *Take 1–5ml tincture in a little water 3 times a day.*

ESSENTIAL OILS

Oils can fight infection, reduce bacteria, promote healing, and reduce inflammation.

Palmarosa is antiseptic and also helps to balance sebum production and hydrate the skin.
Bergamot helps balance oily skin and its uplifting effect alleviates depression. Avoid sun exposure after use.
➥ *Add 2 drops of any of the above oils to 5ml jojoba oil and massage into the face; or add 5 drops oil to 5ml base lotion for use on the body.*

➤ CONTINUED...

Tea tree is antimicrobial and well known for treating acne. It combines effectively with rosehip oil.
➥*See remedy, below.*

Lavender is antiseptic, healing, and anti-inflammatory, helping to calm and soothe the skin. Avoid with epilepsy.
➥*Add 2 drops to 10ml wheatgerm oil and massage into the skin.*

FOOD

Nutrients can boost resistance to the acne-linked *Propionibacterium acnes* and *Staphylococcus epidermidis* bacteria. Plus staying well hydrated with water and herbal teas helps to flush out toxins from the body more efficiently.

Legumes, such as chickpeas and lentils, as well as spinach, asparagus, and Brussels sprouts are all high in folate, which helps to boost red cell production and oxygenate cells.
➥*Add pulses to salads and meals and eat other sources regularly.*

Flaxseed is high in omega-3, which helps to reduce the inflammation that can accompany some types of acne.
➥*Add ground flaxseeds to salads, soups, or bakes.*

Coconut oil is a potent antibacterial. It can be helpful internally, and studies also show that applied externally it inhibits *Propionibacterium acnes*.
➥*Use 1–2 tbsp a day in cooking or dab onto skin.*

WHAT TO AVOID

Sugary, processed foods. Some people benefit from avoiding dairy products.

SUPPLEMENTS

Antioxidants and gut-friendly probiotics aid skin health and reduce inflammation.

Vitamin C is anti-inflammatory, immune-boosting, and vital for collagen repair.
➥*Take 1g daily.*

Zinc aids repair and boosts immunity.
➥*Take up to 40mg in divided doses daily.*

Probiotic supplements with prebiotic fibre replenish good gut bacteria to increase immunity.
➥*Look for one that supplies up to 10 billion live organisms per dose.*

LIFESTYLE

20–30 minutes of sunshine a day without sunscreen helps tackle acne.
Relaxation and sleep boost skin health.

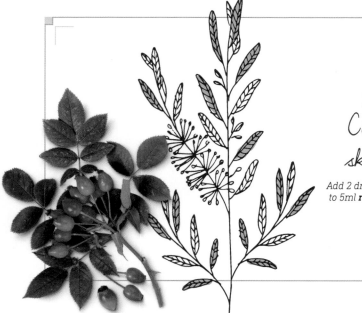

REMEDY

Cleansing skin blend

*Add 2 drops **tea tree** essential oil to 5ml **rosehip oil** and massage into the skin.*

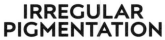

IRREGULAR PIGMENTATION

Two conditions that cause irregular skin pigmentation are vitiligo and melasma. Vitiligo is an auto-immune skin disease in which loss of the pigment melanin creates irregular white patches. Melasma is the dark skin colouration that appears on sun-exposed areas of the face. Both can be managed but not cured.

HERBS

Antioxidant herbs limit skin damage from ageing and UV exposure. Combine herbs that nourish with ones that cleanse and help eliminate waste to revitalize tissues.

Ginkgo biloba is immune-supporting and antioxidant. Avoid in pregnancy, if breastfeeding, and with anticoagulants and antiplatelet medication.
➥*Take 40mg in a capsule 3 times daily.*

Rosehip seeds produce an antioxidant oil with vitamins and essential fatty acids to reduce hyperpigmentation.
➥*Use 2–3 times daily for a few months.*

Gotu kola is detoxifying, stimulates cellular regeneration, and is effective against UV-induced pigmentation. Avoid in pregnancy and with epilepsy. May cause skin sensitivity.
➥*Infuse 1–2 tsp dried gotu kola in 175ml (6fl oz) boiling water and drink 3 times daily. Can also be used externally in creams.*

ESSENTIAL OILS

Use essential oils to help rejuvenate the skin and improve skin tone.

Lemon helps to even skin tone and brighten the complexion.
➥*Add 4 drops to 20ml (⅔fl oz) apricot oil and massage into the affected skin.*

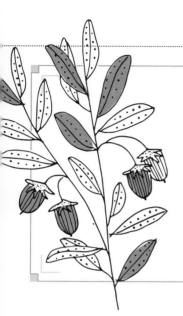

REMEDY

Skin-toning blend

*Add 4 drops **rose** essential oil to 20ml (⅔fl oz) **jojoba oil** and massage into the affected skin.*

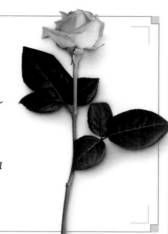

Sandalwood helps to diminish skin discolouration.
➡*Add 4 drops to 20ml (⅔fl oz) argan oil and massage into the affected area on the body.*

Rose brightens and rejuvenates the skin, helping to even skin tone.
➡*See remedy with jojoba oil, above.*

FOOD

Foods won't halt vitiligo, but certain nutrients support and improve overall skin tone. Eat foods that provide beta-carotene, a carotenoid that is converted into skin-friendly vitamin A in the body, and other essential vitamins.

Liver from beef, pork, and poultry is a natural source of retinol (vitamin A1), which helps to promote healthy skin pigmentation.
➡*Eat a maximum one portion a week.*

Carrots, broccoli, sweet potato, butter, kale, and peas are all good sources of antioxidant carotenoids.
➡*Stir-fry or steam vegetables to preserve nutrients and add a knob of butter to dishes to aid absorption.*

WHAT TO AVOID

Processed foods and, for vitiligo, blueberries. pears, wheat, and coffee, which have hydroquinone, a de-pigmenting agent.

SUPPLEMENTS

Addressing deficiencies of folic acid, vitamin B12, or trace elements can help to support melanin production in the skin.

B vitamins (B12 and folic acid) together with phototherapy – a type of light therapy for skin conditions – may help to restore skin pigmentation in cases of vitiligo.
➡*Take a good-quality B complex daily.*

Copper promotes melanin production. Melasma sufferers should avoid this, but those suffering with vitiligo may benefit from additional copper.
➡*Take up to 900mcg daily.*

Betaine HCl is sometimes recommended for vitiligo when this is caused by low stomach acid.
➡*Take as directed.*

Pine bark extract is a powerful antioxidant that helps to protect melasma sufferers from the effects of UV radiation.
➡*Take 25mg 3 times daily.*

LIFESTYLE

Avoiding direct sunlight and/or using sunscreens with an SPF factor 50 daily is essential for protecting the skin. Also avoid skin products with harsh chemicals and colourants.

ECZEMA

Also referred to as dermatitis, this describes the itchy and uncomfortable skin condition, which can lead to broken, weepy skin.

HERBS

Eczema responds well to healing and anti-inflammatory herbs as well as ones that help to inhibit the itching, known as antipruritic herbs. Taking herbs internally is especially effective for treating eczema and any underlying causes.

Heartsease, or viola, is a traditional remedy to relieve inflammation.
➡*Take 1–2ml tincture in a little water 3 times a day, or add to a neutral base cream to apply externally.*

Chickweed cools and relieves inflamed skin to help ease itching.
➡*Apply a chickweed-based ointment or take 1–2ml tincture in a little water daily. Fresh chickweed can also be enjoyed in salads, stir-fries, or as an alternative to sprouting seeds in sandwiches.*

Cleavers cools and tones the skin, helping it to heal.
➡*Infuse 2 tsp dried cleavers in 175ml (6fl oz) boiling water, cool, and use to wash the skin.*

BETTER BOILED

Boiling carrots makes the carotenoid beta-carotene (which converts to vitamin A in the body) more readily available to the body.

➤ CONTINUED...

REMEDY

Skin-calming infusion

Infuse 1 tsp each dried **red clover** and **heartsease** in 175ml (6fl oz) boiling water and drink 3 times daily, or add the infusion to a warm bath.

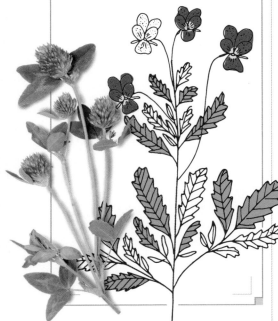

Red clover is calming and balancing; combine with heartsease. Avoid in pregnancy or with anticoagulants.
➼*See remedy, above.*

ESSENTIAL OILS

Anti-inflammatory, healing, and de-stressing essential oils are beneficial for eczema. Do not apply to broken skin.

Lavender relaxes and relieves itching.
➼*Dilute 5 drops in 10ml whole milk and add to a warm bath.*
Helichrysum is analgesic and calming.
➼*Add 2 drops to 5ml base ointment and apply to the affected area.*

German chamomile has an anti-inflammatory component, a-bisabolol.
➼*Add 2 drops to 5ml base ointment and apply to the affected area.*

FOOD

A varied wholefood diet supplies the broad range of nutrients needed to fight infection and maintain a healthy skin barrier.

Oily fish, such as salmon, are high in anti-inflammatory omega-3, which helps maintain moisture balance.
➼*Eat 2–3 servings a week.*
Apples contain a bioflavonoid quercetin, a natural anti-inflammatory and antihistamine. Other good fruit sources include blueberries and cherries.
➼*Eat an apple daily.*
Buckwheat is gluten-free and rich in anti-inflammatory mucilaginous fibre, which helps remove waste efficiently.
➼*Eat in cereals, as a side dish, or use the flour in baking.*

SUPPLEMENTS

Vitamins that strengthen skin and immunity can minimize eczema's impact.

Evening primrose oil reduces itching and encourages healing.
➼*Take 1–3g daily.*
Vitamin C with added bioflavonoids can act as a natural antihistamine.
➼*Take up to 3g in three divided doses per day.*
Vitamin D can significantly reduce eczema symptoms.
➼*Take 2000iu vitamin D3 for 4 weeks.*

LIFESTYLE

Yoga and meditation help to reduce the stress that often accompanies eczema, helping to cope with itching.
Keep showers and baths short, and warm, not hot; avoid overusing soaps and detergents; and moisturize often.

PSORIASIS

This is caused by the immune system mistakenly attacking healthy skin cells as if there was an infection. Psoriasis results in scaly, silvery patches of skin that occur most commonly on the elbows, knees, shins, scalp, and lower back.

HERBS

Choose herbs to support the liver, the body's main eliminatory organ, anti-inflammatory herbs to soothe skin, and calming herbs to help reduce the anxiety and stress that can accompany symptoms.

Yellow dock root is a bitter that works on the liver and has a gentle laxative action, helping the liver to eliminate waste effectively. Avoid in pregnancy and if breastfeeding.
Sarsaparilla is an anti-inflammatory ideal for chronic skin conditions.
Figwort is diuretic and can help calm chronic irritated skin conditions. Avoid with heart medication.
➼*For an effective tonic, combine all three herbs. Take a combined tincture (make yourself or ask a herbalist to make one up for you) with 1.5ml of each of the above herbs in a little water 3 times daily.*

ESSENTIAL OILS

Immune-boosting, healing essential oils help to calm and relieve inflamed skin.

Yarrow has soothing and healing properties for the skin.
➼*Add 4 drops to 20ml (⅔fl oz) calendula macerated oil and massage into the skin.*
Patchouli relieves inflammation and redness on the skin.
➼*Add 4 drops to 20ml (⅔fl oz) sweet almond oil and massage into the skin.*

Geranium can be used to stimulate new cell growth.

➡ *Add 4 drops to 20ml (⅔fl oz) base lotion and apply to the affected area.*

FOOD

Adequate protein helps ensure the strength and integrity of skin. Try to obtain protein from a variety of sources and eat more plant-based proteins.

Vegetable proteins include soya, legumes, and pulses.

➡ *Add daily to salads, stews, and stir-fries.*

Animal protein from organic and/or pasture-fed livestock has more skin-supporting fats such as omega-3 fatty acids than non-organic meat.

➡ *Eat no more than 2–3 90–120g (3–4oz) portions of meat a week.*

Garlic has a systemic cleansing effect.

➡ *Use in cooking and raw in dressings.*

Olive oil lubricates skin from the inside.

➡ *Take 1 tbsp of olive oil each day on its own or add to salad dressings.*

SUPPLEMENTS

A broad range of nutrients is needed to support skin health and immunity.

Multi-vitamins and minerals are essential for skin health.

➡ *Take a daily supplement.*

Vitamin D deficiency may be associated with psoriasis.

➡ *Take up to 1600iu vitamin D3 daily.*

Omega-3 marine oil is a strong anti-inflammatory that speeds healing.

➡ *Take 1–2g daily from plant or marine sources.*

Betaine HCl is helpful if low stomach acid is stopping the efficient absorption of nutrients from food.

➡ *Take 1–3 capsules with each meal.*

LIFESTYLE

Use a soap substitute and avoid overusing detergents. Moisturize regularly and try to get out in sunlight for 20 minutes each day when possible as sunlight helps to treat psoriasis.

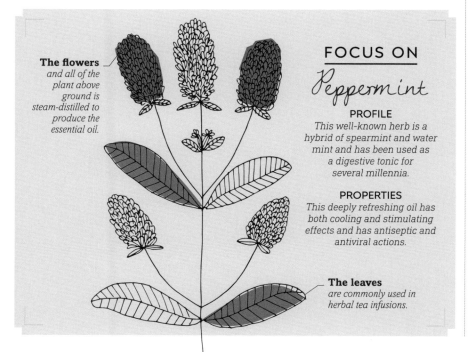

The flowers *and all of the plant above ground is steam-distilled to produce the essential oil.*

FOCUS ON
Peppermint

PROFILE
This well-known herb is a hybrid of spearmint and water mint and has been used as a digestive tonic for several millennia.

PROPERTIES
This deeply refreshing oil has both cooling and stimulating effects and has antiseptic and antiviral actions.

The leaves *are commonly used in herbal tea infusions.*

URTICARIA

Also known as hives or prickly heat, this rash usually affects the trunk, thighs, upper arms, or face. It can be caused by heat from sunlight, allergy, insect bites and stings, food additives, medications, and stress. If onset is rapid with swelling of the mouth and throat, seek urgent medical help.

HERBS

Anti-inflammatory and anti-allergenic herbs are effective when taken internally. Herbs can also be used topically to soothe itching, cool skin, and reduce redness.

Nettles have an anti-allergenic and anti-inflammatory action and are high in blood-boosting minerals.

➡ *Take in an infusion or tincture: infuse 1–2 tsp dried nettle in 175ml (6fl oz) boiling water, or take 5–10ml tincture in a little water, 3 times daily. In season, sauté with onions and garlic, add natural yogurt, and purée into a cooling soup.*

Witch hazel is one of the most effective herbs for relieving itchy skin.

➡ *Apply witch hazel gel to affected areas as needed.*

Chickweed is cooling and moisturizing, relieving itching and calming rashes.

➡ *Infuse 1–3 tsp dried chickweed in 175ml (6fl oz) boiling water and add to a tepid bath. Or cool and dab on the affected area.*

ESSENTIAL OILS

Anti-inflammatory and soothing essential oils ease itching.

Peppermint contains a high percentage of cooling menthol. See box, left.

➡ *Make a cold compress: add 5 drops to cold water and place on the skin for up to 20 minutes.*

➤ CONTINUED…

German chamomile is a well-known anti-inflammatory that can be used to help calm skin.
➡ *Add 5 drops to 10ml jojoba oil and apply to the skin.*

Lavender helps to soothe itching and calm the skin.
➡ *Add 5 drops to a bath dispersant and add to a warm bath.*

SUPPLEMENTS

Anti-inflammatory supplements and ones that act as natural antihistamines can be useful if you suffer frequently with hives.

Quercetin is a natural antihistamine and anti-inflammatory, helping to calm allergic reactions.
➡ *Take 1–2g daily.*

Evening primrose oil is rich in gamma-linolenic acid (GLA), an anti-inflammatory that is thought to be useful for hives caused by sun allergy.
➡ *Take 1–3g daily in split doses.*

Vitamin C acts as an antihistamine, reducing itching and rashes.
➡ *Take 1g daily with food.*

LIFESTYLE

Wear light layers made from natural fabrics such as cotton and silk.

Avoid heavy creams and ointments.

> "*Anti-inflammatory essential oils can be effective for soothing sun-related hives.*"

ROSACEA

This is characterized by inflamed skin on the face, which leads to red patches and bumps that are similar in appearance to eczema. Eventually broken capillaries or spider veins appear on the face. Rosacea occurs more commonly in women than in men.

HERBS

Cooling, astringent herbs are the most beneficial and can be used both topically and internally. Anti-inflammatory herbs and bitter digestive herbs also help to reduce heat.

Witch hazel has a cooling, astringent effect on the skin.
➡ *Steep leaves in warm water for 24 hours, strain, and use topically when required. Refrigerate for a maximum of 2 days, then discard.*

Rose is a gentle, fragrant astringent, which helps to cool and soothe skin and tighten capillaries, in turn helping to tone the skin.
➡ *Apply rose water directly to the skin as a toner or a facial spritz.*

Mahonia is a bitter herb that helps to promote healthy liver function and it is linked to a healthy complexion. Avoid in pregnancy.
➡ *Take 1–3ml tincture in a little water 3 times daily.*

ESSENTIAL OILS

These are effective for reducing inflammation and redness.

Rose is especially beneficial for sensitive skin, working as a strengthening tonic and astringent on the capillaries.
➡ *Add 4 drops to 20ml (⅔fl oz) rosehip seed oil and massage into the skin.*

Helichrysum helps to reduce swelling and inflammation where skin is irritated and red.

Roman chamomile is extremely soothing and calming, making it especially beneficial for treating sensitive, red skin.
➡ *Add 4 drops of either helichrysum or chamomile essential oils to 20ml (⅔fl oz) base lotion and massage into the affected area of skin.*

FOOD

Eating anti-inflammatory, alkaline, and mostly plant-based foods and increasing your daily consumption of raw foods can help to calm skin and provide a balance of nutrients to boost general skin health.

Sprouted seeds, beans, and grains are easy to digest and contain vital nutrients to help support skin health.
➡ *Add sprouting alfalfa, broccoli, kamut, spelt, or mung beans to salads, stir-fries, and juices.*

Citrus fruits, although thought of as acidic, actually have an alkaline effect inside the body, helping to balance stomach acids. They are also high in skin-supporting vitamin C.
➡ *Start each day with fresh grapefruit juice or lemon juice and hot water.*

WHAT TO AVOID
Acidic foods and drinks, such as alcohol, grains (excepting millet and

FREE FROM CHEMICALS

If sprouting seeds, buy ones produced specifically for this purpose, which will be free from chemicals used on seeds for outside plants.

quinoa), vinegar, eggs, oils, nuts, seeds, sugar, and soya are thought by some to exacerbate rosacea. Meat and fish can also be acid-forming in the body, but small amounts eaten with plenty of vegetables are fine.

SUPPLEMENTS

Taking vitamin and mineral supplements alongside other treatments can support healthy blood vessels.

Vitamin C can help to reduce the inflammation of rosacea and also strengthens capillaries.
➡*Take up to 2g daily in split doses with food.*
Vitamin A is commonly used for the treatment of skin disorders and helps skin tissue synthesis. Avoid during pregnancy.
➡*Take 15,000iu retinoic acid daily for 3 months. Thereafter, reduce to 10,000iu daily.*
Methylsulfonylmethane (MSM) can help to treat rosacea.
➡*Apply topically to the affected areas or take internally as a supplement at the recommended dose.*
Zinc is well known for promoting tissue repair and zinc deficiencies, though rare, often manifest as skin rashes.
➡*Take up to 30mg daily. Try zinc gluconate lozenges to improve uptake.*

LIFESTYLE

Protect skin from the sun's harmful UV rays. Always wear a SPF factor 50 sunscreen and stay out of the sun in the warmer months at the time when the sun is at its strongest, between 11am and 3pm.
Use clean cosmetics made from organic and natural ingredients only.
Reduce stress and insomnia by addressing any problems and learning relaxation techniques such as yoga and meditation.

ATHLETE'S FOOT, RINGWORM, AND JOCK ITCH

These infections are caused by fungi called dermatophytes that live on the skin, hair, and nails and thrive in warm, moist areas. They are highly infectious and can be very persistent unless caught early.

HERBS

Antifungal herbs used externally are helpful for tackling infections. And herbs used internally can focus on deep-cleansing as well as help strengthen immunity, improving skin health and resistance to infections.

Calendula is antifungal and immune-boosting, as well as supportive of the liver and lymphatic system, and can be used internally and externally.
➡*Clean and dry the affected area and apply a calendula-based cream or ointment twice daily.*
Gotu kola is balancing and healing. Like calendula, it can be used both internally and topically. Avoid internal use during pregnancy and with epilepsy. May cause skin sensitivity.
➡*Take 1–5ml tincture in a little water 3 times daily. Can be combined with other recommended herbs.*
Myrrh is antifungal and improves immunity. It works well with calendula, increasing the benefits of both herbs. Avoid internal use during pregnancy.
➡*See remedy, right.*

ESSENTIAL OILS

Oils that have anti-inflammatory and antifungal properties can help to treat the symptoms such as itching and pain.

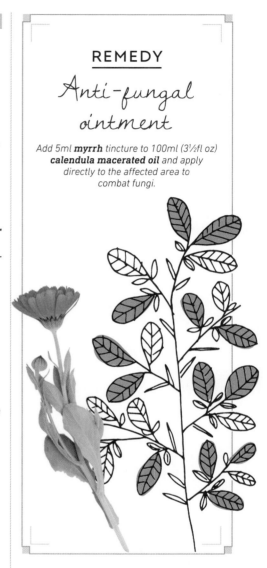

REMEDY
Anti-fungal ointment

Add 5ml **myrrh** tincture to 100ml (3½fl oz) **calendula macerated oil** and apply directly to the affected area to combat fungi.

Tea tree is antifungal, making it highly effective for treating fungal infections topically.
➡*Add 2 drops to 5ml neem oil and massage into the affected area.*
Myrrh is both antifungal and anti-inflammatory and is an effective skin-healing remedy.
Lavender has analgesic properties and is also healing.
➡*Add 2 drops of either myrrh or lavender oils to 5ml base ointment and massage into the affected area.*

➤ CONTINUED...

FOOD

Foods can help to strengthen the skin barrier and boost immunity. Aim for over half of your diet to be fresh and organic, with plenty of raw produce and more vegetables than fruit.

Fermented foods such as sauerkraut, kimchi, kefir, and natural yogurt help to populate the gut with healthy bacteria to fight infections.
➡ *Eat as a side dish or condiment and include yogurt in your diet daily, with cereals, porridge, in smoothies, or added to meals.*
Coconut oil is a strong antifungal.
➡ *Take 1 tbsp 1–2 times a day. Eat on its own, in smoothies, or use for cooking.*
WHAT TO AVOID
Sugary foods, including refined carbohydrates and alcohol, which the body converts to sugar.

SUPPLEMENTS

A diet deficient in vitamins and a weak immune system encourages the growth of fungus. It's best to get nutrients from food, but short-term supplements can help.

Zinc boosts immunity to help fight infection.
➡ *Take 8–11mg daily.*
Probiotic supplements help rebalance the gut with beneficial bacteria.
➡ *Supplements should contain up to 10 billion live organisms per dose.*
Garlic is powerfully antifungal, but gentle on beneficial gut organisms.
➡ *For persistent infection, take 200mg of garlic oil 3 times daily.*

LIFESTYLE

Don't share towels and wash bed linen regularly at a high temperature. Dry between the toes and in skin creases and wear natural fabrics and sandals in summer. Lose weight if overweight.

CORNS AND CALLUSES

Corns and calluses, thickened areas of skin, often on the feet, are caused by regular friction, for example from ill-fitting or high-heeled shoes, which triggers accelerated skin growth as a protective measure.

HERBS

Herbs can help to reduce inflammation, cool the skin, and soothe pain and discomfort. Some herbs help to stimulate circulation to promote healing.

Bay leaf is a traditional remedy used topically to relieve swelling and pain.
➡ *Dab neat tincture on the affected area as required.*
Chickweed cools and soothes, helping to relieve itching and irritation.
➡ *Make a poultice with a small handful of chopped, fresh herbs, or 2–3 tbsp dried chickweed to cover the affected area.*
Prickly ash boosts circulation to the feet. Avoid with anticoagulant medication.
➡ *Take 1–5ml tincture in a little water 3 times daily.*

ESSENTIAL OILS

Look for oils that are pain-relieving and anti-inflammatory.

German chamomile has analgesic properties.
➡ *Add 3 drops to 5ml castor seed oil – which is pain-relieving and boosts skin-cell renewal – and massage in.*
Tagetes works as an anti-inflammatory.
➡ *Add 5 drops to a warm footbath and soak to soften the calluses and corns.*
Peppermint is strongly analgesic.
➡ *Add 3 drops to 5ml jojoba oil and gently massage into the feet.*

HERPES INFECTION

Herpes is a family of viruses, which form part of the community of micro-organisms in our bodies. When we are run down these can become active. Cold sores are the most common manifestation, but herpes infections can also present as genital herpes, chickenpox, and shingles. Infections can appear as pimples, rashes, or blisters, can cause tingling, itching, and burning, and are highly contagious.

HERBS

Antiviral and immune-boosting herbs can be used internally to help fight herpes infections. Use these alongside anti-inflammatory herbs, applied topically, to reduce discomfort.

Echinacea supports and boosts the immune response and promotes skin healing. Avoid with immunosuppressant medication.
➡ *Take 1–5ml tincture in a little water 3 times daily.*

"Immune-boosting, anti-inflammatory herbs and essential oils help to reduce discomfort."

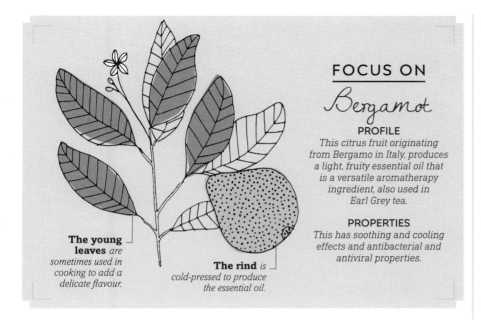

FOCUS ON
Bergamot
PROFILE
This citrus fruit originating from Bergamo in Italy, produces a light, fruity essential oil that is a versatile aromatherapy ingredient, also used in Earl Grey tea.

PROPERTIES
This has soothing and cooling effects and antibacterial and antiviral properties.

The young leaves *are sometimes used in cooking to add a delicate flavour.*

The rind *is cold-pressed to produce the essential oil.*

Lemon balm, also known as melissa, is specifically active against the herpes virus. Avoid with hypothyroidism.
➡ *Infuse 2 tsp dried lemon balm or 1 tsp tincture in 175ml (6fl oz) boiling water and drink 3 times daily. Or add 1 tsp tincture to an ointment base and apply externally to the affected area.*

St John's wort is anti-inflammatory and antiviral, and also helps to heal and soothe nerve damage. Avoid internally in pregnancy and high doses in strong sunlight. Taken internally, interacts with many prescription medicines.
➡ *Infuse 2 tsp dried St John's wort in 175ml (6fl oz) boiling water and drink 3 times daily. Or use in an ointment with aloe vera gel.*

ESSENTIAL OILS

Antiviral, anti-inflammatory, and analgesic oils help to relieve the viral symptoms.

Bergamot is antiviral and uplifting. Avoid sun exposure after use. See box, above.
➡ *Use a cotton bud to apply neat onto blisters. In addition, add 3 drops to a diffuser to help lift spirits.*

Lavender soothes irritation and pain. Avoid with epilepsy.
➡ *Add 2 drops to 5ml lotion and apply to the area after the blisters have gone.*
Lemon balm is an effective antiviral oil.
➡ *Add 2 drops to 5ml lotion and apply to the affected area.*

FOOD

Herpes viruses can become active in a body that is undernourished so ensure your diet provides a range of nutrients.

Fresh fruits and leafy green vegetables are rich in vitamin C, which improves resistance and aids healing.
➡ *Eat several portions of raw fruit and vegetables each day.*
Dairy products such as yogurt, milk, and cheese are high in lysine, which helps prevent cold sore breakouts.
➡ *Natural yogurt topped with fruit makes a nutritious breakfast or snack.*
Avocados are abundant in skin-healing vitamin E and also have a favourable lysine to arginine ratio (see following).
➡ *Add to a salad, or mash and spread on wholewheat toast.*

WHAT TO AVOID
Foods with high levels of the amino acid arginine, such as nuts, seeds, and pulses can prompt herpes outbreaks, especially if your diet is low in lysine.

SUPPLEMENTS

Supporting immunity with supplements can increase your resistance to herpes infections and help to fight them off more effectively when they do occur.

Vitamin C fights cold sores by inactivating the herpes simplex virus.
➡ *Take a minimum of 1g a day. When you feel symptoms developing, up the dose to 3g, in split doses with food.*
Zinc can reduce the frequency, duration, and severity of both herpes and shingles infections.
➡ *Take 30mg a day during active infections.*
Lysine supplements can be helpful in treating active cold sores, shingles, and chickenpox.
➡ *Take 500mg to 1g of L-lysine daily on an empty stomach.*

LIFESTYLE

Practise yoga and meditation to help manage stress. Managing stress is important as stress is known to trigger herpes outbreaks and can make existing infections worse.

ZINC TOP UP
For stubborn cold sores, taking 15–20mg zinc lozenges every 3 hours for up to 3 days during the infection may be more effective than a daily supplement.

5

RECIPES FOR WELLNESS

OVERNIGHT OATS

Kick-start your metabolism with these antioxidant-rich oat and fruit compote combos. Combine the oats and milk and soak overnight. Cook the compote ingredients in a pan for 10 minutes on a low heat, until the fruit is soft but not mushy. Serve the oats with the compote spooned on top.

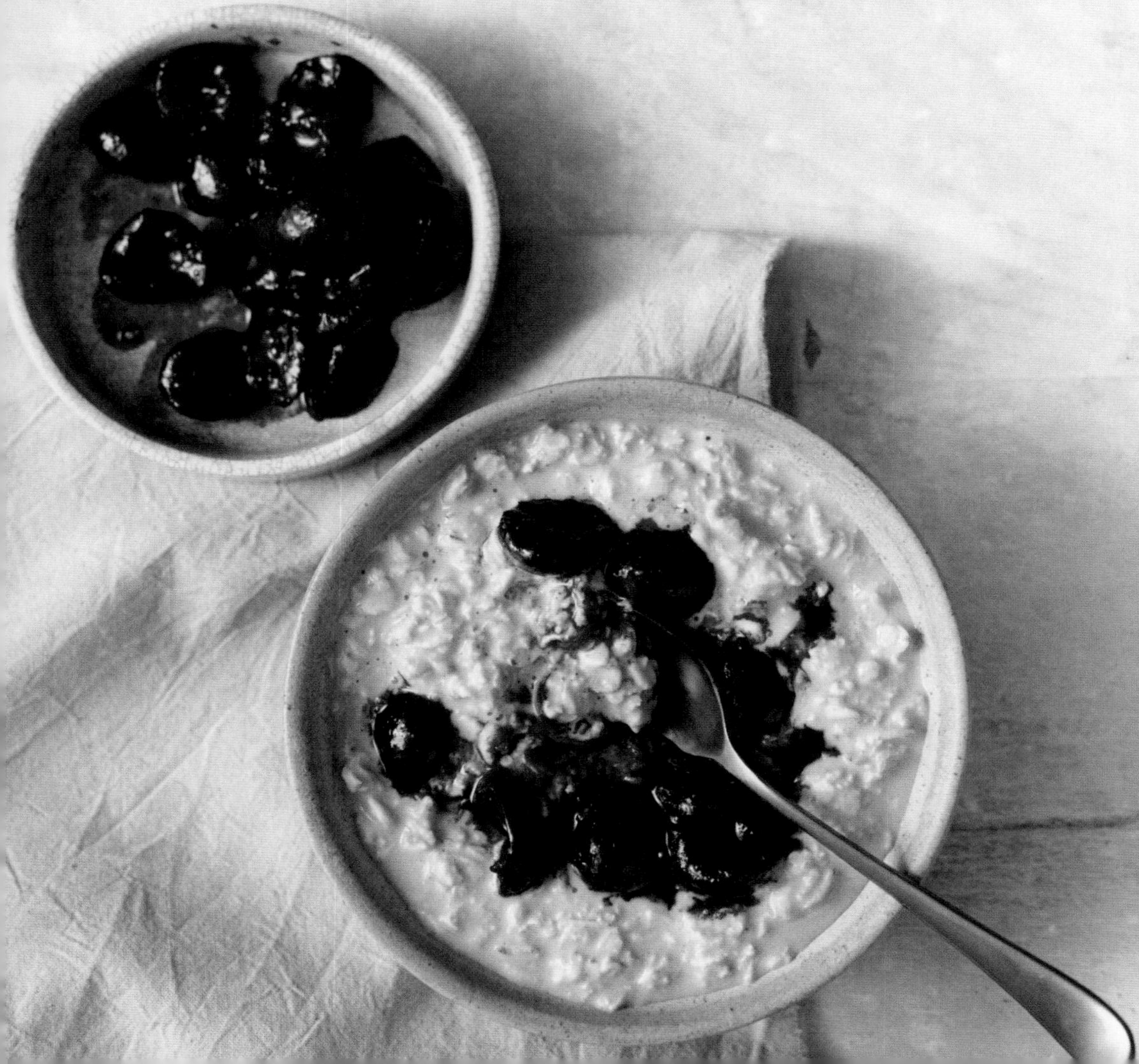

1

OATS WITH CHERRY COMPOTE

Cherries are an excellent source of antioxidant anthocyanins, thought to support cardiovascular health, as well as relaxing melatonin.

SERVES 1 • PREP TIME 15 MINS, PLUS SOAKING

60g (2oz) jumbo rolled oats

120ml (4fl oz) hazelnut, almond, or organic cow's milk

For the compote

115g (4oz) pitted cherries

1½ tbsp lemon juice

¼ tsp cinnamon

1½ tsp runny honey

Nutritional info per serving:
Kcals 410 Fat 7g Saturated fat 1g Carbohydrates 75g Sugar 30.5g Sodium 65mg Fibre 7g Protein 8g Cholesterol 0mg

2

OATS WITH APPLE AND BLUEBERRY COMPOTE

Tasty and sweet, apples are abundant in protective antioxidants to boost blood vessel health, as well as dietary fibre to control cholesterol. Blueberries contain eye-supporting carotenoids lutein and zeaxanthin, important for the health of the retina.

SERVES 1 · PREP TIME 15 MINS, PLUS SOAKING

60g (2oz) jumbo rolled oats

120ml (4fl oz) hazelnut, almond, or organic cow's milk

For the compote

175g (6oz) apple, peeled, cored, and thickly sliced

1 tbsp runny honey

½ tsp cinnamon

30g (1oz) blueberries

30g (1oz) raisins

Nutritional info per serving:
Kcals 565 Fat 8g Saturated fat 1.5g Carbohydrates 110g Sugar 65g Sodium 85mg Fibre 9g Protein 9g Cholesterol 0mg

3

OATS WITH MANGO AND PEACH COMPOTE

Sweet mangoes have more than 20 vitamins and minerals, including flavonoids such as beta-carotenes, converted into vision- and skin-enhancing vitamin A in the body, while peaches are a good source of potassium, vital for nerve and cell health.

SERVES 1 · PREP TIME 15 MINS, PLUS SOAKING

60g (2oz) jumbo rolled oats

120ml (4fl oz) hazelnut, almond, or organic cow's milk

For the compote

200g (7oz) mango, peeled, pitted, and chopped

1 peach, pitted and chopped

1 tbsp lemon juice

¼ tsp fresh ginger, peeled and diced

2 tbsp chia seeds

Nutritional info per serving:
Kcals 685 Fat 16.5g Saturated fat 2g Carbohydrates 106.5g Sugar 43g Sodium 74mg Fibre 25g Protein 15g Cholesterol 0mg

4

OATS WITH STRAWBERRY COMPOTE

Strawberries are abundant in anti-inflammatory antioxidants, one of the top sources of vitamin C, and a good source of manganese and potassium, helping to regulate blood pressure and providing cardiovascular benefits.

SERVES 1 · PREP TIME 15 MINS, PLUS SOAKING

60g (2oz) jumbo rolled oats

120ml (4fl oz) hazelnut, almond, or organic cow's milk

For the compote

115g (4oz) strawberries, quartered

60g (2oz) blueberries

1 tbsp runny honey

2 tbsp water

Nutritional info per serving:
Kcals 461 Fat 7.5g Saturated fat 1g Carbohydrates 85g Sugar 35g Sodium 68mg Fibre 10.5g Protein 9g Cholesterol 0mg

5

OATS WITH PEAR, CINNAMON, AND GINGER COMPOTE

Fibre-rich pears are given an intense flavour kick with cinnamon – high in potent anti-inflammatory polyphenols – and ginger, which has immune-boosting properties.

SERVES 1 · PREP TIME 15 MINS, PLUS SOAKING

60g (2oz) jumbo rolled oats

120ml (4fl oz) hazelnut, almond, or organic cow's milk

For the compote

200g (7oz) pear, peeled, cored, and chopped

½ tsp fresh ginger, peeled and diced

¼ tsp cinnamon

1 tsp runny honey

1 tbsp water

Nutritional info per serving:
Kcals 458 Fat 7g Saturated fat 1g Carbohydrates 86g Sugar 36g Sodium 66mg Fibre 10.5g Protein 8g Cholesterol 0mg

WARTS AND VERRUCAS

Warts – small lumps on the skin – and verrucas – which are warts on the feet – are relatively harmless but highly contagious. They can be caused by any one of several strains of the human papilloma virus (HPV).

HERBS

Using herbs with antiviral properties directly on the skin helps to fight the infection, while immune-boosting herbs offer support when taken internally. Calming herbs that ease stress and anxiety can be beneficial, too.

Greater celandine, a traditional remedy for warts and verrucas that is applied topically to the affected area, contains substances that appear to inhibit the HPV virus.
➡ *Apply a tincture directly to the affected area after gently scraping the wart or verruca.*

"Antimicrobial essential oils such as lemon and tea tree help to promote healing to tackle stubborn warts and verrucas."

Thuja is an effective antiviral herb for the treatment of warts and verrucas.
➡ *Use tincture neat on hands and feet. Dilute in 5ml water for genital warts. Use 2–3 times a day for up to 3 months.*

Echinacea works as an all-round immune-boosting herb. Avoid with immunosuppressant medication.
➡ *Take 1–5ml tincture in a little water 1–3 times daily.*

ESSENTIAL OILS

Antiviral essential oils can be used to help tackle stubborn warts and verrucas, helping to speed the rate of healing.

Lemon is a potent antimicrobial essential oil, which also has effective astringent properties.

Tea tree is powerfully antimicrobial and also an excellent essential oil to promote healing.
➡ *Using a cotton bud, apply 1 drop of either lemon or tea tree essential oils directly on to the wart or verruca, taking care to avoid skin on the surrounding area.*

FOOD

Eating a mainly vegetarian diet, which includes plenty of fresh, whole foods that are high in essential vitamins and minerals will support your immune system and help to fight stubborn viruses such as HPV.

Red peppers actually contain more vitamin C than many fruits and, similar to other highly coloured foods, they are rich in protective, skin-supporting antioxidants such as beta-carotene, which converts to vitamin A in the body.
➡ *Try peppers baked, stuffed with brown rice, and served with a rainbow of other vegetables; snack on raw pepper sticks; or enjoy them with a healthy hummus dip.*

ALL THE GOODNESS

Sweet potatoes have a higher concentration of fibre, potassium, and beta-carotene in their skins so lightly scrub only and eat with the skins on.

Sweet potato is also high in the antioxidant carotenoid beta-carotene, to provide skin-supporting vitamin A. Beta-carotene also increases T-cell activity – the white cells that play a role in the immune response – to help fight infection.
➡ *Eat baked or add to casseroles and stir-fries.*

SUPPLEMENTS

If your diet is lacking key nutrients or you are under high levels of stress it can be helpful to boost your nutrient intake to support the immune system.

Multi-vitamins provide essential micronutrients. Look for a multi-vitamin supplement that contains good levels of vitamins A, C, and E, and the B complex vitamins.
➡ *Take a multi-vitamin daily.*

LIFESTYLE

Hygiene is extremely important to stop warts and verrucas spreading on your own body or infecting others. Wash your hands regularly, avoid sharing towels or clothes, and wash bed linen on the highest possible temperature.

Practise relaxation techniques such as yoga and meditation if you think that chronic stress is compromising your immune system.

CELLULITE

Cellulite occurs when fat pushes closer to the skin's surface in uneven patches, resulting in a dimpled "orange rind" appearance. Cellulite is more common in women, whose skin is thinner and has a weaker underlying support structure.

HERBS

Stimulating and circulatory tonic herbs help to flush body fluids through tissues to promote cleansing. Diuretic herbs support the elimination of waste from the body.

Horse chestnut tones capillaries and stimulates circulation. Avoid with anticoagulant medication. If irritant to the stomach when taken internally, take with soothing limeflower.
➡️*See remedy, right.*
Prickly ash is a circulatory stimulant and helps to increase sweating. Avoid with anticoagulant medication.
➡️*Take 1–5ml tincture in a little water 3 times daily.*
Parsley is warming and diuretic. Avoid with inflammatory kidney conditions.
➡️*Take as an infusion or take 1–5ml tincture in a little water 3 times daily.*

ESSENTIAL OILS

Oils can detoxify and stimulate the lymphatic system and act as diuretics.

Grapefruit is a lymphatic stimulant and acts as a diuretic.
➡️*Add 5 drops to 10ml wheatgerm oil and massage into the skin.*
Cypress helps to stimulate circulation.
➡️*Add 5 drops to 10ml base lotion and massage into the skin.*
Juniper berry is a strong detoxifier.
➡️*Add 5 drops to 10ml rosehip oil and massage into the skin.*

FOOD

A low-carbohydrate, nutrient-dense diet with healthy fats can prevent cellulite from becoming worse. Staying well hydrated with water and herbal teas is also vital to improve skin tone and support kidney function to remove waste.

Seaweeds, such as wakame and bladderwrack, are full of nutrients, including antioxidant carotenoids, and have excellent detoxifying properties.
➡️*Use the flakes as a seasoning for soups, stir-fries, salads, and dressings. Carotenoids need fats to aid absorption so eat with healthy fats.*
Green tea raises metabolic rates, helping to speed up fat oxidation to reduce the risk of, or improve, cellulite.
➡️*Drink 3–4 cups a day. Or try adding powdered forms of green tea such as sencha and matcha to bakes, dressings, and soups.*

SUPPLEMENTS

Supplements that help the body to burn fat more efficiently can support other methods of keeping cellulite under control, such as massage and body brushing.

Brown seaweed supplements derived from kelp and wakame contain fucoxanthin, a marine carotenoid that helps the body burn fat over time.
➡️*An effective daily dose is 5mg.*
Chromium helps to regulate the metabolism.
➡️*Take 50–500mcg daily. Chromium picolinate and pidolate are the most efficiently absorbed forms.*

LIFESTYLE

Exercise regularly, with a focus on strength training to help replace fat with muscle, and also keep an eye on your weight.
Skin brushing helps to stimulate the lymphatic and immune systems and improves skin tone.

OTHER THERAPIES

Hydrotherapy – saunas followed by a cold shower or alternating hot and cold sitz baths – can improve circulation, which in turn boosts skin tone.
Deep tissue massage can be beneficial, supporting lymphatic drainage to help minimize the buildup of cellulite.

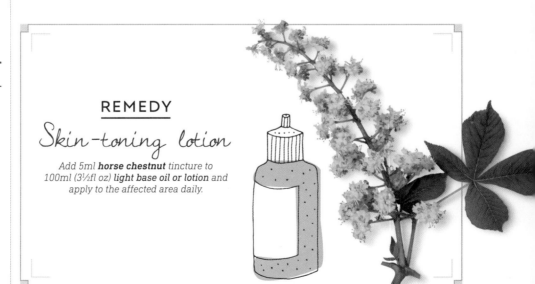

REMEDY
Skin-toning lotion

Add 5ml **horse chestnut** tincture to 100ml (3½fl oz) **light base oil or lotion** and apply to the affected area daily.

STRETCH MARKS

Stretch marks result from tearing of the dermis – the middle layer of skin. They can be caused by sudden weight gain, for example during pregnancy, and intense weight training.

HERBS

Herbs can promote cell replication, stimulate circulation, and strengthen the underlying connective tissue, all of which help to reduce the appearance of stretch marks and support new skin formation.

Gotu kola stimulates collagen formation and blood vessels to nourish and promote skin regeneration. Avoid during pregnancy and with epilepsy. May cause skin sensitivity.
➡ *Infuse 1½ tsp dried gotu kola in 175ml (6fl oz) boiling water and drink daily.*
Calendula promotes skin healing by conditioning and restoring skin. It also has an anti-inflammatory action.
Comfrey heals rapidly. It promotes tissue growth in the epidermis – the outer skin layer – and its underlying connective tissue. Avoid on deep or infected skin lesions as comfrey heals rapidly so could trap bacteria.
➡ *Apply both calendula and comfrey externally in an infusion or cream: either infuse 1½ tsp dried herb in 175ml (6fl oz) boiling water, cool, and dab on to the skin with a cotton wool pad or add the infusion to a warm bath; or add quarter of the infusion to a base lotion.*

ESSENTIAL OILS

Massaging stimulating essential oils into the skin can help to reduce the appearance of stretch marks over time.

Neroli stimulates new cell growth to help rejuvenate skin.
➡ *Add 10 drops to 20ml (⅔fl oz) wheatgerm oil and massage into the skin.*
Mandarin has a stimulating action, helping the skin cells to regenerate.
➡ *Add 10 drops to 20ml (⅔fl oz) argan oil and massage into the skin.*
Frankincense encourages cell rejuvenation.
➡ *Add 10 drops to 20ml (⅔fl oz) avocado oil and massage into the skin.*

SUPPLEMENTS

Stretch marks are hard to eradicate completely, but you can help to minimize their appearance by ensuring that you are getting adequate levels of skin-supporting nutrients. Supplements can support a varied diet to nourish skin when it is under stress.

Zinc is needed by the body to generate collagen, the protein that supports the underlying structure of the skin and helps skin elasticity.
➡ *Men should get a minimum of 11mg daily and women 8mg daily.*
Vitamin E is a skin-protecting antioxidant that helps to maintain the health of skin tissues and skin membranes.
➡ *Take up to 1000iu daily.*

EXCESSIVE SWEATING

Perspiration is natural, especially during exercise, when under stress, or in hot weather. Some people, though, sweat excessively, known as hyperhidrosis, typically in the palms, armpits, groin, and feet. Excessive sweating can be due to an overactive thyroid so get this checked if you think it could be the root cause.

HERBS

Herbs can help to control sweating where this is caused by excessive activity in the nervous system – they work to balance this activity and in turn relieve the impact of stress and anxiety on the body. In addition, astringent herbs can be used topically to dry and tone the skin.

Sage is a cooling and astringent herb. It is particularly useful for sweating caused by hormonal changes during the menopause. Avoid therapeutic doses during pregnancy and with epilepsy and avoid taking for prolonged periods of time.
➡ *Infuse 1–2 tsp dried sage in 175ml (6fl oz) boiling water and drink 3 times daily. Also look for a gentle deodorant that contains natural sage extract.*

HARDY HERB

Fresh sage can be stored in the fridge for up to 5 days. A hardy herb, it can be wrapped loosely in a paper towel and placed in a sealed container before chilling.

"Skin-supporting nutrients are needed to generate collagen, the protein that supports skin structure."

Lemon balm is effective in reducing sweating caused by nervous anxiety. Avoid with hypothyroidism.
➥*Infuse 1–2 tsp dried lemon balm in 175ml (6fl oz) boiling water and drink 3 times daily.*

Astragalus can relieve the effects of stress, raise vitality, and reduce excessive sweating. Avoid using with acute infections such as colds and flu.
➥*Infuse 1–2 tsp dried astragalus in 175ml (6fl oz) boiling water 3 times daily or take 2–4ml tincture in a little water. Or add the powder to soups and smoothies.*

ESSENTIAL OILS

Cooling, refreshing, and deodorizing essential oils can be effective in helping to control excessive sweating.

Cypress is astringent and deodorizing.
➥*Add 5 drops to a foot bath for excessively sweaty feet.*

Lemon is an excellent detoxifier, and is a cooling and drying oil.
➥*Make a body spritz with 15 drops added to 50ml (2fl oz) water.*

Petitgrain refreshes the skin, helping to minimize the effects of sweating.
➥*Add 10 drops together with 100ml (3½fl oz) cider vinegar to a bath.*

LIFESTYLE

Wear light layers of clothing made from natural fabrics such as cotton, linen, and silk.

Avoid foods that promote sweating, such as chillies and cinnamon, and also avoid alcohol, which encourages sweating, and very hot tea and coffee.

OTHER THERAPIES

Acupuncture, biofeedback (increasing awareness of bodily functions), and hypnosis can all be used to calm the nervous system and in turn help reduce sweating.

DANDRUFF

The characteristic flakes of dead skin occur when skin cells on the outer scalp layer are shed at a faster than normal rate. It can be caused by sensitivity to products, fungal infection, or dietary deficiencies.

HERBS

Astringent and emollient herbs calm irritation, and circulatory and antimicrobial ones boost circulation and scalp health.

Rosemary stimulates circulation and is antimicrobial. It can be combined with apple cider vinegar for a conditioning scalp rinse. Avoid therapeutic doses internally in pregnancy.
➥*See remedy, right.*

Sage is antimicrobial and astringent, cleansing and soothing the scalp. Avoid therapeutic doses internally in pregnancy and with epilepsy.

Elderflower is emollient and antimicrobial when used topically, calming and soothing skin.
➥*Use a strong infusion of either sage or elderflower as a final rinse. Don't rinse out and leave to dry naturally.*

ESSENTIAL OILS

Maintain a healthy scalp and help to condition hair by massaging essential oils into the scalp.

Cedarwood, a traditional treatment for scalp conditions, heals and soothes.
➥*Add 5 drops to 10ml coconut oil and massage into the scalp. Leave for 1–2 hours or overnight, then wash out.*

Rosemary works to cleanse the scalp. Avoid with epilepsy.
➥*Add 20 drops to 40ml (1½fl oz) water for a final rinse. Apply, avoiding the eyes, then leave the hair to dry.*

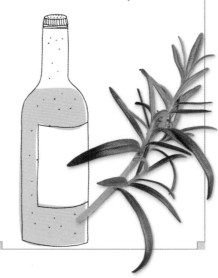

REMEDY

Conditioning scalp rinse

*Steep 2.5g dried **rosemary** in 500ml (16fl oz) **apple cider vinegar** for 2 weeks. Strain into a clean bottle then add 1–2 dessertspoons to 1 litre (1¾ pints) water, rinse into just-washed hair, then leave to dry.*

Tea tree is a traditional dandruff remedy.
➥*In a bain-marie, warm 30ml (1fl oz) olive oil and add 15 drops tea tree. Massage into the scalp, leave for up to 5 hours, then shampoo and rinse hair.*

FOOD

People whose diets are low in zinc and B vitamins and high in saturated or trans fats may be more prone to dandruff.

Turkey and chicken contain useful amounts of vitamin B6, a deficiency of which can cause the scalp to dry. Other useful sources of the vitamin are avocados and wholegrains.
➥*Enjoy a turkey and avocado sandwich on wholemeal bread.*

➤ CONTINUED...

Oily fish, such as sardines, mackerel, and salmon, contain nourishing omega-3 fats that help to keep the skin on the scalp well hydrated and less prone to flaking.
➡ *Eat 2–3 times a week.*

Oysters contain more zinc per serving than any other food.
➡ *Eat raw or try them smoked on a wholegrain cracker.*

WHAT TO AVOID
Saturated fats, because these can encourage the overgrowth of malassezia, the fungi that is associated with dandruff.

SUPPLEMENTS

Dandruff can point to nutrient deficiencies in essential fatty acids and trace elements.

Omega-3 marine oil, from fish or plant sources, may relieve a dry, itchy scalp.
➡ *Take 1g daily with food.*

Zinc is essential to the maintenance of healthy skin, scalp, hair, and nails. Flaking can be a sign of a deficiency.
➡ *Take 11mg daily for men and 8mg for women.*

LIFESTYLE

Check hair products. Reactions to products can cause flakes so avoid using lots of different products and/or try switching your shampoo.

THINNING HAIR

Some hair loss each day is normal and hairs are usually replaced, but sometimes regrowth slows or stops completely, or hair loss accelerates. Hair loss can be caused by factors such as stress, shock, infection, and sometimes poor thyroid function.

HERBS

Herbs can boost the circulation to the scalp, providing oxygen and essential nutrients. They can also treat underlying hormonal issues, ease stress and tension, and many are potent antioxidants to help counter the ageing process.

Nettle root helps to balance hormones to reduce hair loss, while nettle leaf supports the circulation and is mineral-rich, strengthening hair and scalp health.
➡ *Take 1–5ml of nettle leaf tincture in a little water 3 times daily.*

Rosemary boosts circulation to the head to support hair health and is strongly antioxidant. Avoid therapeutic doses internally in pregnancy.
➡ *Infuse 1–2 tsp dried rosemary in 175ml (6fl oz) boiling water, cool, and use as a final rinse, or use daily between hair washes. Leave to dry on the hair.*

Saw palmetto has a balancing action on hormone levels, helping to slow hair loss, and may also increase existing hair density in both men and women.
➡ *Infuse 1–2 tsp dried saw palmetto in 175ml (6fl oz) boiling water daily or take 160mg capsules twice daily.*

ESSENTIAL OILS

Using stimulating oils in a scalp massage boosts circulation to the scalp, stimulating the hair follicles and promoting hair growth.

Rosemary helps increase cellular metabolism, encouraging hair growth. Avoid with epilepsy.
➡ *Add 4 drops to 8ml jojoba oil and massage into the scalp. Leave for 1–2 hours, or overnight, then rinse out.*

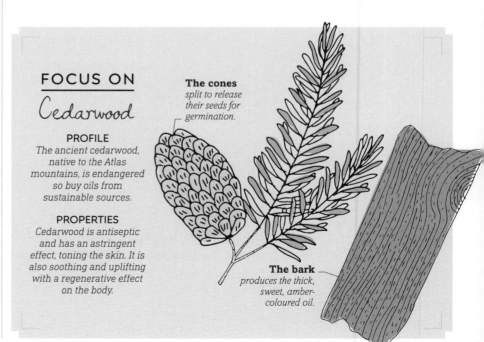

FOCUS ON
Cedarwood

PROFILE
The ancient cedarwood, native to the Atlas mountains, is endangered so buy oils from sustainable sources.

PROPERTIES
Cedarwood is antiseptic and has an astringent effect, toning the skin. It is also soothing and uplifting with a regenerative effect on the body.

The cones *split to release their seeds for germination.*

The bark *produces the thick, sweet, amber-coloured oil.*

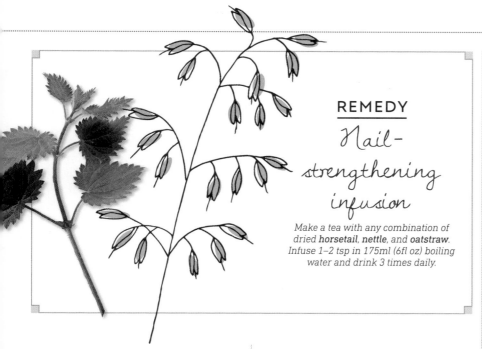

If nails are brittle or splitting, this can indicate that overall health and vitality are low. Persistently soft nails can be a symptom of another condition such as anaemia, diabetes, or heart or lung conditions, so consult your doctor if concerned.

HERBS

Nutrient-rich herbs, particularly ones with calcium and silica, improve the strength and condition of nails. In addition, herbs that help to improve peripheral circulation can increase the blood supply to the fingers and nails.

Horsetail is a traditional remedy for nail growth. It is high in silica, which converts to calcium in the body, vital for strong, well-conditioned nails. Avoid with diabetes, kidney disease, gout, or heart disease.

Nettles are a good source of calcium and silica to nourish nails, and have a tonic effect on the whole body.

Oatstraw provides calcium and biotin, promoting nail and bone growth. Avoid with gluten sensitivity.
➥*See remedy for horsetail, nettle, and oatstraw tea, above.*

ESSENTIAL OILS

Massaging essential oils into nails helps to boost their health and in turn improve their appearance.

Myrrh has moisturizing properties that help prevent nail and cuticle breakage.
➥*Add 4 drops to 8ml olive oil and massage into the nails and cuticles.*

Lavender helps to strengthen nails.
➥*Add 4 drops to 8ml wheatgerm oil and massage into nails and cuticles.*

REMEDY

Nail-strengthening infusion

*Make a tea with any combination of dried **horsetail**, **nettle**, and **oatstraw**. Infuse 1–2 tsp in 175ml (6fl oz) boiling water and drink 3 times daily.*

Cedarwood stimulates the hair follicles. See box, opposite.
➥*Add 4 drops to 8ml jojoba oil and massage into the scalp. Leave for 1–2 hours, or overnight, then rinse out.*

Sage helps to balance oils, toning the hair and scalp. An antifungal action helps prevent infections that can contribute to thinning hair. Avoid in pregnancy.
➥*In a bain-marie, warm 10ml coconut oil, add 5 drops sage essential oil, and massage into the scalp. Leave for 1–2 hours, or overnight, then rinse out.*

SUPPLEMENTS

These address nutritional deficiencies to support hair growth.

Iron deficiency can lead to hair loss.
➥*Take 20–40mg daily in a ferrous, not ferric, form, or take an iron water supplement as directed.*

Vitamin E in the form of mixed tocotrienols may reduce hair loss.
➥*Take 1000iu daily.*

Zinc supports the hair follicle and can help reverse hair loss if there is a deficiency.
➥*Take 10mg daily. Do not exceed recommended dose as an excess may aggravate hair loss.*

LIFESTYLE

Avoid or reduce your use of hair gels and other chemical-containing hair products that can weaken the hair. Also limit blow-drying, drying hair naturally whenever possible, and don't brush hair when it is wet.

Exercise at least 30 minutes a day to help lower stress levels.

" *Herbs with stimulating effects help to boost circulation to the scalp, nourishing hair follicles and promoting growth.* "

➤ CONTINUED...

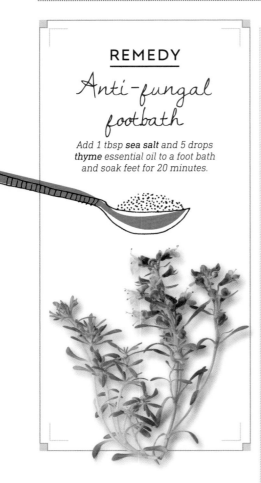

REMEDY

Anti-fungal footbath

Add 1 tbsp **sea salt** and 5 drops **thyme** essential oil to a foot bath and soak feet for 20 minutes.

Lemon helps to brighten and condition dull-looking nails.
➼ *Add 4 drops to 8ml jojoba oil and massage into the nails and cuticles.*

FOOD

Nails are made from a protein called keratin so adequate amounts of protein in the diet are necessary to keep nails strong and looking healthy. Many foods that are a source of protein are also rich in iron and the amino acid cysteine, both of which are vital for healthy nails.

Liver and kidneys, especially from lamb and chicken, are rich sources of protein and iron.
➼ *Try chicken livers on toasted ciabatta or in a salad.*

Eggs are a great source of high-quality protein and the egg white – albumen – is high in the nail-boosting amino acid cysteine.
➼ *Have a boiled egg daily – for breakfast, in a salad, or as a snack.*

SUPPLEMENTS

A daily multi-vitamin and mineral supplement can help to boost dietary sources to support strong nail growth when nails are in poor condition. There are also specialist supplements to help boost nail health.

Biotin, a B vitamin, can reduce the tendency of nails to split.
➼ *Take 100mcg daily for 6–9 months.*
Colloidal silicon has been shown to strengthen brittle nails.
➼ *Take 10–30ml daily of silicic acid or 10ml daily of orthosilicic acid.*

LIFESTYLE

Wear gloves when gardening and also for housework to keep your hands dry and protected from harsh chemicals and products.
Avoid nail polishes, varnishes, veneers, and nail hardeners as these can all exacerbate brittle nails.
Massage a lanolin-based lotion into the nail beds each day to condition and strengthen flaky nails.

THE EGG TEST

Test how fresh your egg is! Gently place it in a bowl or saucepan of water. The freshest eggs will stay on the bottom, while older, less fresh ones will rise to the top.

FUNGAL NAIL INFECTION

Also known as onychomycosis, fungal nail infections start on the rim of the nail, which turns whitish–yellow, brown, or green. Fungal infections are highly contagious so require prompt treatment.

HERBS

Antifungal herbs are used topically. Support these by taking immune-boosting and tissue-strengthening herbs internally to help improve overall nail health.

Calendula is antifungal and promotes cell regeneration.
Myrrh is antifungal, toning, and anti-inflammatory.
➼ *Apply 5ml combined calendula flower and myrrh tinctures to the area twice daily: for at least 3 months for fingernails and at least 6 months for toenails.*
Horsetail boosts immunity and is rich in silica to promote healthy nails. Avoid with gout, diabetes, or with kidney or heart disease.
➼ *Infuse 1–2 tsp dried horsetail in 175ml (6fl oz) boiling water. Drink 1–3 times daily, with a week's break after 4 weeks. Or add a strong infusion to a foot bath.*

ESSENTIAL OILS

Oils that are antifungal and healing can help tackle infections.

Tea tree is one of the most effective antifungal oils.
➼ *Add 5 drops to 5ml sweet almond oil and apply to the affected area regularly.*
Myrrh is healing and anti-inflammatory.
➼ *Add 5 drops to 5ml coconut oil and apply to the affected area regularly.*
Thyme has fungicidal properties.
➼ *See remedy with sea salt, left.*

> " *Anti-fungal herbs can help to tone the nails, while herbs that are high in silica can be used to improve the health of nails.* "

SUPPLEMENTS

As well as a multi-vitamin supplement, it is worth taking supplements with other specific nutrients that can help to fight off invasion by fungi, improving nail health and also giving the body a boost.

Multi-vitamins help to support the health of nails, leaving nails strong, glossy, and less vulnerable to infections.
➡ *Take a daily supplement.*
Vitamin B12 deficiency can weaken nails, leaving them vulnerable and allowing an infection to take hold.
➡ *Take up to 50mcg daily.*
Biotin (vitamin B7) can help prevent splitting, which makes it harder for any fungi that is present to take hold.
➡ *Take 30mcg daily.*

LIFESTYLE

Wear protective gloves when doing household chores or gardening.
Avoid nail polish and nail polish remover, which can damage nails, letting fungi take hold.

INGROWING NAILS

Ingrown toenails curve and grow into the skin causing discomfort, pain, and infection. Wearing tight-fitting shoes increases the risk of nails growing inwards.

HERBS

Anti-inflammatory herbs can be used to help reduce the discomfort and swelling that occurs around an ingrowing toenail, while antiseptic herbs help to keep the toenail and the surrounding tissue free from infection.

Calendula is anti-inflammatory to help reduce pain, and is also is antiseptic and promotes rapid healing.
St John's wort is anti-inflammatory and relieves nerve pain.
➡ *The classic ointment or cream, hypercal, combines calendula and St John's wort. Apply as needed.*
Golden seal is a potent antimicrobial and skin-healing herb.
➡ *Apply a cream, ointment, or tincture.*

ESSENTIAL OILS

The pain and swelling associated with ingrowing nails can be soothed using analgesic and anti-inflammatory oils.

Eucalyptus works as a soothing analgesic oil. See box, below.
➡ *Add 5 drops to 5ml coconut oil and gently massage around the area.*
Lavender has pain-relieving, anti-inflammatory, and healing properties that all work to relieve the discomfort of ingrown nails. It can also help to ward off infection where skin is broken and vulnerable.
➡ *Add 5 drops to 5ml base ointment and gently massage into the area.*
Myrrh is well known for its antimicrobial and anti-inflammatory actions.
➡ *Add 5 drops to 1 tbsp sea salt or Epsom salts and add to a foot bath. Soak feet for 20 minutes.*

LIFESTYLE

Wear properly fitting shoes and cut toenails straight across and not too short. If the area becomes infected, get medical advice.

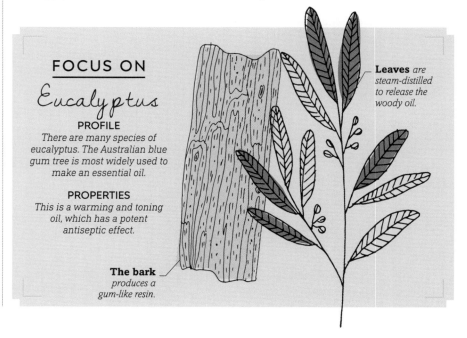

FOCUS ON
Eucalyptus

PROFILE
There are many species of eucalyptus. The Australian blue gum tree is most widely used to make an essential oil.

PROPERTIES
This is a warming and toning oil, which has a potent antiseptic effect.

Leaves *are steam-distilled to release the woody oil.*

The bark *produces a gum-like resin.*

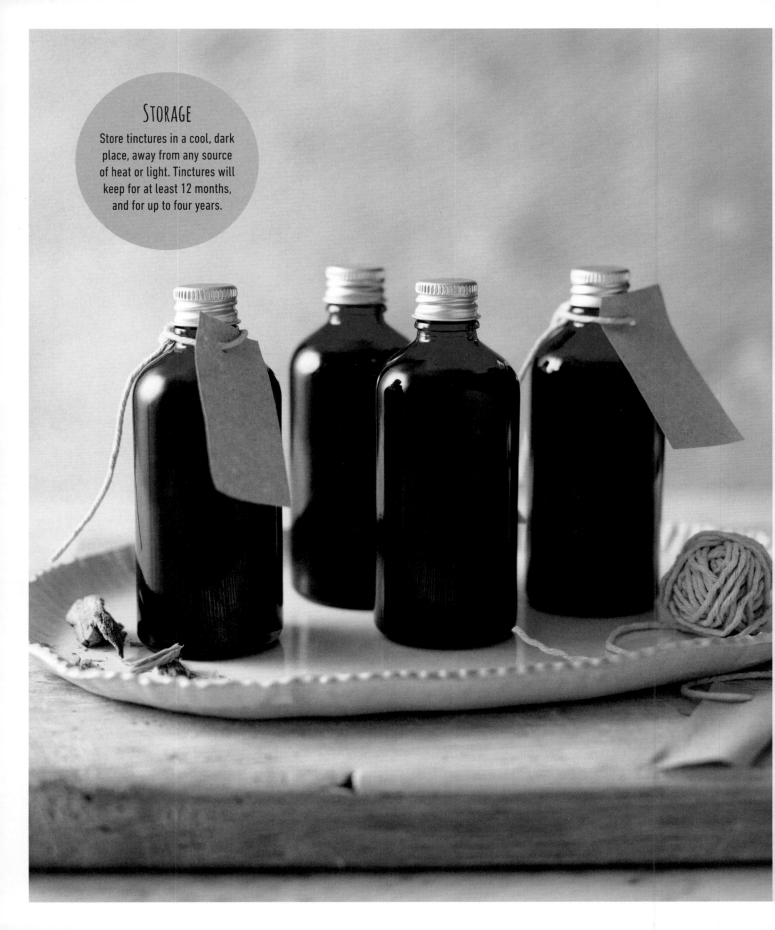

STORAGE

Store tinctures in a cool, dark place, away from any source of heat or light. Tinctures will keep for at least 12 months, and for up to four years.

HOW TO MAKE
A TINCTURE

Alcohol can be used to extract active constituents from herbs to create easy-to-administer medicinal tinctures. Alcohol also acts as a preservative, so tinctures have a long shelf life. Tinctures are stronger than other herbal preparations, such as infusions and decoctions, so only small amounts are used. Dosages are either one part fresh herb to three parts vodka, or one part dried herb to five parts vodka.

Makes about 1 litre (1³/4 pints)

YOU WILL NEED

200g (7oz) dried herbs, or 330g (11oz) fresh herbs, chopped

1 litre (1¾ pints) 37.5% vodka

kilner, or fermentation jar, plus jar for pouring if needed

bowl

muslin cloth

fruit/wine press (optional)

paper coffee filter (optional)

dark glass bottles with screw caps

labels

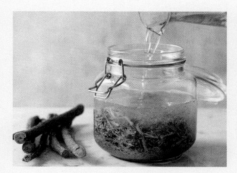

1 Sterilize the jars, bowl, and storage bottles: wash thoroughly then dry in an oven at 140°C (275°F) or in a microwave for 30–45 seconds. Place the herbs in the jar and pour over the vodka. Seal, shake well, label, and store in a cool, dark place for 2–3 weeks. Shake every other day.

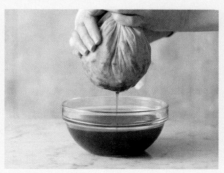

2 With clean hands, or wearing sterile rubber gloves, strain the herb mixture into a bowl, squeezing it through a muslin cloth, or, if avilable, use a fruit press. If you wish, filter the herbs again through a paper coffee filter.

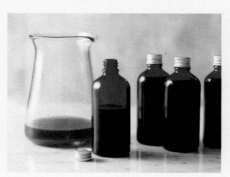

3 Pour the strained liquid into dark glass bottles, seal with a screw cap, and label with the herb and date.

EYES AND EARS

Sight and hearing are two of our most valued senses, playing a vital role in how we experience the world and relationships. Explore how a nutrient-dense diet can be key to preserving and optimizing the health of these important senses as we age, and how nourishing and revitalizing herbs and essential oils provide support. When problems do affect the eyes and ears, find out how natural remedies and key micronutrients can play a part in restoring function and health.

STAYING WELL
EYES AND EARS

Some eye conditions, including glaucoma and cataracts, are associated with ageing, but these aren't inevitable. A healthy diet and lifestyle from a young age can help ensure good eyesight well into our later years. Likewise for hearing, a nutrient-dense diet and healthy lifestyle can ensure lifelong clear hearing. Both eye and ear health can be greatly enhanced by well-chosen natural remedies.

FOOD

A diet abundant in antioxidants and key nutrients to boost circulation and immunity and reduce free radical damage helps protect and optimize eye and ear health.

PROTECTIVE ANTIOXIDANTS

Antioxidants help to prevent or slow down tissue and nerve damage from free radicals that can be a significant factor in declining eye and ear health. This protection can delay the onset of cataracts and may slow the progress of existing ones. Eat at least five portions of fruit and vegetables daily for an antioxidant boost.

FOODS TO SUPPORT CIRCULATION

Good circulation is essential for eye and ear health. Beetroot, kale, and collard greens contain circulation-boosting antioxidants and dietary nitrates, which enrich blood with oxygen, increasing micro-circulation to the tiny blood vessels in and around the eyes and in the ears. Healthy fats also support circulation. Two to three servings a week of oily fish, such as salmon, trout, or mackerel, provide omega-3 fatty acids to boost eye and ear health.

NATURAL IMMUNE BOOSTERS

Some foods strengthen resistance to eye and ear infections. Garlic has antimicrobial properties, with raw garlic being most potent. Elderberries, another traditional immune booster, are usually taken in syrup form to ward off infection in both adults and children.

IRON-RICH FOODS

Adequate levels of iron are important for women during menstruation or in pregnancy to avoid dark under-eye circles. Dark circles become more pronounced if levels of iron are low because insufficient oxygen, carried by iron, reaches the cells around the eyes. Boosting your protein intake with some lean red meat and plenty of pulses will bolster iron levels, also helping to

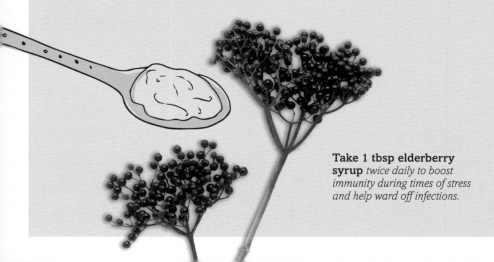

Take 1 tbsp elderberry syrup *twice daily to boost immunity during times of stress and help ward off infections.*

Take 1–3ml ginkgo biloba tincture *in a little water 3 times daily to boost circulation to the eyes and ears.*

energize you and avoid the fatigue that can lead you to rub your eyes and exacerbate dark circles. Vitamin C aids iron absorption, so eat foods such as citrus fruits alongside iron sources.

Herbs

Antioxidant and nourishing herbs counter the effects of stress and ageing to help optimize vision and hearing

Protective herbs

Antioxidant herbs can lessen the effects of stress and ageing on the eyes and ears. A member of the blueberry family, bilberries are a traditional herbal remedy for boosting micro-circulation in the eye area, helping to nourish and protect the eyes and prevent them from drying out. Along with other purple foods, bilberries are rich in anthocyanin, an antioxidant pigment, which helps protect delicate cells in the eyes and ears from oxidative stress.

Circulation boosters

Effective circulation to the ears helps to keep hearing clear as you get older. Ginkgo biloba helps to boost circulation to the extremities; passionflower also aids circulation, toning and relaxing nerves to aid sound transmission through the ear canals.

Revitalizing tonic herbs

Nourishing herbs such as schisandra revitalize and act as a strengthening tonic to reduce eye fatigue. Also, as we age, our eyes take longer to adjust when we move from bright to dim light, or vice versa, and night vision can deteriorate. Schisandra's tonic properties also help to improve night vision and retinal sensitivity.

Clearing herbs

It's important to keep the ear passages clear to optimize hearing. Anticatarrhal herbs and those that restore nerve tissue and improve blood flow are effective decongestants.

Make a bilberry decoction *with 1–2 tsp bilberries to 250ml (9fl oz) boiling water. Drink up to 3 times a day.*

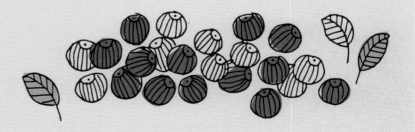

Herbs to ward off infection

Many herbs have powerful anti-infective properties to ward off infections. Chamomile is antimicrobial and anti-inflammatory and can be used to calm and soothe dry, sore eyes and so reduce the risk of infection. One of the most popular immune-boosting herbs, echinacea, has antibiotic and anti-inflammatory properties to help optimize immune system function and ward off infections.

Essential oils

These gently soothe and revitalize, helping to moisturize the eyes and keep the ears clear. They must not be used neat on the skin near the eyes, but benefits are gained from steam inhalations, compresses, and diffusions.

Eye-soothing oils

When eyes are under strain, for example during stressful periods at work, they are more susceptible to dryness and itching, and in turn more vulnerable to infection. Relaxing essential oils, well diluted in hot and cold compresses, can be extremely beneficial for revitalizing the eyes and preventing them from drying out. Lavender, a deeply relaxing oil with a cooling and soothing effect, is a perfect pick-me-up for tired, overworked eyes.

Anti-inflammatory oils

Anti-inflammatory oils can be restoring. Chamomile is a gentle anti-inflammatory, and when used in a light massage can boost recovery after an ear infection in both adults and children.

Rehydrating oils

Late nights and hectic days can result in dark under-eye rings and puffiness around the eyes. Oils used in steam inhalations and compresses moisturize and hydrate the delicate eye skin to counter and prevent these problems. Gently rehydrating oils such as rose, or moisturizing oils such as sandalwood, revitalize eyes, while German chamomile is effective for preventing puffiness.

Clearing oils

Decongesting oils, such as lemon verbena and angelica, help to clear the sinuses in the cold and flu season and support hearing.

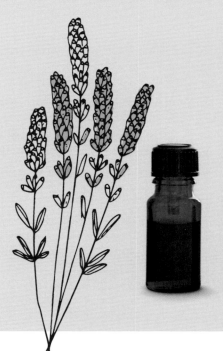

Add 3 drops lavender essential oil *to a bowl of hot water, soak a flannel in the water, wring this out, and lay it over your closed eyes. Relax for 10 minutes to revitalize the eyes. Use only the gentlest essential oils, such as lavender and rose, on the eye area.*

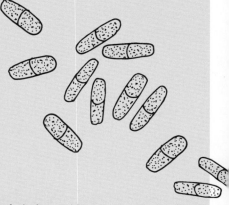

Supplements

Certain nutrients help to optimize eye and ear health, so supplementing the diet can be beneficial.

Preventative supplements

A daily multi-vitamin and mineral supplement ensures that your body is receiving adequate amounts of vital nutrients and is a simple and effective way to boost eye health and reduce the risk of developing cataracts.

Eye-protecting phytonutrients

Certain nutrients are key to eye health and maintaining healthy, well-functioning vision. Carotenoids, pigments found in brightly coloured foods, protect the body from the effects of free radicals, which can damage the lens of the eye as we age. Lutein and zeaxanthin are the only carotenoids found in the retina of the eye. These phytonutrients support eye health and boost vision and our eyes need a constant supply of them to stay healthy. Taking a supplement helps to top up levels of these essential nutrients.

Eye lubricants

Fish oil supplements with the long chain fatty acids eicosapentaenoic acid (EPA) and docosahexaenoic acid (DHA) support eye health. Eyes need to be kept constantly moist, ensured by secretions from the lacrimal glands coating the eyes in a moisture film. Fish oils boost tear function, lubricating eyes so they are less vulnerable to damage and vision is clearer.

Probiotic protectors

Probiotic supplements with *Lactobacillus* and *Bifidobacterium* strains can protect young children against recurrent ear infections, and zinc supports a healthy immune response in adults and children, reducing the risk of infection.

Antioxidants for hearing

Coenzyme Q10 (CoQ10) is an antioxidant produced in the body that supports hearing cells. Levels decrease with age, increasing the risk of hearing loss. Supplementing may protect hearing and slow the pace of hearing loss. Studies also show that antioxidant vitamins C and E, taken together, can help prevent, or repair, some damage from hearing loss due to loud noises.

"Our eyes need a constant supply of phytonutrients to support eye health and boost vision."

TREATMENTS
EYES AND EARS

We often take our eyesight and hearing for granted, but these important senses can be vulnerable to damage and infection, especially as we get older. Healing herbs and essential oils can help to support many eye- and ear-related conditions. There's also increasing evidence that key micronutrients are vital for eye and ear health. For eyes, regular checkups are crucial.

DRY EYES

Scratchy, uncomfortable dry eyes are increasingly common due to factors such as overuse of contact lenses and excessive screen time. Dry eyes are more common with increasing age, and can be caused by medications and hormonal changes, or accompany conditions such as rheumatoid arthritis, where the immune system attacks tear glands.

HERBS

Herbs that boost overall circulation help to increase the micro-circulation in the tiny blood vessels around the eyes, improving the flow of fluids into the tissues to lubricate, oxygenate, and nourish.

Ginkgo biloba helps increase blood flow to the eye. Avoid during pregnancy and when breastfeeding or taking with anticoagulant and antiplatelet medications.
➦ *Take a 66mg leaf extract capsule, equal to 3300mg, 1–3 times daily.*
Bilberry is antioxidant and strengthens capillaries, improving the blood supply to the eyes.
➦ *See remedy, right.*

Cayenne stimulates micro-circulation in the tiny blood vessels around the eyes to boost the oxygenation of eye tissues and help to produce tears. Avoid with peptic ulcers, reflux, or on broken skin.
➦ *Take 1–2 drops cayenne tincture in a glass of water 3 times daily.*

ESSENTIAL OILS

Dry eyes can be relieved by combining hot and cold water therapies with relaxing, rejuvenating, and soothing essential oils. Do not apply neat directly to the eye area.

Lavender is cooling and soothing, and its calming fragrance helps to relax and ease tension.
➦ *Add 2 drops of oil to a bowl of hot water to steam your face, covering with a towel to prevent steam escaping.*

Rose has anti-inflammatory properties and helps tissue regeneration.
➦ *Soak a cotton wool pad in rose water and apply as an eye mask for up to 10 minutes.*

SUPPLEMENTS

Healthy eyes require a high level of nutrients to help maintain and repair the ocular surface, including antioxidants and healthy fats. Supplements can help to address nutritional deficiencies to support and boost eye health.

Omega-3 marine oil contains the long-chain fatty acids EPA and DHA, which boost the lacrimal tear function to restore moisture balance.
➦ *Take a minimum of 250mg and up to 1g daily.*

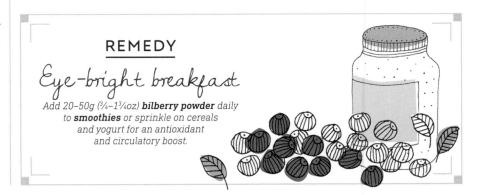

REMEDY

Eye-bright breakfast

Add 20–50g (¾–1¾oz) **bilberry powder** daily to **smoothies** or sprinkle on cereals and yogurt for an antioxidant and circulatory boost.

"Omega-7 fatty acids are anti-inflammatory, helping to relieve itchy, dry eyes and eye strain."

Phytoestrogens can be beneficial where dry eyes are linked to the menopause.
➡ *Try a fenugreek extract – fenugreek contains phytoestrogens and has been shown to support the meibomian glands, which produce a lipid film that keeps eyes from drying out. Take 500–600mg daily.*

Omega-7 palmitoleic acid supplements are usually derived from sea buckthorn, a rich natural source. Sea buckthorn is anti-inflammatory and helps to relieve dry eyes and eye strain.
➡ *Take 1g daily.*

LIFESTYLE

Eyedrops can be effective in the short term, but can make dry eyes worse if used for a long period of time. If you use eye drops, look for ones that contain vitamins A and E and have few preservatives.

Use a humidifier to counter the effects of a dry environment, which can accelerate tear evaporation, at home or during work.

Avoid long hours in front of a computer, too much sun exposure, and smoking or second-hand smoke, all of which can contribute to dry eyes.

EYE STRAIN

Eye strain is a catch-all term to describe symptoms such as burning, itching, eye fatigue from computer strain, and reduced night vision. Often it can be accompanied by tension headaches around the forehead and at the back of the eyes.

HERBS

Nutrient-dense and circulatory herbs can improve eye weakness and poor night vision. Stress can be an underlying cause of eye strain so should also be treated with relaxing and strengthening tonic herbs.

Lycium is a tonic and antioxidant herb. It has beta-carotene, important for eye health. Avoid with digestive irritability.
➡ *Take 3–5ml tincture in a little water 3 times daily.*

Schisandra is a revitalizing tonic herb. It reduces eye fatigue and improves night vision and retinal sensitivity. Avoid with acute infections or with barbiturates.
➡ *Take 2–4ml tincture in a little water 3 times daily.*

Bilberry strengthens the micro-circulation around the eyes. It contains antioxidant anthocyanins, which can help to improve vision.
➡ *Add 20–50g (¾–1¾oz) bilberry powder to smoothies, cereals, or yogurt daily.*

ESSENTIAL OILS

Essential oils, used well-diluted, can soothe tired eyes. Never apply them neat directly to the eye or the eye area.

Chamomile is antioxidant, anti-inflammatory, detoxifying, and has a gentle astringent effect.
➡ *Add 6 drops to alternating warm and cool compresses to reduce tension around the eye area.*

Rose is uplifting and relaxing, helping to relieve stress.
➡ *Add 2 drops to 5ml almond oil and massage gently into the area around the eyes. Follow with a warm compress.*

SUPPLEMENTS

Supporting your diet with supplements that contain nutrients known to boost eye health can help to make eyes less prone overall to eye strain.

Lutein and zeaxanthin are carotenoids that are known to protect eye health. They have been shown to improve night vision, especially helping with contrast and glare, and can give a small boost to blurred vision.
➡ *Take 20mg daily.*

Omega-3 fatty acids may be helpful for relieving eye strain and the associated dry eyes that are caused by long hours in front of a computer.
➡ *Take a daily capsule containing 180mg EPA and 120mg DHA.*

LIFESTYLE

Blink regularly. We tend to blink less when we are looking at computer screens, but the eyes can dry out completely after just 10 seconds of not blinking, increasing the likelihood of eye strain.

Check your posture. Eye strain can be related to other types of muscle strain in the head, neck, and spine.

Amber-tinted computer glasses that block the blue light from computers and other devices may help to reduce eye strain, as well as improve sleep.

Watch your weight. In particular, women who are overweight may have trouble metabolizing the eye-protective carotenoids lutein and zeaxanthin, or may metabolize them more slowly. Vision problems can also be related to conditions such as diabetes so keep this under control.

PUFFY EYES AND DARK CIRCLES

These can be related to poor circulation. Puffy eyes and dark circles often go hand in hand as puffiness can make dark circles appear more pronounced. Both conditions can be caused by too many late nights, computer eye strain, dehydration, food allergies, or simply getting older.

REMEDY

Gentle eye massage

*Add 1 drop **German chamomile** essential oil to 5ml **almond oil** and massage carefully into the bony area around the eye, taking care to avoid the eyelids and the area directly under the eyes.*

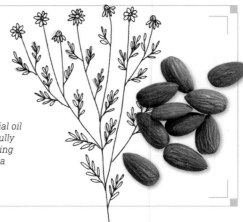

HERBS

Herbs that tone the delicate tissue around the eyes can be effective. Drinking herbal infusions can enhance waste elimination from the body via the urinary system, helping to keep tissues clear and vital.

Cleavers is diuretic and enhances lymphatic drainage, promoting effective fluid circulation and excretion.
➡ *Infuse 1–2 tsp dried cleavers in 175ml (6fl oz) boiling water and drink 3 times daily.*

Schisandra improves kidney and liver function. Its tonic action supports the body's response to chronic stress and anxiety. Avoid with acute infections or if taking barbiturates.
➡ *Take 2–4ml tincture in a little water 3 times daily.*

IN SEASON

Nettles grow abundantly in the wild, making them easy to source. For best use, harvest young leaves in spring and the upper part of the plant when flowering.

Witch hazel is astringent, toning, and cooling when applied topically.
➡ *Infuse 2 tsp dried witch hazel in 175ml (6fl oz) boiling water. Apply as a cool compress.*

Nettle is a blood tonic that is rich in minerals. It improves kidney and liver function, helping to strengthen the whole body.
➡ *Infuse 1–2 tsp dried nettle in 175ml (6fl oz) boiling water. Drink 3 times daily.*

ESSENTIAL OILS

Dark circles and puffiness can be signs of dehydration, so oils that moisturize can be beneficial. Never apply neat essential oils directly to the eye or the eye area.

Rose has rejuvenating properties and helps to keep skin hydrated.

Sandalwood has moisturizing and reviving properties and acts as an anti-inflammatory, helping to reduce puffiness around the eyes.
➡ *Add 2 drops of either rose or sandalwood essential oils to a bowl of hot water, lean over, covering your head with a towel to trap the steam, and inhale until the steam cools.*

German chamomile has anti-inflammatory properties, making it a helpful oil for reducing puffiness in the delicate tissues around the eyes.
➡ *See remedy with almond oil, above.*

FOOD

A diet lacking key nutrients contributes to the tiredness that causes puffy eyes. In particular, a lack of iron is linked to anaemia, which can make dark circles more pronounced during menstruation or in pregnancy. Dehydration can cause sunken eyes with dark circles. Drink 1.5–2 litres (2¾–3½ pints) water daily.

Beef and other meats are a good source of heme iron, which is more readily absorbed than plant-based sources.
➡ *Eat 85g (3oz) up to 2–3 times a week.*

Lentils, kidney beans, and other pulses are an excellent source of plant-based, non-heme iron.
➡ *Add to salads and casseroles.*

"A lack of vital minerals and dehydration can make dark circles around the eyes more pronounced."

Red peppers contain high levels of vitamin C, which is needed to aid the absorption of iron.
➡ *Add chopped peppers to a three-bean salad for a satisfying lunch.*
WHAT TO AVOID
Excess salt causes fluid retention throughout the body, including in the area underneath the eyes. Foods that are high in the compounds phytates and oxalates, such as nuts, chocolate, rhubarb, and soya, can interfere with iron absorption so avoid these with sources of iron.

LIFESTYLE

Get sufficient sleep. Fatigue is the most common cause of dark circles under the eyes.
Allergies to certain foods or chemicals can be at the root of chronic dark circles. If other causes aren't obvious, consider getting tested for allergies.
Avoid smoking or drinking, which can make dark circles more pronounced.
Elevate your head during the night. Two or more pillows can prevent fluid pooling in the lower eyelids.

STYES

A stye is an abscess that occurs around the root of the eyelash and it is usually caused by the *Staphylococcus* bacteria. With the right support, styes can clear up in around seven days, but they can also spread to adjacent hair follicles and become a chronic problem.

HERBS

Immune-boosting herbs enhance immune resistance, while relaxing herbs are calming and strengthening, helping to treat any underlying stress. Anti-inflammatory herbs applied topically can ease discomfort.

Chamomile calms the nerves and has antibacterial and anti-inflammatory properties that can speed healing. Avoid with *Asteraceae* sensitivity.
➡ *Infuse 1–2 tsp dried chamomile in 175ml (6fl oz) boiling water and use the infusion as a warm compress.*

Astragalus is a strengthening tonic, which boosts immunity and supports the body during times of chronic stress. Avoid with acute infections and with immune-suppressant and blood-thinning drugs.
➡ *Take 250–500mg capsules 3 times daily, or take 2–4ml tincture in a little water 3 times daily.*
Elderflower has healing properties; see box, below.
➡ *Brew a strong tea, soak a cotton wool pad in the warm liquid, and use to clean carefully around the eye, or as a warm compress held gently on the eyelid.*
Lavender is both soothing and toning. Its comforting fragrance helps to relieve underlying stress and it has strong healing properties.
➡ *Brew a strong tea, soak a cotton wool pad in the warm liquid, and use as a warm compress.*

LIFESTYLE

Being generally run down makes styes more likely to occur. Ensure you are eating a nutritious, balanced diet and are getting regular and adequate rest to support your body's immune response to bacteria.
Practise good hygiene. Wash your hands regularly and avoid rubbing your eyes as this can not only trigger an infection, but can also spread an existing infection to other hair follicles, creating a more chronic condition. Clean make-up brushes regularly and don't hold on to items such as mascara when they are past their use-by date as bacteria can build up in these cosmetic items over time.

OTHER THERAPIES

Homeopathy can help in the treatment of styes by helping to strengthen the whole body, in turn boosting the immune response.

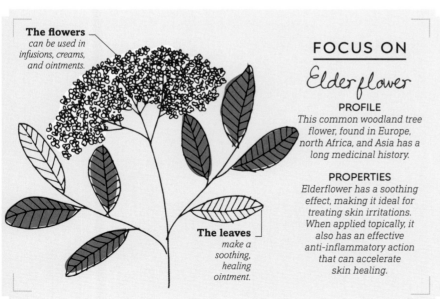

The flowers *can be used in infusions, creams, and ointments.*

The leaves *make a soothing, healing ointment.*

FOCUS ON
Elderflower

PROFILE
This common woodland tree flower, found in Europe, north Africa, and Asia has a long medicinal history.

PROPERTIES
Elderflower has a soothing effect, making it ideal for treating skin irritations. When applied topically, it also has an effective anti-inflammatory action that can accelerate skin healing.

HOW TO MAKE
A MACERATED OIL

A macerated oil is one that is infused with herbs. It can then be applied directly to the skin or can be used as an ingredient in salves, creams, or lotions. Macerates are commonly made by placing the infusion over direct heat, although some delicate flowering herbs, such as mullein and calendula, can also be macerated by sitting the infusion in sunlight for three to six weeks.

Makes 500ml to 1 litre (16fl oz to 1³/4 pints)

YOU WILL NEED

100g (3½oz) dried herbs, or 300g (10oz) fresh herbs, leaves chopped and left for several hours to wilt

500ml to 1 litre (16fl oz to 1¾ pints) organic oil such as olive, sunflower, or almond

bain-marie (heat-proof bowl set over saucepan)

wide-necked jug

muslin cloth

rubber gloves (optional)

dark glass bottle

label

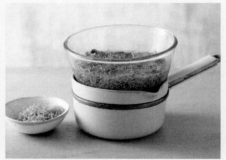

1 Sterilize the bowl, jug, and storage bottles: wash thoroughly then either dry in an oven at 140°C (275°F) or in a microwave for 30–45 seconds. Put the herbs and oil in a bain marie, ensuring the oil covers the herbs, then simmer on a hob at a very low heat for 2–3 hours, topping up the water in the saucepan if needed.

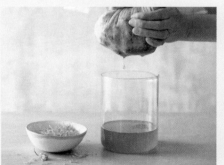

2 Line the mouth of the jug with the muslin. With clean hands, or wearing sterile rubber gloves, carefully transfer the herb and oil mix into the cloth to strain the oil through, gently gathering up the muslin and twisting and squeezing it to press out as much liquid as possible.

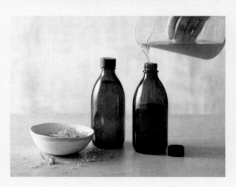

3 If using fresh herbs, allow the oil to sit for a few hours until any water content from the herbs separates from the oil. Carefully pour the oil into a dark glass bottle, leaving behind any water content, and label with the herb and date.

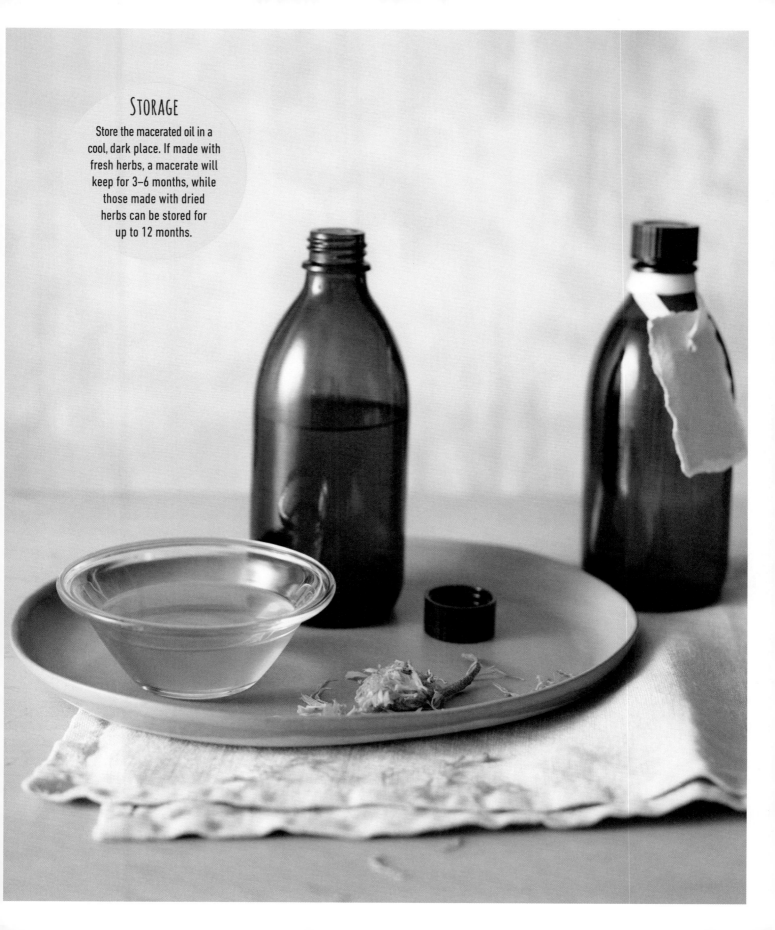

STORAGE

Store the macerated oil in a cool, dark place. If made with fresh herbs, a macerate will keep for 3–6 months, while those made with dried herbs can be stored for up to 12 months.

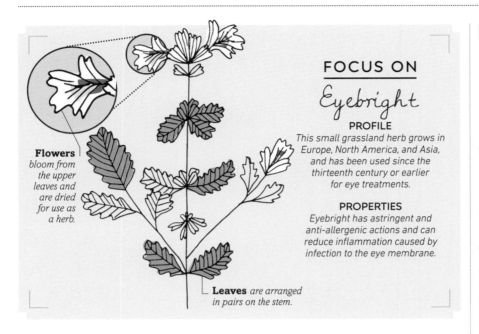

Flowers *bloom from the upper leaves and are dried for use as a herb.*

FOCUS ON

Eyebright

PROFILE

This small grassland herb grows in Europe, North America, and Asia, and has been used since the thirteenth century or earlier for eye treatments.

PROPERTIES

Eyebright has astringent and anti-allergenic actions and can reduce inflammation caused by infection to the eye membrane.

Leaves *are arranged in pairs on the stem.*

CONJUNCTIVITIS

Conjunctivitis – or pink eye – can be caused by infection, an allergic reaction (including to pollen), eye strain, or an irritant such as a stray eyelash. It can be painful, red, and often produces a sticky or watery discharge.

HERBS

Anti-inflammatory herbs ease discomfort, astringent herbs support tissues and calm irritation, and anti-infectives fight infection.

Chamomile is antimicrobial and anti-inflammatory, calming and soothing the eye. Avoid with sensitivity to the *Asteraceae* plant family.

Fennel seed, a traditional eye remedy, is a cooling and cleansing anti-inflammatory herb.
➡️*Infuse 1–2 tsp dried chamomile or fennel seed in 175ml (6fl oz) boiling water, cool, and use as a compress with a cotton wool pad.*

Eyebright helps to soothe sore eyes. See box, above.
➡️*Add 1–2 drops of tincture to boiled cooled water and use for a soothing and calming eye bath.*

LIFESTYLE

Eat a diet that consists primarily of fresh whole foods to provide a range of nutrients that help to support healthy, strong immunity.

Develop a regular sleep pattern. Broken, irregular, or insufficient sleep can lower your defences, leaving you more susceptible to infection.

Pay attention to hygiene. Make sure you wash your hands regularly, and especially after you have touched your eyes, to avoid spreading infection. If the infection is in one eye, avoid touching one eye then the other without washing hands inbetween.

OTHER THERAPIES

Homeopathy helps to support the whole body, which can bolster resistance against infections.

CATARACTS

The eye depends on the surrounding liquid – its aqueous humour – to supply nutrients and remove waste products. If this system fails, then waste products can build up, damaging the lens and causing it to become cloudy and vision to be blurred. Natural remedies can prevent or slow the progress of cataracts.

HERBS

Herbs that have nourishing and cleansing properties and which contain antioxidants help to improve the micro-circulation to the tiny blood vessels around the eye area. This in turn encourages the removal of waste and toxins, promoting eye tissue health and helping to slow the development of cataracts.

Parsley is rich in cleansing chlorophyll and has antioxidants vitamin C and beta-carotene (which converts to vitamin A in the body). All of these nutrients help to purify and revitalize tissues. Avoid with inflammatory kidney conditions.
➡️*Take 1–2ml tincture in a little water 3 times daily, or add chopped parsley to soups, salads, and smoothies.*

Bilberry strengthens the micro-circulation to the tissues around the eyes. It also has antioxidant anthocyanins, which are thought to help improve vision.
➡️*Take 20–50g (³⁄₄–1³⁄₄oz) bilberry powder daily: add to smoothies or yogurt, or sprinkle over cereals or oats.*

Lycium contains antioxidant beta-carotenes, which are supportive for eye health, and it also works as a strengthening tonic herb for the whole body. Avoid with digestive irritability.
➡️*Take 3–5ml tincture in a little water 3 times daily.*

> *"The carotenoids zeaxanthin and lutein are essential for eye health."*

FOOD

A diet rich in antioxidants found in abundance in fresh fruits and vegetables can help delay the onset of cataracts and may also help to slow their progression.

Oranges, grapefruit, papaya, and cantaloupe melons are all excellent sources of vitamin C, which is thought to support retinal health.
➡ *Start your day with a glass of fresh juice or a slice of melon to help meet your daily vitamin C requirement.*

Nuts and seeds are an excellent source of vitamin E, which helps to protect the eye cells.
➡ *Snack on a handful of almonds or other nuts and seeds.*

Kale is one of the best sources of lutein, zeaxanthin, and beta-carotene, all important nutrients to optimize and protect eye health.
➡ *Eat daily – raw, steamed, or added to stir-fries.*

WHAT TO AVOID
Refined carbohydrates. Studies show that diets high in these increase the risk of cataracts developing.

SUPPLEMENTS

As well as antioxidants, it's important to get a full spectrum of nutrients for your body to utilize. Supplements can help to support your dietary intake.

Multi-vitamin and mineral supplements help the body to use other nutrients efficiently. Studies have shown that a daily supplement can lower cataract risk in men.
➡ *Take a daily multi supplement.*

Vitamins C and E combined are a powerful weapon against cataracts. Studies reveal that these two vitamins can help reduce the incidence of "cortical" and "nuclear" type cataracts.
➡ *Ensure you are getting 250mg to 1g of vitamin C and 100–400iu of vitamin E daily.*

Lutein and zeaxanthin are carotenoids found in the eye. They are located mainly in the macula in the centre of the retina, the part of the eye that is involved in detailed vision, and play an important role in vision.
➡ *Taking 6–10mg daily of lutein with added zeaxanthin can help to lower the risk of cataracts.*

LIFESTYLE

Smoking and excessive alcohol consumption both raise the risk of developing cataracts.

Wear sunglasses. Too much UV light exposure is one of the risk factors for developing cataracts.

MACULAR DEGENERATION

This occurs when the cells of the macula in the retina are damaged. Age-related macular degeneration (AMD) is most common. AMD can't be cured, but it is possible to reduce the risk or to slow the disease down.

HERBS

Herbs that contain antioxidants help to counter the ageing process and nutrient-rich herbs support a healthy eye structure. Circulatory herbs strengthen the blood supply to feed eye tissues.

Lycium is a tonic with antioxidant beta-carotenes, which can help to counter the effects of ageing. It combines well with cayenne, below. Avoid with digestive irritability.
➡ *Take 3–5ml tincture in water 3 times daily, or see remedy below.*

Cayenne is a tonic and an effective circulatory stimulant, and is beneficial for boosting blood supply in the aged. Avoid with peptic ulcers, reflux, or on broken skin.
➡ *Take 1–2 drops tincture in water.*

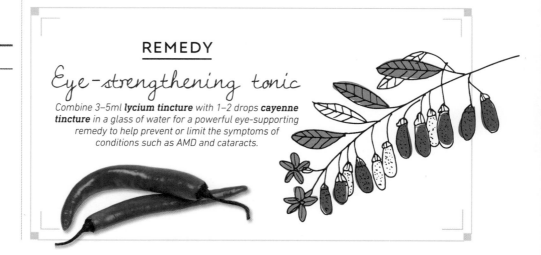

REMEDY

Eye-strengthening tonic

Combine 3–5ml **lycium tincture** with 1–2 drops **cayenne tincture** in a glass of water for a powerful eye-supporting remedy to help prevent or limit the symptoms of conditions such as AMD and cataracts.

➤ CONTINUED...

A SWEET TOUCH

Papaya has a digestive enzyme called papain, which aids nutrient absorption. Add puréed papaya to marinades for a sweet note and digestive boost.

Bilberry strengthens the micro-circulation to the eyes and has antioxidant anthocyanins, which are thought to support vision.
➡ *Add 20–50g (¾–1¾oz) bilberry powder daily to smoothies or yogurt or sprinkle over cereals and oats.*

FOOD

Certain key nutrients play an important role in optimizing eye health.

Spinach and other leafy greens supply the eye-supporting carotenoids lutein and zeaxanthin. Research shows that those who eat spinach daily have 10 per cent less incidence of AMD than those who eat it only occasionally; and for AMD sufferers, eating spinach can help to prevent it worsening.

Papayas, mangoes, and other orange, red, and yellow fruits are high in eye-protecting beta-carotene, as well as providing lutein and zeaxanthin.
➡ *Eat a serving daily to lower your risk of developing AMD.*

Oily fish, such as salmon, trout, and mackerel, eaten more than once a week, can halve the risk of AMD.
➡ *Enjoy 2–3 servings a week.*

Green tea has powerful antioxidants that can help to slow, or even halt, the progression of AMD. Buy unprocessed, preferably organic, loose leaves.
➡ *Drink 1–3 cups daily.*

Turmeric has the active ingredient, curcumin, a powerful antioxidant that has been shown to protect the eye.
➡ *Toss 1 tsp turmeric over roasted vegetables, sprinkle over rice or scrambled eggs, blend into a smoothie, or enjoy a turmeric latte.*

SUPPLEMENTS

Topping up certain nutrients can help to support the diet in protecting eye health.

Lutein and zeaxanthin supplements can lower the risk of macular degeneration by more than 40 per cent.
➡ *Take a daily supplement that contains at least 10mg lutein and 2mg zeaxanthin.*

Vitamin E is a powerful antioxidant, vital for the healthy functioning of the eyes.
➡ *Take 400iu daily.*

Zinc aids the absorption of other nutrients – it's involved in over 100 metabolic processes – and supports proper waste elimination, helping to fight inflammation and cellular damage around the eye.
➡ *Take up to 25mg daily, with supervision from a nutritional therapist.*

LIFESTYLE

Losing weight helps to lower high blood pressure, which in turn benefits eye health. There is also evidence that overweight women have difficulty metabolizing zeaxanthin and lutein, or metabolize these nutrients more slowly.

Remember to blink as this spreads secretions across the eyes to keep them clean and moist. We tend to blink less in front of a computer screen so remind yourself to do this consciously.

Wear sunglasses. Exposure to UV light is a risk factor for AMD. Wear good-quality sunglasses, and if you spend a lot of time on screens, use computer glasses to block out blue screen light.

GLAUCOMA

There are over 20 types of glaucoma, but chronic glaucoma and primary open-angle glaucoma (POAG) are the most common. Glaucoma is a leading cause of blindness and is caused partly by poor circulation to the optic nerve, which increases pressure behind the eye.

HERBS

Herbs that improve the micro-circulation to the eyes, increasing the supply of oxygen and nutrients, and those that are antioxidant and have anti-inflammatory properties can be used to help support chronic glaucoma.

Ginkgo biloba boosts the blood supply to the eyes, which may limit damage to the visual field. Avoid in pregnancy, if breastfeeding, and with anticoagulant and antiplatelet medication.
➡ *Take a 66mg leaf extract tablet, equal to 3300mg whole leaf, 1–3 times daily.*

Rosehip is a source of vitamin C, which has been shown to help lower pressure behind the eye.
➡ *Take rosehip powder in capsule form or add ½ tsp powder to 175ml (6fl oz) boiling water, and drink 3 times daily.*

Bilberry strengthens the micro-circulation around the eyes. It also has antioxidants called anthocyanosides, which are thought to improve vision.
➡ *Take 20–50g (¾–1¾oz) bilberry powder daily in smoothies, yogurt, or on cereals.*

FOOD

Foods that have circulation-boosting nutrients can be helpful. Excess protein can exacerbate glaucoma so a lower protein diet may be beneficial.

Beetroot, kale, and collard greens are rich in dietary nitrates which help oxygenate blood and significantly increase circulation to the eye.

➡ *One serving of beetroot a month has been shown to lower the risk of developing POAG type glaucoma significantly.*

SUPPLEMENTS

Supplements that promote eye circulation and drainage will support eye health.

A multi-vitamin and mineral supplement will ensure that you receive the full range of nutrients to support eye health.

➡ *Take a daily multi supplement.*

Beta-carotene and other carotenoids are essential for a healthy retina and for strengthening the mucous membranes that surround the eye.

➡ *Look for a supplement that provides 15mg mixed carotenoids.*

Vitamin E helps prevent the eye's drainage system from deteriorating and supports healthy cells.

➡ *Take up to 1100iu daily.*

Vitamin B1 (thiamine) is sometimes found to be severely deficient in patients with glaucoma.

➡ *A daily dose of up to 50mg may improve symptoms.*

LIFESTYLE

Health issues such as diabetes and high blood pressure can raise your risk of developing glaucoma so it's important to manage these conditions.

Regular aerobic exercise has been linked with a reduction in intraocular tension – the fluid pressure inside the eye – so this can be a supportive approach to eye health.

OTHER THERAPIES

Acupuncture supports other treatments and may also stimulate enkephalins – which are molecules that are produced naturally by the central nervous system and which have a role in reducing eye-fluid pressure.

Flower remedies can help to cope with the pain and anxiety that can accompany glaucoma.

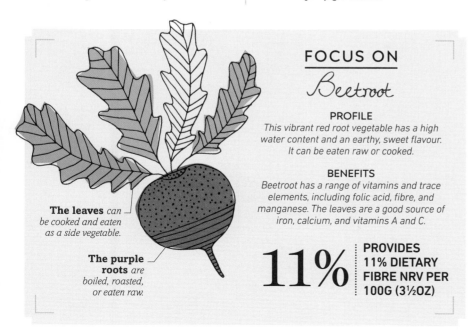

FOCUS ON
Beetroot

PROFILE
This vibrant red root vegetable has a high water content and an earthy, sweet flavour. It can be eaten raw or cooked.

BENEFITS
Beetroot has a range of vitamins and trace elements, including folic acid, fibre, and manganese. The leaves are a good source of iron, calcium, and vitamins A and C.

The leaves *can be cooked and eaten as a side vegetable.*

The purple roots *are boiled, roasted, or eaten raw.*

11%
PROVIDES 11% DIETARY FIBRE NRV PER 100G (3½OZ)

EARACHE

Earache is especially common in children, and can be painful and distressing. Infection of the middle ear – otitis media – may or may not be present. Earache and infections can be caused by inflammation or from a buildup of fluid pressing on the eardrum.

HERBS

Anti-inflammatory and anticatarrhal herbs clear congestion and soothe irritation, pain-relieving herbs soothe, and antibacterial herbs can tackle infections.

Mullein is antibacterial and its mucilage soothes and protects inflamed tissues.

➡ *Apply 2–4 warmed drops mullein macerated flower oil to the outer ear with cotton wool 2–3 times daily.*

St John's wort relieves nerve pain and inflammation. Avoid internally in pregnancy and high doses in sunlight. Taken internally, interacts with many prescribed drugs.

➡ *Apply 2–4 warmed drops St John's wort macerated flower oil to the outer ear with cotton wool 2–3 times daily.*

Chamomile is anti-inflammatory with a mild analgesic action. Avoid with sensitivity to the *Asteraceae* family.

➡ *Infuse 2 tsp dried chamomile in 175ml (6fl oz) water; soak cotton wool in the infusion and apply to the outer ear.*

Echinacea is antibiotic and anti-inflammatory, healing the mucous membranes and boosting immunity. Avoid with immunosuppressants.

➡ *Take 2–3ml tincture in a little water, 3–4 times daily.*

ESSENTIAL OILS

Use pain-killing and antimicrobial essential oils to soothe earache.

➤ CONTINUED...

Tea tree works as an antiseptic.
➥*Add 4 drops to 1 tsp almond or olive oil. Add to a cotton wool ball and dab gently in the external ear opening.*
Lavender is analgesic and anti-inflammatory.
➥*Add 4 drops to a cotton wool ball soaked in warm water for a compress.*
Roman chamomile is gently anti-inflammatory.
➥*Add 2 drops to 5ml coconut oil and massage around the painful area.*

FOOD

Foods with anti-infective properties are supportive when you are run down.

Garlic is a strong antimicrobial.
➥*Use liberally in dressings and food.*
Elderberries are anti-infective.
➥*Buy or make a syrup to take daily, or make into a jam.*

SUPPLEMENTS

These can support a healthy wholefood diet to boost immunity.

Zinc promotes a healthy immune system.
➥*Children can take 2–4mg daily; adults 8–11mg daily minimum.*
Probiotic supplements may reduce the risk of acute otitis media in babies.
➥*Apply drops, or take capsules with 5–10 billion live organisms a dose.*
Vitamin C boosts immunity, and vitamin D helps build resistance with recurrent ear infections.
➥*Give young children chewable vitamin C, 250–500mg daily; or take 1000iu vitamin D daily as drops.*

OTHER THERAPIES

Osteopathy or chiropractic can help built-up fluids drain more freely.
Homeopathy can be used to treat the individual constitutionally and relieve emotional distress.

DIZZINESS AND VERTIGO

Feelings of light-headedness and being off balance can strike anyone, for example, when tired, hungry, over-heated, or when there is a sinus or ear infection. Vertigo is a severe case of dizziness, brought on by a malfunction of the balance mechanism in the inner ear.

HERBS

Herbs that improve the circulation to the peripheral areas of the body will help to increase blood flow to the inner ear, and anti-inflammatory and tonic herbs can support the nervous system.

Ginkgo biloba increases blood supply to the inner ear and is anti-inflammatory, helping to improve vertigo caused by an infection. Avoid in pregnancy, when breastfeeding, and with anticoagulant and antiplatelet medication.
➥*Take a 66mg leaf tablet providing the equivalent of 3300mg whole leaf, 1–3 times daily.*
Wood betony improves circulation to the head and is a relaxing and strengthening cerebral nerve tonic.
➥*Infuse 1–2 tsp dried wood betony in 175ml (6fl oz) boiling water, and drink 3 times daily.*
Rosemary is a tonic herb for peripheral circulation. It soothes the nervous system and is strengthening when feeling weak. Avoid therapeutic doses in pregnancy.
➥*Take 1–2ml tincture in a little water 3 times daily.*

LIFESTYLE

Go fragrance free. Sensitivity to synthetic fragrances are a common cause of dizziness.

Dehydration can lead to dizziness, especially in extreme heat. Always make sure you are well hydrated with plenty of water and herbal teas.
Raise your head while sleeping. If suffering with vertigo, try sleeping with your head slightly raised on two or more pillows to avoid feelings of dizziness when you lie down. Get up slowly from lying down and sit down slowly to give your ears time to adjust.
Regular bouts of dizziness may be a sign of a migraine, anxiety that leads to hyperventilation, or, most commonly with diabetics, low blood sugar, so try to manage these conditions to avoid feelings of dizziness.

OTHER THERAPIES

Chiropractic or osteopathy can be helpful if dizziness is caused by misalignment and/or poor posture.
Craniosacral therapy can be beneficial if misaligned cranial bones are contributing to vertigo.
The Epley manoeuvre – an adjustment of the neck, which helps reposition crystals in the ear that interfere with balance – can help to address chronic vertigo. Conventional practitioners, osteopaths, and chiropractors are all qualified to carry out this procedure.
Hypnotherapy may help for vertigo that is caused by a fear of heights.

GET PICKING

To find fresh elderberries be ready to forage. These richly fruity berries grow wild in hedgerows and are ripe for picking from August to October.

HEARING LOSS

Loss of hearing is more common with age. "Conductive" hearing loss occurs with wax buildup, damage to the eardrum, or arthritis in the inner ear bones. "Sensorineural" hearing loss is caused by nerve damage. Preventative measures are helpful.

HERBS

Herbs that aid the circulation, increasing tissue oxygenation, are beneficial, as well as those that act as a nerve tonic.

Ginkgo biloba boosts circulation to the extremities. Avoid in pregnancy, if breastfeeding, and with anticoagulant and antiplatelet medication.
➧*Take a 66mg leaf tablet, providing the equivalent of 3300mg whole leaf, 1–3 times daily.*
Passionflower boosts circulation and tones and relaxes nerves, which may aid sound transmission in the ear. May cause feelings of drowsiness.
Plantain is astringent, anti-inflammatory, and anti-catarrhal.
➧*Infuse 1–2 tsp dried passionflower or plantain in 175ml (6fl oz) boiling water, and drink 3 times daily.*

ESSENTIAL OILS

Essential oils that have an anti-inflammatory effect can calm where hearing loss is due to infection.

Helichrysum is helpful for those with hearing problems.
➧*See remedy with avocado oil, above.*
Eucalyptus is beneficial with hearing loss that is caused by catarrh. The oil will help to clear the eustachian tubes.
➧*Add 3–4 drops to a bowl of hot water, lean over with a towel over the head, and inhale until the steam cools.*

REMEDY

Hearing-enhancing oil

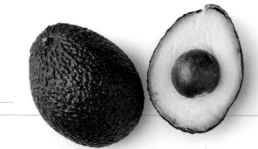

Add 2 drops **helichrysum** essential oil to 5ml **avocado oil**. Rub the oil blend gently behind the ear and down the jaw line.

FOOD

Ears are nourished by the blood supply so eat plenty of whole foods and healthy fats to ensure nutrients circulate to the ears.

Cold-water fish such as salmon, trout, albacore tuna, herring, mackerel, sardines, and anchovies have omega-3 fatty acids to support circulation.
➧*Have 2–3 servings a week.*

SUPPLEMENTS

Supplements with antioxidant and anti-inflammatory properties may protect the ears and slow hearing loss.

CoQ10 can support energy production in hearing cells.
➧*Take 160–200mg daily.*
Alpha lipoic acid is a powerful antioxidant that supports nerve function and plays an essential role in generating mitochondria in the hair cells of the inner ear.
➧*Take 100–300mg daily.*
Folic acid appears to slow hearing loss that commonly occurs with age in people with high levels of the amino acid homocysteine.
➧*Aim for 600mcg daily.*

Vitamins C and E taken together may help to reduce free radical damage to the nerves, in turn helping to prevent or repair damage to hearing due to loud noises.
➧*Take 900iu vitamin E daily, and 1200mg vitamin C daily.*

LIFESTYLE

Earplugs are a must to avoid nerve damage from exposure to continuous loud noise at work or a music festival.
Reduce phone use. Using a phone for 60 minutes or more a day can increase the risk of hearing loss.
Stop smoking. Smokers are nearly twice as likely to experience hearing loss than non-smokers,
Check cholesterol and blood pressure. Hypertension and high cholesterol can contribute to age-related hearing loss.
Reduce salt. Hearing may be improved by reducing salt, which can cause fluids to be retained in the ear.

OTHER THERAPIES

Visit a chiropractor if you have suffered neck or head trauma – treating these problems may prevent hearing loss as you age.

MOUTH AND THROAT

The digestive process begins in the mouth, where food is broken down to help its transit through the body, while the complex anatomy of the throat houses vital parts of the digestive and respiratory systems, passing food to the gut and air to the lungs. Discover how immune-boosting and nourishing foods, herbs, and essential oils strengthen tissue and balance bacteria to keep the mouth and throat healthy, and when illnesses occur, how a holistic approach can fight infection and inflammation to restore health.

STAYING WELL
MOUTH AND THROAT

Looking after the mouth and throat environment helps to strengthen immunity in this part of the body, prevent problems such as inflammation, and is essential for strong and healthy teeth and gums. A diet that is rich in essential nutrients can be supported with immune-strengthening and protective natural therapies to promote healthy bacteria in this important environment, and to boost tissue health, in turn helping to ensure the long-lasting health of the teeth and gums.

FOOD

As well as ensuring you get the essential nutrients, diet can be tailored to provide more of the nutrients that are particularly beneficial for oral and throat health. Avoiding very acidic foods and foods with lingering smells also helps to keep the mouth and teeth healthy.

SLEEP INDUCERS

Studies show that getting sufficient restful sleep is one of the most important factors for good oral health, helping to reduce inflammation and lowering the risk of gum disease, as well as accelerating healing of problems such as painful mouth ulcers.

Foods that contain natural sources of melatonin, the hormone that is responsible for regulating our circadian rhythms, can help to promote sleep. Ensure that your diet contains regular servings of melatonin-rich foods such as tart cherries or cherry juice, tomatoes, chillies, white and black mustard seeds, fenugreek, corn, rice, sprouted seeds, and the grain lupin to aid regular and restful sleep. Including foods that contain the amino acid tryptophan in your evening meal can also help to promote sleep. Tryptophan boosts production of calming serotonin in the body and has a natural sedative effect. Sources of tryptophan include poultry, chickpeas, cottage cheese, and eggs.

PROBIOTIC FOODS

Live or fermented foods such as natural yogurt, sauerkraut, and kimchi, help to neutralize acidic conditions in the mouth and stop unhealthy bacteria forming damaging plaque. These probiotic foods also help balance the natural flora of the mouth to speed the healing of mouth ulcers and reduce the risk of reoccurrence.

INFECTION FIGHTERS

Honey is a traditional and effective throat soother, which can be beneficial when cold and flu viruses are circulating. Honey coats the throat and has anti-inflammatory properties, soothing irritated mucous membranes. It is also antimicrobial, helping to prevent infection taking hold, and its many beneficial substances act as natural antibiotics. Blackcurrants also have soothing anti-inflammatory properties and the diluted syrup can be taken warm or cold if you feel the beginnings of a sore throat.

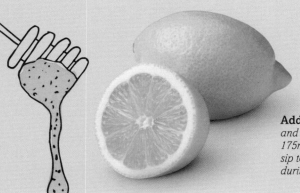

Add a spoonful of honey
and the juice of half a lemon to 175ml (6fl oz) boiling water and sip to help ward off infection during the cold and flu season.

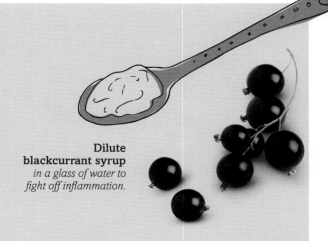

> **"Antibacterial and antiviral herbs can help to support oral health."**

Dilute blackcurrant syrup *in a glass of water to fight off inflammation.*

Another food, garlic, has the sulphur-containing compound allicin, which has antibacterial properties, plus garlic has other potent antibacterial substances. Including garlic regularly in meals and adding raw garlic to dressings can give a boost to immunity that can ward off the viruses that lead to a sore throat.

BREATH FRESHENERS

Just as some foods can cause bad breath, certain foods have a freshening effect. Lemons and chlorophyll-rich foods such as parsley can help to neutralize undesirable odours. Also live foods such as yogurt introduce beneficial bacteria to combat the harmful bacteria that can lead to bad breath. Crunch fruit and vegetables, such as apples, celery, carrots, and cucumber between meals to stimulate saliva production, which helps to keep breath fresh.

ESSENTIAL MICRONUTRIENTS

Several nutrients are key to teeth and gum health. Calcium, found in dairy products and leafy greens, promotes tooth enamel remineralization and strong bones, ensuring a healthy jaw bone to hold teeth in place. Vitamin D, found in eggs and oily fish, is needed for the absorption of calcium, and phosphorous, found in cheese, nuts, pulses, and wholegrains, also aids calcium absorption. Vitamin C, found in citrus fruits, berries, peppers, and sweet potatoes, boosts immunity and promotes collagen synthesis to ensure strong connective tissue in the gums.

HERBS

Antibacterial and antiviral herbs support oral health, while herbs that aid digestion can help prevent bad breath.

TONIC HERBS

Herbs such as dandelion root and psyllium husks act as strengthening tonics for the digestive system, encouraging the transit of waste and promoting healthy liver function. By cleansing and supporting healthy digestive function, the herbs can in turn help to prevent digestive problems that can sometimes contribute to bad breath.

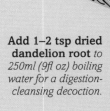

Add 1–2 tsp dried dandelion root *to 250ml (9fl oz) boiling water for a digestion-cleansing decoction.*

Infection-fighting herbs

Echinacea is a key herb for fighting infection and reducing inflammation in the body. When applied topically, echinacea can help to calm gum inflammation, in turn promoting strong gums that are able to do their job of holding and supporting the teeth.

Calendula can be beneficial for soothing the mucous membranes in the mouth and throat, helping to promote tissue health, and both calendula and eucalyptus make excellent mouth rinses that can be used regularly to promote oral hygiene and optimize the health of tissues in the mouth and throat.

Sage is a useful herb for reducing any inflammation in the tissues to promote healthy gums, and also has antibacterial properties that can fight the bacteria that lead to sore throats.

Herbs to support lymphatic health

Certain herbs support the lymphatic system – an essential part of the immune system, which helps the body to fight off invading germs – so improving the body's resilience to debilitating conditions such as glandular fever, which can cause a sore throat among other symptoms. Cleavers, which is known as a common garden weed, also has a strong reputation for promoting lymphatic function and health.

Essential oils

Care needs to be taken when using essential oils around the mouth. However, applied topically in a very dilute form they can be effective. They can also be used in a gargle solution, but should not be swallowed.

Bright and fresh

Peppermint and spearmint are well known for freshening the breath and are included in most mouthwashes and toothpastes.

Lemon essential oil can also be used to promote fresh breath. Lemon has natural brightening properties, too, and can be added to a mouthwash to help teeth look clean and white.

Gum support

Immune-boosting essential oils such as lavender or thyme can help to support immunity throughout the body, in turn supporting oral health. Oils can also be used locally to bolster immunity. For example, oils with antimicrobial properties such as tea tree, can be used in a gargle or soothing gum rub to help prevent and fight gingivitis – gum disease – and keep the gums in good condition.

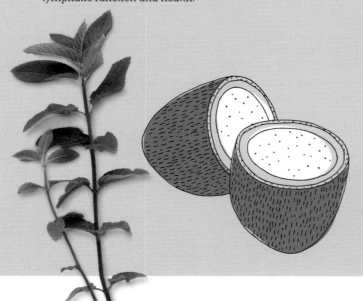

Add 4 drops peppermint essential oil *to 10ml coconut oil. Mix with a little tepid water and wash the solution around the mouth for a few minutes. Spit the mouthwash out then rinse the mouth with water.*

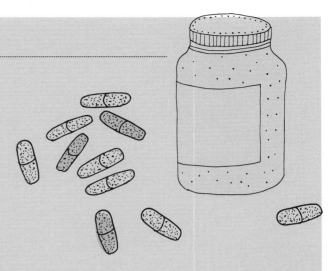

Oils to decongest and protect

A steam inhalation with eucalyptus essential oil makes an effective decongestant remedy for stubborn coughs that persist long after other cold symptoms have subsided. Ginger essential oil is also helpful for loosening mucus in the airways and making coughs more productive.

Lemon, as well as freshening breath, also has antibacterial properties that can help to prevent an infection from taking hold in the first place.

Supplements

While mouth and throat conditions usually heal naturally within a week or so, supplements can help to top up nutrients where levels are low to boost immunity and lower the risk of recurrence.

Getting the basics

Taking a daily high-quality multi-vitamin will ensure that your body is receiving the full range of vital nutrients, which can be especially helpful if you have recurring infections.

Boosting resistance

If levels of the essential mineral zinc are low in the diet, this can lead to reduced immunity. If you have succumbed to an infection, or repeated infections, it can be worth getting your zinc levels checked and taking a supplement if your diet is failing to meet your requirements.

Taking zinc and vitamin C together – preferably in a lozenge form for a steady release of the nutrients – provides powerful immune support to help the body fight infections such as layrngitis and glandular fever.

Beneficial bacteria

Taking a probiotic supplement helps to populate the gut – and the length of the digestive tract from the throat to the intestines – with beneficial bacteria, keeping harmful bacteria such as *Staphylococcus* in check and promoting strong immunity.

Nutrients for gum health

A good-quality B complex supplement taken daily can support tissue health, making it harder for bacteria to take hold in the gums. Also, using mouthwashes fortified with folic acid can help to strengthen gums.

"Supplements can help to boost immunity when nutrient supplies from the diet are low."

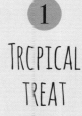

5

RECIPES FOR WELLNESS
SMOOTHIES

Ready in seconds, these hydrating smoothies feature
a medley of fresh produce, delivering an impressive package
of free-radical busting antioxidants and essential nutrients
to boost health throughout the body. Simply peel the fruit and
deseed (if necessary), add any remaining ingredients, and blitz!

1

TROPICAL TREAT

This creamy smoothie has
brain-boosting benefits
from vitamin B6 found in
mangoes and bananas,
while peaches provide
dietary fibre to support
healthy digestion.

SERVES 1–2 ▪ **PREP TIME** 5 MINS

200g (7oz) mango, peeled,
pitted, and chopped into
chunks

1 peach, pitted

1 banana, peeled

5 pitted dates

1 tsp chia seeds

1 tsp hemp powder

1 tbsp lemon juice, pips
removed

200ml (7fl oz) almond milk

Nutritional info per serving:
Kcals 294 Fat 2g Saturated
fat 0.5g Carbohydrates 60g
Sugar 55g Sodium 79mg Fibre
10g Protein 3.5g Cholesterol 0mg

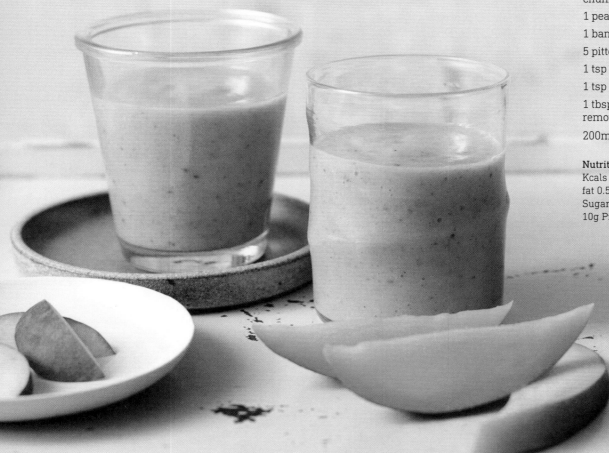

2

SWEET SUMMER BERRIES

Sweet summer berries are bursting with protective antioxidants and essential vitamins, particularly vitamin C, promoting healthy circulation and providing an effective boost to immunity.

SERVES 1–2 • **PREP TIME** 5 MINS

125g (4½oz) blueberries

125g (4½oz) raspberries

60g (2oz) strawberries

1 tsp chia seeds

1 tbsp lemon juice, pips removed

5 ice cubes

200ml (7fl oz) hazelnut milk

Nutritional information per serving:
Kcals 149 Fat 3g Saturated fat 0.5g Carbohydrates 26g Sugar 17g Sodium 56g Fibre 5.5g Protein 2.5g Cholesterol 0mg

3

REFRESHING PINEAPPLE

Pineapple contains beneficial enzymes to support digestion and help eliminate toxins, while vitamin C-rich kiwi fruit boosts immunity throughout the body.

SERVES 1–2 • **PREP TIME** 5 MINS

400g (14oz) pineapple, peeled, core removed, and flesh cut into chunks

1 kiwi fruit, peeled

60g (2oz) strawberries

5 ice cubes

200ml (7fl oz) coconut water

Nutritional info per serving:
Kcals 140 Fat 1g Saturated fat 0.2g Carbohydrates29g Sugar 29g Sodium 116mg Fibre 5g Protein 1.5g Cholesterol 0mg

4

VEGETABLE MEDLEY

This sweet and tangy combo is a nutritional powerhouse. Swiss chard is densely packed with disease-preventing antioxidants, while beetroot has cleansing pigments. You may need to blitz for slightly longer.

SERVES 1–2 • **PREP TIME** 5 MINS

75g (2½oz) Swiss chard, sliced

100g (3½oz) beetroot, peeled and quartered

200g (7oz) pineapple, peeled, core removed, and flesh cut into chunks

5 mint leaves

200ml (7fl oz) coconut water

1 tsp maple syrup

Nutritional info per serving:
Kcals 107 Fat 0.5g Saturated fat 0.2g Carbohydrates 22g Sugar 20g Sodium 224mg Fibre 3g Protein 2.5g Cholesterol 0mg

5

CREAMY FRUIT COMBO

Kefir or natural yogurt promotes a healthy gut flora to boost immunity and supports digestion. Anti-inflammatory pineapple supports joint health while berries provide a host of essential vitamins as well as fibre for healthy digestion.

SERVES 1–2 • **PREP TIME** 5 MINS

150g (5½oz) kefir or natural yogurt

200g (7oz) pineapple, peeled, core removed, and flesh cut into chunks

125g (4½oz) blueberries

75g (2½oz) strawberries

1 tsp chia seeds

5 ice cubes

handful of oats (optional)

Nutritional info per serving:
Kcals 142 Fat 3.5g Saturated fat 1.5g Carbohydrates 21g Sugar 20g Sodium 34mg Fibre 5g Protein 4g Cholesterol 0mg

MOUTH AND THROAT

The mouth and throat have their own unique "ecosystem" of bacteria and viruses, most of which are benign. But when immunity is low and/or nutrition is inadequate, this system can become disrupted, causing a range of uncomfortable conditions. Natural therapies can help to restore harmony and boost immunity.

GINGIVITIS

Gingivitis is an inflammation of the gums that causes swelling and bleeding, and, left untreated, can lead to tooth loss. It is usually caused by a build-up of plaque as a result of inadequate brushing and flossing. Regular brushing and flossing and stopping smoking are important.

HERBS

Antibacterial herbs help to fight infection and anti-inflammatory herbs soothe gums to promote healing. Support these with herbs to boost compromised immunity.

Calendula is anti-inflammatory, antibacterial, and helps rapid healing.
Thyme is antibacterial, soothing, and refreshing.
➡ *Infuse 1–2 tsp of dried calendula or thyme in 175ml (6fl oz) boiling water. Rinse in the mouth 3 times daily; spit out.*
Echinacea is anti-inflammatory and antibacterial when used topically and boosts immunity when taken internally. Avoid using alongside immunosuppressant medication.
➡ *Take 1–5ml tincture in a little water 3 times daily.*

"Certain foods help to neutralize acidity in the mouth and halt plaque-forming bacteria."

ESSENTIAL OILS

Antimicrobial essential oils can be used to help prevent and combat gingivitis.

Tea tree has an antimicrobial action that can help prevent gingivitis.
➡ *Add 2 drops to 5ml coconut oil, rub into the gums twice daily then rinse.*

FOOD

Certain foods help fight plaque-forming bacteria that comes from other foods.

Garlic is antibacterial, helping to lower levels of plaque-forming bacteria in the mouth.
➡ *Use liberally in cooking or add raw to dressings.*
Probiotics in live dairy products neutralize acidic oral conditions and interfere with plaque-forming bacteria.
➡ *Eat natural yogurt, or add probiotic powders to smoothies and juices.*

Green tea has antioxidant polyphenolic compounds called catechins. Two of these, epigallocatechin gallate (EGCG) and epicatechin gallate (ECG), have been shown to combat oral plaque.
➡ *Have 2–3 cups daily.*

SUPPLEMENTS

Certain supplements can support gum tissue health and halt the overgrowth of *Staphylococcus* bacteria.

Probiotic supplements help populate the gut with good bacteria and lower levels of plaque-forming bacteria.
➡ *Look for a supplement with 5–10 billion live organisms per dose.*
B vitamins such as folic acid support tissues, reducing the risk of gingivitis.
➡ *Take up to 400mcg daily, or use a mouthwash containing folic acid.*
CoQ10 is similar to a vitamin and is important for healthy gums.
➡ *Take 20mg daily.*

TOOTHACHE

Pain felt around the teeth or jaw area can be caused by tooth decay, a cracked tooth, loose or broken fillings, teeth grinding, jaw clenching, and sensitivity to hot, cold, or acidic foods. Regular dental check-ups are essential to identify and treat any problems promptly.

HERBS

Herbs that act as anti-inflammatories, muscle relaxants, and analgesics can ease the pain of toothache. Some herbs also act as "antibiotics" to help fight infection.

White willow bark is a powerful anti-inflammatory and analgesic herb that can help to reduce the swelling and discomfort.
➺ *Take 3–5ml tincture in some water 3 times daily, rinsing it around the mouth before swallowing.*

Myrrh is strongly antibacterial and boosts infection-fighting white blood cells. Avoid in pregnancy and with inflammatory kidney disease. Avoid if breastfeeding.
➺ *Take 1–4ml tincture in a little water 3 times daily.*

Peppermint has antibacterial properties and mild analgesic and sedative actions that help to calm and relieve pain gently. Avoid if you have oesophageal reflux.
➺ *Make a strong peppermint infusion in a closed teapot to capture the essential oils, and sip to relieve discomfort.*

ESSENTIAL OILS

Oils with anaesthetic properties can help to numb the pain of toothache.

Clove contains a compound eugenol, which has powerful anaesthetic properties.
➺ *Make a compress by adding 3 drops clove oil to 2ml olive oil. Soak a cotton wool ball in the blend and hold gently on the affected area. Rinse the mouth with water after use.*

LIFESTYLE

Relaxation techniques or counselling can help to deal with any possible causes of stress and anxiety that may have contributed to tooth grinding and jaw clenching.

Use a soft toothbrush and brush more gently for longer to avoid over-zealous brushing wearing down tooth enamel.

Visit the dentist regularly.

REMEDY

Minty breath freshener

Mix 2 drops **peppermint oil** with 1 tbsp **vegetable glycerine** and 1 tsp **salt** and add to a glass of water. Use as a breath-freshening mouth rinse when required.

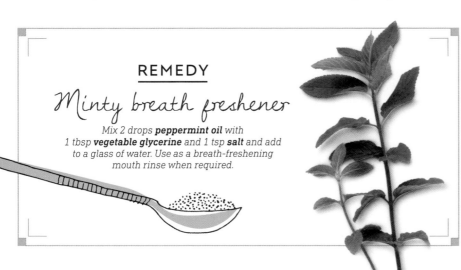

HALITOSIS

Bad breath affects most people at some point. It can be caused by a specific food or from bacteria in the mouth, in particular sulphur-producing bacteria that sits at the back of the tongue.

HERBS

Herbs that boost liver function, stimulate digestion, and encourage regular bowel movements can help prevent halitosis by ensuring a healthy, clean, and well-functioning digestive tract. Gut-cleansing herbs also support healthy gut function.

Dandelion root stimulates the liver and kidney function and gently promotes regular bowel movements. Avoid taking with gallstones.
➺ *Drink dandelion root coffee daily.*

Peppermint is carminative and gently stimulating for the gut. Its aromatic oils help sweeten breath. Avoid with oesophageal reflux.
➺ *Drink a peppermint infusion during the day, especially after meals.*

Psyllium husks cleanse the colon and stimulate peristalsis, promoting bowel movements. Avoid with conditions causing intestinal blockage such as inflammation, hernias, or Crohn's.
➺ *Add 1 heaped tsp psyllium husks to 150ml (5fl oz) cold water, stir, and drink immediately, just before bed.*

ESSENTIAL OILS

Mint oils are the gold standard for freshening breath and are found in most mouthwashes and toothpastes, and in chewing gums.

Peppermint and spearmint are natural breath fresheners.
➺ *See remedy, left.*

➤ CONTINUED...

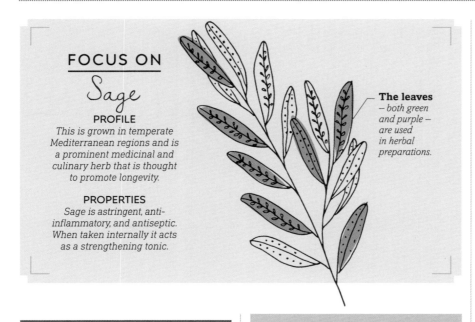

FOCUS ON
Sage

PROFILE

This is grown in temperate Mediterranean regions and is a prominent medicinal and culinary herb that is thought to promote longevity.

PROPERTIES

Sage is astringent, anti-inflammatory, and antiseptic. When taken internally it acts as a strengthening tonic.

The leaves
– both green and purple – are used in herbal preparations.

FOOD

Certain foods can neutralize odours or stimulate saliva production to help combat a dry mouth, which can be a breeding ground for the sulphur-producing bacteria that affects breath.

Parsley is rich in chlorophyll, which helps to neutralize bad breath.
➥*Eat some after meals or add to salads, juices, and smoothies.*

Lemons are natural deodorizers and also stimulate saliva production.
➥*Suck on a lemon slice after a meal or squeeze a fresh lemon into a glass of water, and sip during the day.*

Drinking more water helps to combat a dry mouth linked to bad breath.
➥*Drink 1.5–2 litres (2¾–3½ pints) daily.*

LIFESTYLE

Brush your tongue to reduce levels of bacteria. Use a "tongue" brush or a scraper and rinse well afterwards.

Floss regularly to prevent bacterial build-up and visit the dentist – chronic bad breath may be a symptom of an underlying problem, such as gum disease or tooth decay.

MOUTH ULCERS

Mouth ulcers are small blisters that appear on the inside of the cheek. They are slightly more common in women than in men and can be very painful. If an ulcer persists for more than three weeks, consult your doctor.

HERBS

Topical remedies can ease the discomfort and help to improve the health of the lining of the mouth. Herbs also support general health in order to prevent a recurrence.

Calendula is anti-inflammatory and aids rapid healing of mucous membranes.
➥*Add 1–2ml tincture to a little water, rinse around the mouth, and then spit out. Repeat this 4–5 times daily.*

Sage helps to tone and heal the mucous membranes. See box, above. Avoid therapeutic doses in pregnancy and with epilepsy. Avoid taking for prolonged periods of time.
➥*Add 2–4ml tincture to a little water, rinse around the mouth, and then spit out. Repeat around 3 times daily.*

Nettles are highly nutritious and rich in iron, helping to strengthen and improve general health.
➥*Infuse 1–2 tsp dried nettle in 175ml (6fl oz) boiling water. Drink 3 times daily.*

ESSENTIAL OILS

Anti-inflammatory and antimicrobial essential oils can help to tackle painful mouth ulcers and speed healing.

Tea tree is effective for supporting all-round oral health.
➥*Add 2 drops to 1 tsp table salt and dissolve in warm boiled water. Swish around the mouth before spitting out.*

FOOD

Include foods in your daily diet that have immune-boosting properties.

Garlic has natural antibacterial and antiviral properties that may help to heal and prevent mouth ulcers.
➥*Use liberally in cooking and add raw to dressings.*

Green tea is antibacterial and antiviral.
➥*Drink 1–2 cups daily to promote healing and prevent recurring ulcers.*

Probiotics found in live dairy products help balance the mouth flora and speed recovery.
➥*Eat natural yogurt, or add probiotic powders to smoothies and juices.*

SUPER MATCHA

Matcha powder is derived from green tea leaves, but is more potent nutritionally than green tea. Add boiling water to the powder and whisk thoroughly for an antioxidant boost.

"Herbs can help to boost your general health and prevent a recurrence of mouth ulcers."

WHAT TO AVOID

Acidic, salty, or hard foods aggravate mouth ulcers and increase pain.

SUPPLEMENTS

Mouth ulcers usually heal within 7–10 days on their own, but supplements can boost immunity to help prevent a recurrence of ulcers.

A multi-vitamin and mineral supplement will ensure that you are getting adequate levels of all the essential nutrients.
➡ *Take daily with food.*

B vitamins help support immunity. Some people with recurrent mouth ulcers may be deficient in vitamin B12.
➡ *Take a liquid B12 supplement with 50mcg per dose last thing at night.*

Iron levels may be low when mouth ulcers are recurring.
➡ *Men take up to 11mg and women up to 18mg daily.*

LIFESTYLE

Toothpastes may contain harsh detergents that can disturb the natural flora of the mouth. Try switching to a sodium lauryl sulphate (SLS)-free toothpaste to lower the risk of recurrent mouth ulcers.

SORE THROAT AND TONSILLITIS

A sore throat is usually caused by a viral infection. If it spreads to the glands at the back of the throat – the tonsils – it is called tonsillitis. With rest and support to help deal with any pain and discomfort, both conditions will usually clear up within a week or so.

HERBS

Astringent herbs can be beneficial to help calm inflammation and soothe sore throats. Herbs can also help to clear infection and cleanse the lymph system, and immune-boosting herbs avoid recurrent infections.

Sage is astringent, helping to soothe sore throats, and is anti-infective to fight infection. Avoid therapeutic doses during pregnancy and with epilepsy. Avoid taking sage for prolonged periods of time.
➡ *Infuse 1–2 tsp dried sage in 175ml (6fl oz) boiling water, gargle, then swallow. Repeat 3–4 times daily.*

Elderberry is antiviral and anti-inflammatory.
➡ *Buy, or make your own, elderberry syrup then add ½ tsp syrup to water, gargle, and swallow. Do this 4 times daily at the first sign of a sore throat.*

Boneset helps to boost immunity and acts as a strengthening tonic herb for the mucous membranes. Boneset can also be used to relieve pain, which makes it especially effective for treating the discomfort and pain that accompanies tonsillitis.
➡ *Take 2–4ml tincture in a little water 3 times daily.*

WHAT TO AVOID

Siberian ginseng, astragalus, panax ginseng, and angelica senensis.

ESSENTIAL OILS

These are very beneficial for treating the pain of a sore throat as well as the root cause of an infection.

Juniper is antibacterial and excellent for relieving inflammation.
➡ *Add 2 drops to 1 tsp table salt, add to warm water, and use to gargle.*

Thyme is antioxidant, antimicrobial, and strengthens the immune system.

Ginger helps loosen and remove mucus.
➡ *Add 4–5 drops thyme or ginger to a bowl of hot water, lean over, covering your head with a towel to trap the steam, and inhale until it cools.*

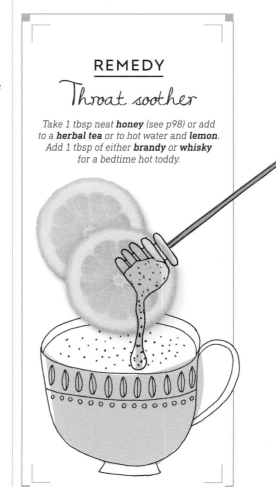

REMEDY

Throat soother

*Take 1 tbsp neat **honey** (see p98) or add to a **herbal tea** or to hot water and **lemon**. Add 1 tbsp of either **brandy** or **whisky** for a bedtime hot toddy.*

➤ CONTINUED...

FOOD

Certain foods can soothe the throat to help speed recovery. Staying hydrated also helps to thin secretions to soothe irritation – hot fluids such as tea or soup can feel good.

Honey is a traditional throat soother. All honeys, but especially Manuka honey, have excellent antibacterial, anti-inflammatory, and antiviral properties to help speed healing.
➡ *See remedy, p97.*

Garlic is antibacterial and antiviral to fight infection.
➡ *Take 1 tsp crushed garlic with honey in hot water every hour for an antiviral punch.*

Blackcurrants are packed with vitamin C to help combat a sore throat or cold.
➡ *Dilute the juice or cordial in a little warm water and sip slowly.*

WHAT TO AVOID
Dry, hard foods are painful to swallow.

SUPPLEMENTS

Supporting your diet with supplements can help to boost immunity.

Vitamin C supports the immune system and helps to fight off infection.
➡ *During an active infection, take 1g 3 times a day with food.*

Zinc works with vitamin C to support immunity. In lozenge form it is soothing and can speed recovery.
➡ *Take a 15–20mg lozenge every 3 hours for up to 3 days.*

LIFESTYLE

Change your toothbrush regularly as bacteria and viruses can build up.

OTHER THERAPIES

Homeopathy can help to strengthen your entire system, thereby helping to strengthen immunity.

LARYNGITIS

The viral infections that cause colds or sore throats can lead to laryngitis – an inflammation, or irritation, of the voice box (larynx) and vocal cords. The throat may feel sore and the voice is hoarse or lost. If voice loss persists beyond 4 weeks consult a doctor.

HERBS

Soothing astringent herbs that are anti-inflammatory and antimicrobial help to treat a sore, swollen, infected larynx.

Sage is astringent, anti-inflammatory, and toning; its volatile oils are antibacterial. Avoid therapeutic doses internally in pregnancy and with epilepsy. Avoid taking for prolonged periods of time.
➡ *Infuse 1–2 tsp dried sage in 175ml (6fl oz) boiling water; gargle as required.*

Thyme is antimicrobial and astringent. Avoid in pregnancy.
➡ *Add 2–4ml tincture to a little water, gargle, and swallow 3 times daily.*

Self-heal (Prunella) helps to protect inflamed tissues with its soothing properties; see box, below.
➡ *Use a few sprigs of the fresh herb to make a throat-soothing infusion. Gargle the infusion first and then swallow. Repeat this 3 times daily.*

ESSENTIAL OILS

Therapeutic essential oils can help to fight infection as well as soothe discomfort. Make sure you don't swallow essential oils when gargling.

Cedarwood is soothing and has antiseptic properties.
➡ *Add 2 drops to a bowl of hot water, lean over, covering your head with a towel to trap the steam, and inhale until the steam cools.*

Peppermint can help relieve the symptoms of an allergy, including a scratchy throat.
➡ *Add 1–2 drops to 1 tsp of honey or vegetable glycerine, then add the mixture to a small tumbler full of warm, boiled water and use as a throat-soothing gargle.*

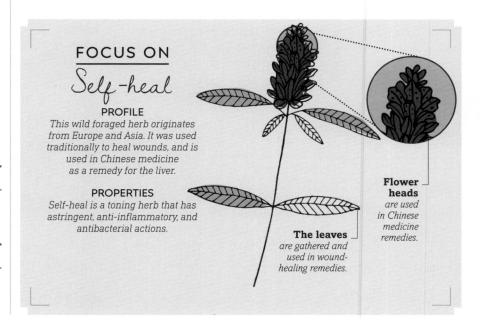

FOCUS ON
Self-heal

PROFILE
This wild foraged herb originates from Europe and Asia. It was used traditionally to heal wounds, and is used in Chinese medicine as a remedy for the liver.

PROPERTIES
Self-heal is a toning herb that has astringent, anti-inflammatory, and antibacterial actions.

Flower heads *are used in Chinese medicine remedies.*

The leaves *are gathered and used in wound-healing remedies.*

FOOD

It can be hard to eat a lot of solid foods with a sore throat, but soothing liquids can help to calm inflammation.

Honey is a traditional remedy for soothing a sore or irritated throat.
➥*Add to a herbal tea or warm boiled water with lemon juice; see remedy, p97.*

SUPPLEMENTS

Most cases of laryngitis resolve themselves with sufficient rest and time, but supplementation, especially liquid supplements or lozenges, can be supportive of the healing process.

Multi-vitamin supplements ensure that you get a broad spectrum of essential nutrients, particularly if you are eating less solid food.
➥*Look for easy-to-swallow liquid supplements or water-soluble tablets.*
Zinc lozenges – sucking on these can improve symptoms.
➥*Take a 15–20mg lozenge every 3 hours for up to 3 days.*

LIFESTYLE

Rest your voice for at least a week. Don't attempt to whisper as this puts more strain on the vocal chords.
Avoid alcohol and cut down or, if possible, quit smoking completely – smoking and alcohol consumption worsen laryngitis.
Practise relaxation techniques such as yoga and meditation daily – anxiety can sometimes lead to laryngitis-like symptoms or to lowered immunity that makes you vulnerable to viruses.

OTHER THERAPIES

Homeopathy is used to strengthen your entire system.

GLANDULAR FEVER

Also called infectious mononucleosis, glandular fever is caused by the Epstein-Barr virus, a relative of the virus that causes herpes and chicken pox. Symptoms include extreme exhaustion, swollen glands, sore throat, fever, fatigue, and weight and appetite loss, and can last for weeks.

HERBS

Antiviral herbs can help to fight the acute infection and immune-boosting herbs offer long-term support.

Wild indigo is antimicrobial and useful for treating fevers and inflamed glands. A strong herb not suitable in pregnancy; do not exceed recommended dose.
➥*Take 1ml tincture in a little water 3 times daily.*
St John's wort has antiviral ingredients hypericin and pseudohypericin. Avoid in pregnancy or high doses in sunlight. Taken internally, interacts with many prescription drugs.
➥*Take 2–4ml tincture in a little water 3 times daily.*
Echinacea boosts resistance. Avoid with immunosuppressant medication.
➥*Take 2–3ml tincture in water, gargle, and swallow. Repeat 4 times daily.*
Cleavers relieves swollen glands and is a lymphatic-cleansing and tonic herb.
➥*Make a cooling decoction with the fresh herb in springtime.*

ESSENTIAL OILS

These can be used to support immunity and relieve pain.

Lavender has analgesic properties for aching muscles.
➥*Add 5 drops to 10ml almond oil for an immune-stimulating massage blend.*

IMMUNE-BOOSTING KICK

Add a garlic clove or chunk of grated fresh ginger to fruit and vegetable juices to give your immune system an extra boost.

Eucalyptus is an effective decongestant, relieving a blocked nose and coughs.
➥*Add 5 drops to hot water, lean over, covering your head with a towel to trap steam, and inhale until the steam cools.*

FOOD

Eat nutrient-dense, easy-to-digest foods, or prepare foods so that nutrients are easy to absorb. Stay hydrated to help control fever.

Juicing boosts nutrients easily. Apple, carrot, and orange or kale, tomato, and celery are immune-supporting combos.
➥*Drink a juice combo daily.*
Slow-cooking helps to release nutrients.
➥*A clear broth makes an extra-nourishing meal when convalescing.*
Camu camu is an Amazonian superfood rich in immune-supporting vitamin C.
➥*Add to juices and smoothies.*

SUPPLEMENTS

Supplementing certain key nutrients is helpful if appetite is low.

Magnesium is key for cellular energy production and helps combat fatigue.
➥*Take 300mg magnesium citrate (the most easily absorbed) twice daily.*
Vitamin C and zinc are both critical for a well-functioning immune system.
➥*Take 1g vitamin C and around 11mg of zinc daily.*

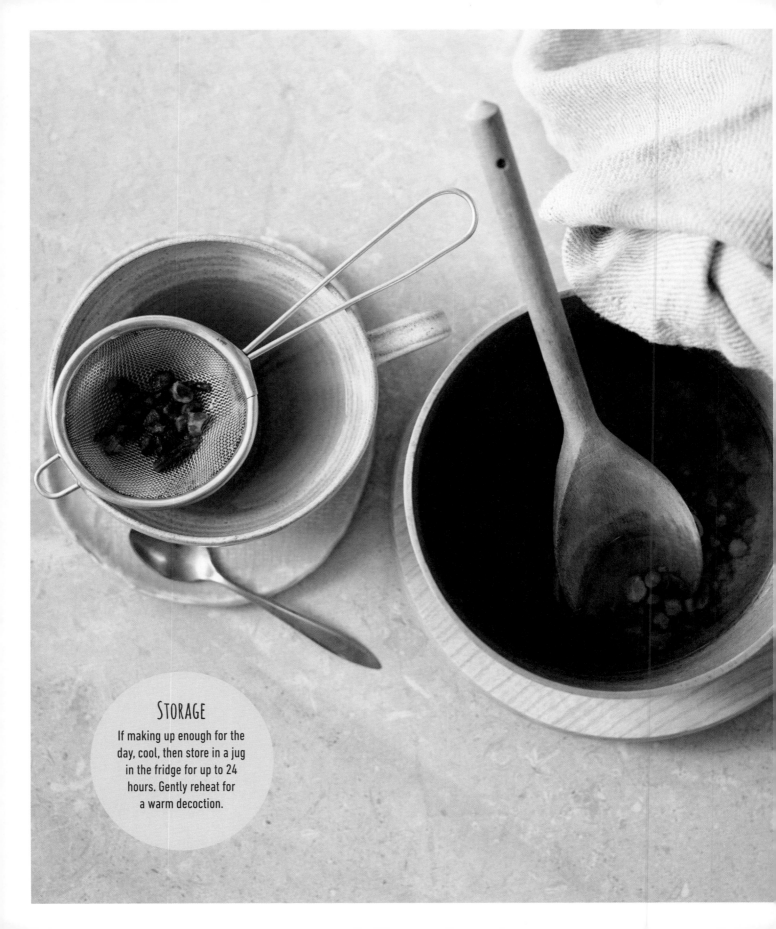

STORAGE

If making up enough for the day, cool, then store in a jug in the fridge for up to 24 hours. Gently reheat for a warm decoction.

HOW TO MAKE
A DECOCTION

Decoctions are herbal water extracts that are made from the tougher parts of a herb, such as the berries, roots, bark, or seeds. Boiling and simmering helps to extract more of the active constituents from these more fibrous, woody ingredients. Decoctions can be made using either fresh or dried herbs, and a regular dose is three cups a day.

Makes 1 large cup, or multiply ingredients for a bigger batch

YOU WILL NEED

1 tsp dried herbs, or 3 tsp fresh herbs; berries, root, bark, or seeds

250ml (9fl oz) water, tap or filtered

saucepan with lid

strainer

teacup

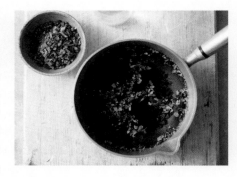

1 Place the dried or fresh berries, root, bark, or seeds in the saucepan with the water. If you wish, treble the ingredients to make enough for a day's dosage. Place a lid on the saucepan, then transfer to the hob and bring to the boil. Keeping a lid on prevents water evaporating and the loss of active herbal constituents in the steam.

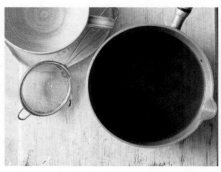

2 Reduce the heat and simmer for 15–30 minutes, depending on the plant material – harder materials such as bark take the longest – until the water is infused with the plant material. If blending herbs, add any leafy herbs when removing from the heat so these can infuse while the extract is cooling.

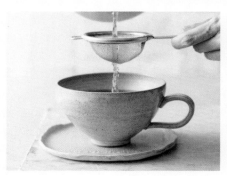

3 Strain the mixture into a teacup and drink warm or leave to cool, as required.

DIGESTIVE SYSTEM

A smoothly functioning digestive system is able to absorb the nutrients the body needs to function well, providing a boost to overall health and wellbeing. Here we explore how gut-balancing foods, tonic herbs, and therapeutic oils help to keep the digestive system in peak health. When problems such as sluggish digestion, stomach upsets, and gut sensitivities do make us feel below par, we look at how a holistic path to healing can soothe and balance the gut to revitalize digestion and restore vitality.

STAYING WELL
DIGESTIVE SYSTEM

A healthy digestive system – which includes the stomach, liver, and gallbladder – metabolizes food, especially fats, efficiently, absorbing essential nutrients and ensuring the smooth transit of waste. Here we explore the key ingredients to optimize digestion, nutritionally by getting the right nutrients, and therapeutically, with herbs and oils, helping to maximize energy and vitality throughout the body.

FOODS

Many foods have key nutrients and substances that help to keep the digestive system working smoothly.

BALANCING THE GUT

The importance of a balance of good and bad gut bacteria as a precursor to overall good health is increasingly recognized. Fermented foods such as live yogurts, sauerkraut, kimchi, and kefir, prompt the production of digestive enzymes and contain natural probiotics, beneficial bacteria that top up gut-friendly "good" bacteria to help optimize and balance digestive health.

"Prebiotics" are a natural partner to probiotic foods. A type of fibre, these feed and encourage the growth of good bacteria already present in the gut. Leeks, onions, garlic, asparagus, and bananas will all ensure you receive a good supply of prebiotics. Try to include a helping of at least one of these in your daily diet.

FOODS TO CALM DIGESTION

Foods with anti-inflammatory properties soothe digestion where there is a tendency to gut irritability. Oily fish, such as mackerel, salmon, and trout, contain essential fatty acids, in particular anti-inflammatory omega-3, which is also thought to aid digestion by supporting a variety of intestinal bacteria. Oily fish are also a good source of high-quality, easily digestible protein.

DIGESTION-SUPPORTING NUTRIENTS

Fresh produce is hugely beneficial for digestive health, providing vital fibre to ensure that the gut is functioning optimally, so it's important to eat plenty of fresh fruit and vegetables.

Various types of seaweed are rich in micro-nutrients such as manganese and soluble fibre, which support digestion and the efficient elimination of waste. Some foods have certain substances that support specific areas of digestion. For example, artichokes contain cynarin and silymarin, substances that increase bile production and help prevent gallstones.

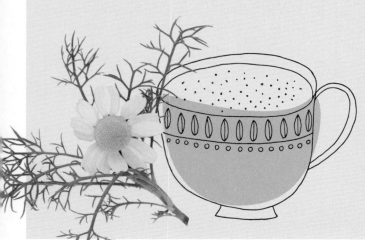

Infuse 1–2 tsp dried chamomile *in 175ml (6fl oz) boiling water, leave to cool a little, and drink as an after-dinner digestive tonic.*

> *"Herbs have a long tradition as aids to digestion, supporting healthy digestive function."*

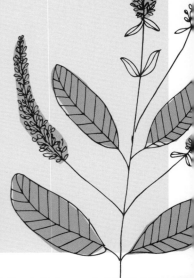

Add a handful of summer berries *to 175ml (6fl oz) natural yogurt and blitz for a gut-supporting smoothie.*

FOODS TO PROTECT THE GUT

The digestive system is vulnerable to germs and bacteria. Berries of all types contain antimicrobial and digestive-soothing substances that protect the digestive system. Fresh and dried berries are beneficial, so their benefits can be enjoyed all year round, added to cereals, smoothies, or simply eaten as a snack.

HERBS

Herbs make natural digestive aids, and herbal remedies have a long tradition of supporting digestion.

RELAXING HERBS

Herbs with anti-inflammatory and soothing antispasmodic properties can relax the smooth muscle in the digestive tract and help to prevent digestive symptoms such as cramps and wind. A cup of chamomile tea is an ideal digestive tonic after meals.

APPETITE STIMULANTS

Herbs can stimulate a waning appetite. Fennel, used as a herb and a vegetable, is a key herb for digestive function. As well as stimulating the appetite, it is also a carminative herb – helping to prevent or relieve intestinal gas and symptoms of nervous indigestion such as wind and cramping, which can be brought on by a rushed meal or emotional upset. Fennel also relieves bloating that can occur around the time of menstruation.

TUMMY-SOOTHING HERBS

Plants such as ginger and peppermint are naturally calming for digestion. Ginger is one of the best-known natural remedies for alleviating feelings of nausea, for example when travelling, and is especially soothing for digestion that is unsettled from stress or over-indulgence. It also has antiseptic properties that boost digestive immunity by helping to fight the bugs and bacteria that can cause nausea and stomach upset. A ginger infusion can be a helpful preventative measure to ward off feelings of nausea.

Infuse ½ tsp each fennel seeds and dried peppermint leaves *in 500ml (16fl oz) boiling water. Add a pinch of salt and honey to taste and sip throughout the day.*

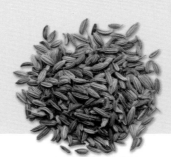

Digestive tonics

Bitter herbs such as chicory, dandelion root, and burdock leaf are well-known digestive tonics, used to support the liver, gallbladder, and pancreas. Dandelion and chicory also make effective coffee substitutes to help you reduce your daily caffeine intake.

Essential oils

Soothing, cleansing, and stimulating compounds in essential oils make these therapeutic essences, used externally, excellent and effective digestive aids. Essential oils should not be ingested.

Stimulating and soothing oils

Oils such as peppermint, mandarin, neroli, fennel, lemon, dill, verbena, and chamomile are popular remedies to provide relief from symptoms such as cramping, bloating, and nausea. As well as calming digestive problems, peppermint also helps to stimulate the digestive process and can be used effectively both in abdominal massage or a steam inhalation to support overall digestion function and prevent digestive upsets occurring.

Cleansing and calming oils

Certain oils are natural cleansers, supporting the health of the liver, and have anti-inflammatory properties that can soothe irritations when these occur in the digestive tract. Rosemary and cardamom can be both cleansing, helping to revitalize the liver, and also work as liver tonics, to strengthen liver function.

Stress-busters

It's common to suffer occasional bouts of constipation, which can be brought on by stress and lifestyle factors. Citrus oils, such as sweet orange, are especially effective for relieving trapped wind and avoiding uncomfortable blockages and can be used preventatively to help stimulate digestion. Citrus oil is also uplifting, helping to relieve the stress that can slow digestion down – its cheery aroma is especially appealing to children.

Oils to promote bowel movements

Sweet marjoram, an aromatic, relaxing, and warming oil, has a long history of therapeutic use for stimulating peristalsis, the wave-like contractions that help to move food along the digestive tract to remove waste efficiently. It also has an antispasmodic action that helps to relieve trapped wind and soothe digestion.

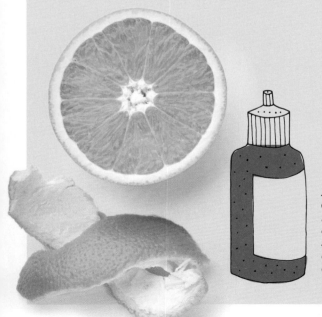

Add 5 drops sweet orange essential oil *to 10ml grapeseed oil and massage into the stomach in a clockwise direction to stimulate digestion.*

"A supplement regime can support the diet to help optimize digestive function."

SUPPLEMENTS

Supplements taken alongside a healthy diet can support digestion, accelerating healing after a period of unsettled digestion and optimizing function.

GUT-BALANCING PROBIOTICS

After a period of illness or a course of antibiotics, both good and bad bacteria are stripped from the gut, leaving the body more vulnerable to infection. Taking a probiotic supplement can be an important restorative measure for the digestive tract during these times, helping to reboot digestive health by replenishing good gut bacteria and restoring a healthy balance to the gut flora. This in turn strengthens the gut and ensures that it is well-equipped to fight future infection-causing germs.

ESSENTIAL MINERALS

Zinc and magnesium are crucial micronutrients for digestive health. These two key minerals promote the production of digestive enzymes, which efficiently extract and absorb nutrients from the food we eat to help fuel the entire body. Zinc can also help to repair any damage to the gut that has been caused by inflammation after a period of digestive irritation or upset, helping to restore the gut to optimal health. Magnesium, as well as boosting digestive enzymes, also plays a role in helping to relax the bowels and draw water into them, which ensures the smooth transit of waste through the digestive tract.

COLLAGEN-BOOSTING VITAMIN C

The protein collagen is vital for healthy digestive tissue. Vitamin C promotes collagen synthesis throughout the body, specifically supporting tissue repair and health in the gut. A regular standard dose of vitamin C can help to heal uncomfortable digestive inflammation and promote a healthy and efficient digestive tract.

STIMULATING ALOE VERA

Certain supplements have a natural laxative action, which can be helpful if you are prone to blockages. A short course of aloe vera, taken either as a juice or in capsule form, can be effective. Aloe vera works by breaking down waste to help move it along the digestive tract, which in turn can avoid bouts of constipation, for example, where there is a tendency towards these around the time of menstruation.

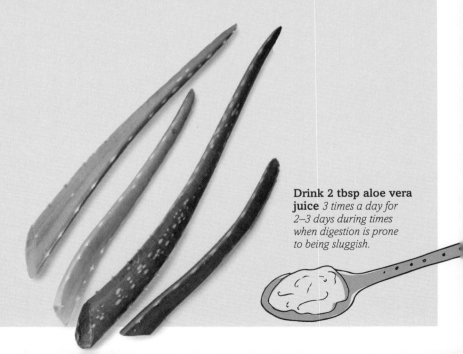

Drink 2 tbsp aloe vera juice *3 times a day for 2–3 days during times when digestion is prone to being sluggish.*

TREATMENTS
DIGESTIVE SYSTEM

An efficient digestive system that absorbs nutrients to fuel the body is essential for vitality, wellbeing, and overall health. Lifestyle, stress, and emotional shock can cause digestive upsets and destroy healthy gut flora. Natural remedies can soothe and stimulate to help restore gut health. Consult your doctor about any prolonged bout of digestive symptoms or change of bowel habits to rule out a serious underlying cause.

CONSTIPATION

This common concern is the inability to have a bowel movement or to empty the bowels fully. Often it is a symptom of another health issue or a lifestyle aspect, such as a lack of exercise or a low-fibre diet.

HERBS

Herbs help to regulate bowel movements gently and effectively. Some stimulate the colon, while others soften stools to help relieve constipation.

Dandelion root is a bitter herb that is a strengthening tonic, gently stimulating digestive health to encourage bowel regularity. Avoid with gallstones.
➡*Make a decoction with 1 tsp dried dandelion root in 250ml (9fl oz) water and drink 3 times daily, or try dandelion coffee.*

Psyllium husks are mucilaginous, providing soluble fibre to soften stools and regulate the colon. Avoid with intestinal obstructions such as inflammation, hernias, and Crohn's.
➡*Make a bedtime drink. Add 1 heaped tsp dried psyllium husks to 150ml (5fl oz) water, stir, and drink immediately.*

Senna pods stimulate the bowel to contract to relieve constipation. Avoid during pregnancy or when breastfeeding and with intestinal obstructions such as inflammation, hernias, and Crohn's. Do not use long term. Can cause abdominal cramps.
➡*Steep 3–6 pods in 175ml (6fl oz) boiled water with a slice of ginger root for 6–12 hours; drink before bedtime.*

ESSENTIAL OILS

Massaging the abdomen with essential oils is an effective way to treat constipation.

Sweet marjoram stimulates peristalsis, the wave-like intestinal movements.
➡*Add 2 drops to 5ml coconut oil and massage into the abdomen in a clockwise motion.*

Cinnamon works as a gastro-intestinal stimulant.
➡*Add 2 drops to 10ml grapeseed oil and massage into the abdomen in a clockwise motion.*

FOOD

A varied diet ensures a good soluble fibre and nutrient intake to ease constipation. Insufficient fluids can exacerbate constipation so stay well hydrated, drinking 1.5–2 litres (2¾–3½ pints) of water daily.

Seeds, particularly mucilaginous seeds – ones that help to lubricate the gut – such as linseeds or chia, will help to move waste along the intestines.
➡*Grind before use to get the full benefit of their lubricating properties.*

Seaweeds of all types are rich in nutrients and soluble fibre. Oats also provide soluble fibre.
➡*Add dried or powdered seaweeds to soups and salads. Eat oats regularly.*

Prunes – sometimes called dried plums – have an abundance of fibre as well as sorbitol, a type of carbohydrate that has a laxative effect. Prunes are a tried-and-tested remedy for mild to moderate constipation.
➡*Drink prune juice as needed, or add soaked dried fruit to salads, cereals, or eat as a snack.*

A CRISP BITE

Crispy nori seaweed sheets are great for snacking on but can quickly lose their bite in humid conditions. Once opened, store packets in airtight containers in a cool, dark place.

SUPPLEMENTS

Certain supplements support digestion and the movement of food through the gut.

Magnesium relaxes the bowel and draws water into it, softening stools.
➼*For occasional constipation take a 250mg magnesium citrate tablet daily. Add one 250mg dose every 3 days until the condition eases. Don't increase the dose too quickly, as this increases the laxative effect.*

Aloe vera is considered a powerful laxative that works by stimulating bowel muscle contractions. Avoid long-term use of aloe vera because the body will develop a tolerance to it and will need ever greater quantities to achieve the same effect.
➼*Take a 50–200mg capsule of aloe latex, or 75–100ml (2½–3½fl oz) juice daily for a maximum of 10 days.*

LIFESTYLE

Avoid an over-reliance on certain drugs. Drugs, such as painkillers (particularly those with codeine, such as co-codamol, or very strong painkillers, such as morphine), some antacids and antidepressants (including amitriptyline), and iron tablets can all cause constipation.

Regular exercise, including yoga, can help to combat constipation. Exercise stimulates intestinal contractions, helping to move waste through the digestive tract more rapidly.

OTHER THERAPIES

Homeopathy treats constipation as part of a larger picture of health concerns. A consultation with a homeopath can help to tailor a remedy most suited to your symptoms and lifestyle.

Hypnosis has been shown to be useful for treating constipation in those suffering from IBS.

DIARRHOEA

This uncomfortable condition can be caused by either bacteria, which can lead to food poisoning, or a virus. It can also be a symptom of chronic anxiety, a food intolerance, or caused by drinking too much alcohol. It usually requires a watch-and-wait approach, however, in children it can quickly lead to dehydration so it's important to keep them well hydrated and seek medical advice if in doubt.

HERBS

The choice of herbal remedy depends on the underlying cause. Antimicrobial herbs can be used to help fight infections if these are the underlying cause, while certain herbs are used to treat gut sensitivities. Herbs are also used to tone the gut lining, soothing irritation and inflammation to help calm diarrhoea, and these are especially helpful for treating children.

Agrimony is a digestive tonic that tones and heals inflamed gut tissue and has a history as a traditional remedy for treating diarrhoea.
➼*Infuse 1–2 tsp dried agrimony in 175ml (6fl oz) boiling water and drink 3 times daily.*

Meadowsweet tones and soothes the gut lining to help calm diarrhoea. See box, right. Avoid during pregnancy and with a sensitivity to salicylates.
➼*Infuse 1–2 tsp dried meadowsweet in 175ml (6fl oz) boiling water and drink 3 times daily.*

Catmint – also referred to as catnip – is relaxing and toning for the digestive system, helping to ease upset stomachs, and is an especially useful remedy to give to children.
➼*For children, infuse ½–1 tsp dried catmint in 175ml (6fl oz) boiling water and drink 3 times daily.*

ESSENTIAL OILS

Gently massaging the abdomen with an essential oil massage blend is an effective way to deliver the therapeutic benefits of essential oils to calm diarrhoea.

Ginger has a spicy, warm, grounding aroma that helps to reduce the feelings of nausea and light-headedness that can accompany diarrhoea.

Black pepper can help to ease stomach cramps associated with diarrhoea.

FOCUS ON

Meadowsweet

PROFILE
Grown widely in Europe and western Asia, this was originally used as honey wine, or mead. It is used commonly as an antacid remedy.

PROPERTIES
As well as being an antacid, this has anti-inflammatory and soothing properties that help to calm digestive upsets.

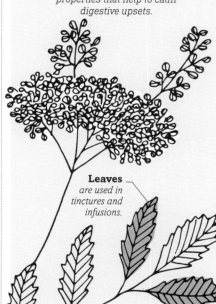

Leaves *are used in tinctures and infusions.*

➤ CONTINUED…

"Healing liquids can provide essential nutrients when appetite wanes during a digestive upset."

Chamomile has a calming effect and can alleviate stomach cramps when massaged gently into the stomach.
➤*Add 2 drops of black pepper, ginger, or chamomile oil to 5ml grapeseed oil and gently massage into the abdomen in a counter-clockwise motion.*

FOOD

Appetite is likely to wane with diarrhoea, so focus on healing liquids and light bites.

Blackcurrant juice has an anti-diarrhoeal action.
➤*Drink hot or cold blackcurrant syrup (widely available in shops) throughout the day. Dilute to taste: usually 1 part syrup to 4 parts water.*
Dried blueberries, or bilberries, can be brewed for an anti-diarrhoeal tea. The sweet taste is appealing to children.
➤*Use 1 tsp dried fruit per 250ml (9fl oz) hot water. Leave to brew for around 10 minutes.*
Carob powder, ground from the seeds, is a traditional remedy for diarrhoea.
➤*Combine 1 tsp carob powder or cinnamon powder with 125ml (4½fl oz) hot water. Allow to cool before drinking. Add a pinch of cinnamon to help fight bacteria. Carob powder can also be added to apple sauce and eaten throughout the day.*

GAS AND BLOATING

Digestion normally produces some gas in the gut, but if excessive gas is produced it can lead to an uncomfortable bloating sensation and increased flatulence. Changes in diet and eating too much or too quickly are common causes of gas and a feeling of being bloated.

HERBS

Carminative herbs – which ease flatulence – have aromatic volatile oils that act on the gut lining. They also soothe colic, tone the digestive canal, and aid assimilation of food.

Fennel seed is carminative with an aniseed-like flavour that will gently relax the gut and disperse colic.
➤*Infuse 1 tsp crushed seeds in 175ml (6fl oz) boiling water, or chew on the fresh seeds after a meal.*

Peppermint has volatile oils that have refreshing aromatic properties and an antispasmodic action to ease bloating and improve digestion. Avoid with oesophageal reflux.
➤*Infuse 1–2 sprigs fresh mint in 175ml (6fl oz) boiling water. Drink after meals.*
Chamomile is mildly bitter, carminative, and a relaxing tonic for the gut, helping to ease spasms and relieve discomfort. Avoid with sensitivity to the *Asteraceae* plant family.
➤*Infuse 1–2 tsp dried chamomile in 175ml (6fl oz) boiling water and drink after meals.*

ESSENTIAL OILS

Aromatic essential oils with carminative properties will help to settle the digestive system. Using the oils in a therapeutic stomach massage is especially beneficial.

Orange helps to settle the digestive system.
Sweet fennel is used to help reduce excessive flatulence.

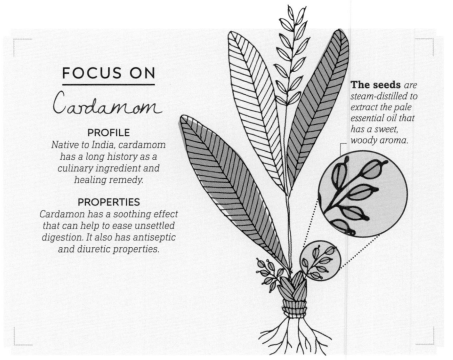

FOCUS ON
Cardamom

PROFILE
Native to India, cardamom has a long history as a culinary ingredient and healing remedy.

PROPERTIES
Cardamon has a soothing effect that can help to ease unsettled digestion. It also has antiseptic and diuretic properties.

The seeds *are steam-distilled to extract the pale essential oil that has a sweet, woody aroma.*

Cardamom is a general digestive tonic. See box, opposite.
➥*Add 5 drops of any of the above essential oils to 10ml grapeseed oil and massage gently into the abdomen in a clockwise direction.*

SUPPLEMENTS

Supporting a healthy diet with certain key supplements can help to target specific aspects of digestion and reduce symptoms of gas and bloating.

Probiotic supplements can help to rebalance the natural bacteria in the gut, helping to boost gut health and, in turn, improve digestion.
➥*Look for a supplement that guarantees 10 billion live organisms per dose and which states that it resists stomach acid.*

Betaine HCl can top up stomach acid. Low stomach acid with ageing can cause bloating, pain, and gas. Avoid with anti-inflammatory drugs such as aspirin and ibuprofen, as this increases the risk of gastrointestinal bleeding.
➥*Take as directed before meals.*

Activated charcoal is often recommended to help reduce excessive flatulence. Avoid during pregnancy or when breastfeeding.
➥*Take as directed. Do not take over a long period of time, which could cause constipation and black stools.*

LIFESTYLE

Wind and bloating can be caused by a sluggish gallbladder. If you are concerned consult your doctor and refer to page 119 for gallstone treatments.

Check for food intolerances. These can cause symptoms of bloating and discomfort. Keep a food diary, detailing what you eat and any corresponding symptoms to identify foods to avoid.

Drink plenty of water to promote efficient digestion.

HICCUPS

A hiccup is an involuntary contraction, known as a "myoclonic jerk", of the diaphragm – the thin layer of muscle that separates your chest cavity from the abdomen. Short bouts of hiccups are common. These usually have no apparent cause and clear up fairly rapidly of their own accord. Hiccups that last beyond 48 hours may need investigating.

HERBS

Antispasmodic herbs help to relax the stomach and diaphragm, while herbs that ease bloating and flatulence can improve digestion and ease any irritation that may be causing bouts of hiccups.

Ginger is carminative, antispasmodic, and anti-inflammatory, working to calm and relax the gut. Avoid with peptic ulcers and gallstones.
➥*Infuse a little thinly sliced ginger root in 175ml (6fl oz) boiling water and drink every 2 hours.*

Fennel seed is carminative and relaxing, easing tension in the digestive and respiratory systems.
➥*Infuse 1 tsp crushed seeds in 175ml (6fl oz) boiling water and drink as required.*

Cramp bark is antispasmodic, relaxing both nerves and muscles, which in turn can help to calm the diaphragm and relieve chronic hiccups. Avoid during pregnancy and when breastfeeding.
➥*Take 3–5ml tincture in a little water 3–4 times daily.*

ESSENTIAL OILS

Choose essential oils that are antispasmodic to help relax the muscles of the diaphragm and bring relief.

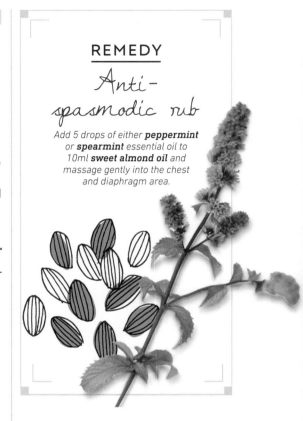

REMEDY

Anti-spasmodic rub

*Add 5 drops of either **peppermint** or **spearmint** essential oil to 10ml **sweet almond oil** and massage gently into the chest and diaphragm area.*

Spearmint and peppermint are both antispasmodic oils, which can help to relieve hiccups. Spearmint has a more gentle action than peppermint.
➥*See remedy with almond oil, above. Or add 2 drops to a tissue to inhale.*

LIFESTYLE

Eat slowly and have regular, smaller meals. Eating a large meal or eating too quickly can sometimes cause bloating, which can bring on hiccups.

Practise stress-reduction techniques daily, such as yoga and meditation. Stress, fear, or emotional excitement can sometimes bring on a bout of hiccups.

Try the "valsalva" manoeuvre. This technique may help to "reset" the diaphragm. Pinch the nostrils closed and keeping the lips closed try to exhale gently into the mouth.

INDIGESTION

Known medically as dyspepsia, this covers a range of symptoms, including gas, heartburn, and acid reflux. It can be caused by a variety of factors including what, and how much, you eat and your lifestyle. Left untreated, acid reflux – when stomach acid travels back up the throat – can damage the sensitive mucosal lining of the oesophagus, leading to a chronic condition, gastroesophageal reflux disease (GORD).

HERBS

Carminative herbs can ease flatulence, bloating, and discomfort, while relaxing, antispasmodic herbs relieve spasm and griping pains. Soothing herbs will protect and calm irritation and inflammation.

Caraway seed is carminative, astringent, and anti-inflammatory.
➡ *Take 1ml tincture in a little water before meals, or add the seeds to sauerkraut and main meals.*
Fennel seed has aromatic volatile oils, which are carminative, antispasmodic, and ease irritation and inflammation.
➡ *Infuse 1 tsp crushed seeds in 175ml (6fl oz) boiling water. Drink after meals.*
Marshmallow root soothes and protects the mucosal lining, reducing inflammation and discomfort. Take separately from other medications as it may impede their absorption.
➡ *Make a decoction: add 1 tsp dried marshmallow root per 250ml (9fl oz) boiling water; stand overnight. Take 130–250ml (4½–9fl oz) 4 times daily.*
Aloe vera juice eases bloating and balances stomach acidity. Its soothing action protects and heals inflamed tissues. Avoid during pregnancy.
➡ *Take 15ml aloe vera juice 2 times daily.*

ESSENTIAL OILS

These can be inhaled, directly from the bottle or via a diffuser, to ease the symptoms of indigestion.

Spearmint is a digestive stimulant.
Mandarin helps with the secretion of bile, which increases the absorption of fats.
Petitgrain is antispasmodic, aiding digestion.
➡ *Add 2 drops of any of the above oils to a tissue or diffuser and inhale.*
Sweet fennel is used as a stomachic – a digestive aid – to relieve a feeling of fullness and bloating.
➡ *See remedy with sunflower oil, below.*
Sweet marjoram stimulates and strengthens peristalsis, the wave-like contractions in the intestines.
➡ *Add 5 drops to 10ml coconut oil and massage into the abdomen in a clockwise direction.*

REMEDY

Stomach soother

Add 5 drops **sweet fennel** essential oil to 10ml **sunflower oil** and massage into the abdomen in a clockwise direction.

FOOD

Certain foods can help to balance acids to support digestion. Foods can also help to balance good and bad bacteria in the gut to promote a healthy gut flora.

Almonds have an alkalizing effect that can ward off heartburn. Almond milk is more acidic and will not have the same effect.
➡ *Snack on a handful of nuts.*
Apple cider vinegar actually has an alkalizing effect to help balance stomach acids.
➡ *Take 15ml in 125ml (4½fl oz) water before meals.*
Fermented foods such as sauerkraut, kefir, and natural yogurt aid digestion.
➡ *Include in your diet daily.*
WHAT TO AVOID
Spicy foods, chocolate, alcohol, citrus juices, carbonated beverages, and caffeine, can all irritate an inflamed oesophagus. If reflux is a problem, also try to avoid eating high-calorie and high-fat foods as well as large, heavy meals that are hard to digest.

SUPPLEMENTS

Certain supplements can bring relief by rebalancing stomach acid and supporting healthy digestion.

Magnesium can stimulate peristalsis and elimination.
➡ *Take 420mg for men, 320mg for women, daily.*
Vitamin C and selenium may help lower the risk of GORD.
➡ *Look for antioxidant supplements that contain 100 per cent of your daily value for these nutrients with a mixture of other antioxidants such as grape seed extract and mixed carotenoids.*
Digestive bitters help stimulate the digestive juices and acid production.
➡ *Take a tincture in a little water before meals.*

> *"Herbs that are antispasmodic help to relieve the spasms and griping pains of indigestion."*

Betaine HCl can help boost stomach acid if low acid is a problem. Avoid with anti-inflammatory drugs such as aspirin and ibuprofen, as this increases the risk of gastrointestinal bleeding.
➡ *Take as directed before meals.*

LIFESTYLE

Eat lightly cooked, rather than raw, foods and chew thoroughly. Avoid lying down within three hours of eating, and elevate your head at bedtime to prevent symptoms during sleep.
Gentle regular exercise reduces symptoms. Avoid vigorous forms of activity, such as cycling or running, which can make symptoms worse.
Abdominal breathing exercises, practised daily, tone the muscle to help prevent reflux.
Stress-reduction techniques such as meditation and yoga can help stress-related indigestion.
Try chewing gum for an hour after a meal to stimulate saliva and aid the digestive process.

OTHER THERAPIES

Acupuncture can stimulate the movement of food through the digestive tract, which can be inefficient in cases of chronic acid reflux.

NAUSEA

Nausea occurs with motion sickness and is also a common symptom of early pregnancy. Combined with vomiting, it can indicate gastroenteritis infection (see p116). Consult your doctor if symptoms are prolonged.

HERBS

Herbs can calm nausea. Aromatic, relaxing herbs with volatile oils ease vomiting, and antimicrobial herbs help combat infection.

Lemon balm is aromatic with volatile oils that help relax and soothe the gut and have an antimicrobial action. Avoid with hypothyroidism.
➡ *Infuse 1 tsp dried lemon balm or a fresh shoot in 175ml (6fl oz) boiling water and sip as required.*
Agrimony is astringent and anti-inflammatory to tone and calm the stomach, and also relaxes the gut. Avoid with constipation.
➡ *Infuse 1 tsp dried agrimony in 175ml (6fl oz) boiling water and sip slowly as required.*
Ginger, a well-known remedy for nausea linked to pregnancy and motion sickness, calms the stomach. Avoid with peptic ulcers and gallstones.
➡ *Infuse some sliced ginger root in 175ml (6fl oz) boiling water and sip slowly, as required. Or take powdered dried root in 0.25–1g capsules, before and during travelling.*
Meadowsweet is an antacid, soothing the stomach lining. Avoid in pregnancy and with sensitivity to salicylates.
➡ *Take 2–4ml tincture in a little water as needed.*

ESSENTIAL OILS

Oils can soothe the digestive system to ease nausea and vomiting.

Peppermint is helpful for travel sickness.
➡ *Add 2 drops to a tissue or diffuser and inhale.*
Ginger stimulates the digestive system.
➡ *Add 3 drops to a bowl of warm water. Soak a flannel to make a warm compress to apply to the stomach.*
Orange helps to calm digestion.
➡ *Add 2 drops to a tissue and inhale, or add 2 drops to 10ml sunflower oil and apply to pulse points.*
Roman chamomile is a mild oil, helpful for treating children.
➡ *Add 2 drops to a tissue and inhale, or add 2 drops to 10ml sunflower oil and apply to pulse points.*

LIFESTYLE

Rest – over-activity can worsen nausea.
Avoid triggers. Cooking smells, perfume, smoke, stuffy rooms, heat, humidity, flickering lights, and driving are all possible triggers for nausea.
Eat bland, easily digested foods such as crackers or toast. Build up to cereal, broths, rice, and cooked fruit. Avoid solids for six hours after vomiting.

OTHER THERAPIES

Acupuncture may help with nausea.
Homeopathy can be effective for nausea.
Flower remedies, such as Rescue Remedy, can calm the distress that can increase feelings of nausea.

GINGER KICK
Grating or finely chopping ginger root increases its potency. Store fresh ginger in the fridge, unpeeled, for up to three weeks.

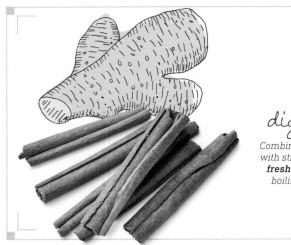

REMEDY

Soothing digestive tonic

Combine digestion-enhancing ginger with strengthening cinnamon: infuse **fresh ginger root** *in 175ml (6fl oz) boiling water and add a pinch of* **cinnamon**.

FOOD POISONING

This can be caused by eating food that has been contaminated with bacteria – commonly the *Salmonella* or *E.coli* bacteria – or by a virus or parasite. Food poisoning can be very uncomfortable, causing nausea, vomiting, and diarrhoea, but usually it is not serious. Most people recover within a few days with rest and supportive treatments.

HERBS

A variety of herbs have antimicrobial actions and are effective in treating food-borne pathogens. Combine antimicrobial herbs with ones that ease gastric discomfort and promote and restore healthy digestion.

Golden seal is effective in fighting the effects of many food-borne pathogens. It repairs and restores the gut lining and is a strengthening liver tonic. Do not take internally for prolonged periods of time. Avoid in pregnancy, if breastfeeding, and with hypertension.
➡ *Take 1ml tincture in a little water 4 times daily.*

Ginger is effective against *E. coli*, *Shigella* and *Salmonella*. It is also a carminative and anti-inflammatory herb, helping to soothe the digestive tract. Avoid with peptic ulceration and gallstones.
➡ *Infuse some thinly sliced ginger root in 175ml (6fl oz) boiling water and drink every 2 hours.*

Cinnamon strengthens digestion weakened from food poisoning and is antimicrobial and antiparasitic, helping to fight infections and speed recovery. Avoid therapeutic doses during pregnancy.
➡ *See remedy, above. Or take ¼ tsp powder in a little water 3 times daily.*

ESSENTIAL OILS

Oils can be effective in helping to alleviate nausea and calm the pain and cramping associated with food poisoning.

Ginger has a spicy, warm, grounding aroma that helps to reduce the feelings of nausea and light-headedness that can accompany diarrhoea caused by food poisoning.

Chamomile has a calming effect on digestion. When massaged gently into the stomach it can help to alleviate stomach cramps.

Lavender is relaxing and soothing and can promote restful sleep, helping to speed recovery. It also has antiseptic properties.
➡ *Mix 2 drops of any of the above essential oils with 5ml grapeseed oil and gently massage into the abdomen in a clockwise motion.*

FOOD

Eating will be the last thing on your mind if you are suffering with food poisoning, but when you are able to tolerate eating, certain foods can help speed recovery. Water is essential to replace fluids lost through vomiting and diarrhoea. Aim to drink 2–3 litres (3½–5¼ pints) daily. If urine is pale, this indicates sufficient fluids.

Apples are easy to digest, hydrating, and nutrient-dense, so a good food choice for recovery.
➡ *Try stewed apple or grate some apple and leave it to sit for 1 hour to turn brown before eating it – this eases diarrhoea and is easy to digest.*

Natural yogurt contains good bacteria that helps restore balance to the gut.
➡ *Eat some daily.*

" Antimicrobial herbs, together with herbs that reduce gastric discomfort, can help to restore and promote healthy digestion."

GASTRITIS

Gastritis is inflammation or irritation of the stomach lining, often caused by the bacteria *H. pylori* or excessive alcohol intake and smoking. Left untreated, a stomach, or gastric, ulcer can develop. Symptoms include indigestion, nausea, vomiting, and upper abdominal pain. If pain persists and/or there is difficulty swallowing or weight loss, see a doctor at once.

HERBS

Astringent and anti-inflammatory herbs soothe the stomach lining; mucilaginous herbs protect the mucous membranes to promote healing; and relaxing and tonic herbs support the underlying stress and anxiety that can accompany gastritis.

Meadowsweet is astringent and anti-inflammatory, helping to soothe and calm irritation and protect the stomach lining. Avoid in pregnancy and with sensitivity to salicylates.
➥ *Infuse 1–2 tsp dried meadowsweet in 175ml (6fl oz) boiling water and drink 3 times daily.*

Marshmallow root, a healing mucilaginous herb, is antibacterial and helps to reduce inflammation. Take separately from other medications as it may impede their absorption.
➥ *Make a decoction: add 1 tsp dried marshmallow root per 250ml (9fl oz) boiling water; stand overnight. Take 130–250ml (4½–9fl oz) 3 times daily.*

Liquorice is anti-inflammatory and antibacterial, helping to combat the effects of *H. pylori* to heal the mucous membranes. It also supports the adrenal glands. Avoid in pregnancy and with hypertension. Do not take large doses for prolonged periods.
➥ *Add a pinch of ground liquorice to a meadowsweet or marshmallow infusion.*

WHAT TO AVOID
Saponin-containing herbs, such as gotu kola, horse chestnut, and sarsaparilla.

ESSENTIAL OILS

Soothing essential oils can help to relieve symptoms of gastritis and related symptoms such as anxiety.

Peppermint has analgesic and anti-inflammatory properties.
Frankincense helps to reduce emotional stress and anxiety.
➥ *Add 4 drops of either of the above to a bowl of hot water, lean over, covering your head with a towel to trap the steam, and inhale until it cools. Or add 2–3 drops of either oil to a diffuser and inhale.*

FOOD

Gastritis and stomach ulcers cause inflammation, which in turn generates damaging free radicals that attack the stomach walls. Foods rich in antioxidants can help reduce the damage. Drinking water can ease the symptoms of gastritis, indigestion, and ulcers. Aim to drink 1.5–2 litres (2¾–3½ pints) daily.

Cranberries contain antioxidant anthocyanins, which have shown an antibacterial action against *H. pylori*. See box, below.
➥ *Drink cranberry juice daily to take the best advantage of its healing powers.*
Broccoli contains sulphoraphane, a nutrient shown to kill *H. pylori* bacteria. Broccoli sprouts are the richest source of this nutrient, containing 20 to 50 times more sulphoraphane than the mature plant.
➥ *Drink a shot of broccoli sprout juice every day to repair and protect your stomach lining.*
WHAT TO AVOID
Coffee, chocolate, hot chilli peppers, and, for some, dairy products, all of which can exacerbate the symptoms. Also avoid alcohol and smoking, two of the most common causes.

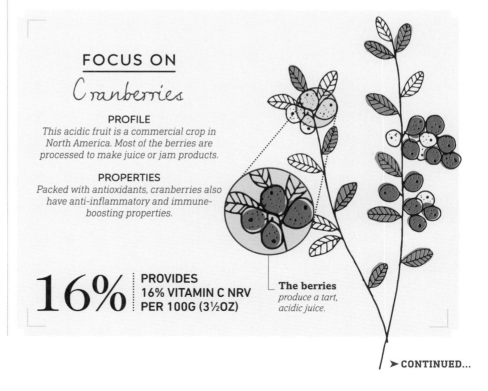

FOCUS ON
Cranberries

PROFILE
This acidic fruit is a commercial crop in North America. Most of the berries are processed to make juice or jam products.

PROPERTIES
Packed with antioxidants, cranberries also have anti-inflammatory and immune-boosting properties.

16% PROVIDES 16% VITAMIN C NRV PER 100G (3½OZ)

The berries *produce a tart, acidic juice.*

➤ CONTINUED...

SUPPLEMENTS

Supporting your diet with supplements that have a proven track record for protecting and healing the gut wall can be beneficial.

Zinc can help to mitigate some of the damage to the intestinal wall caused by inflammation.
➡*For chronic symptoms take up to 40mg daily.*

Carnosine is a molecule produced naturally in the body from the amino acids beta-alanine and histidine. It is a potent antioxidant and works best against gastritis when taken as a zinc–carnosine combination – commonly called zinc L-carnosine.
➡*Take 100–150mg daily.*

Iron deficiency can encourage *H. pylori*, allowing it to take hold.
➡*A daily multi-vitamin with added iron may be sufficient. Ensure you are getting 18mg iron daily.*

Garlic is highly effective against *H. pylori*. Not everyone with gastritis can tolerate the fresh bulb, so supplements can be a good way to obtain its benefits.
➡*Start with low doses and, as you heal, gradually build up tolerance: take 200–400mg 3 times daily.*

LIFESTYLE

Avoid large meals – eat smaller, more frequent meals during the day to take the pressure off your stomach.

Avoid late-night eating and lying down for about two hours after you eat. Gravity can help to keep stomach acid in the stomach and assists the flow of food and digestive juices from the stomach to the intestines.

Avoid non-steroidal anti-inflammatory drugs (NSAIDs), such as ibuprofen, naproxen, and aspirin. These are a significant cause of gastritis and ulcers that can damage the stomach and intestinal lining.

GASTROENTERITIS

Usually viral-related – caused by rotavirus in children and norovirus or food poisoning in adults – this flares up within a day of infection, causing vomiting and diarrhoea.

HERBS

Antimicrobial herbs help fight infection and anti-inflammatory and astringent herbs soothe irritation and calm the gut.

Chamomile is anti-inflammatory, easing discomfort, and antibacterial. Avoid with *Asteraceae* sensitivity.
➡*Take 1–5ml tincture in a little water 3 times daily.*

Agrimony is astringent and relaxes the gut. Avoid with constipation.
➡*Infuse 1–2 tsp dried agrimony in 175ml (6fl oz) boiling water 3 times daily.*

Golden seal is a potent antimicrobial and anti-inflammatory, healing the mucosa. Do not take internally for prolonged periods. Avoid in pregnancy, if breastfeeding, and with hypertension.
➡*Take 1ml tincture in a little water 3 times daily, or combine with chamomile tincture.*

WHAT TO AVOID
Horseradish and saponin-containing herbs such as gotu kola, horse chestnut, and sarsaparilla.

ESSENTIAL OILS

Anti-inflammatory oils can be effective for soothing digestion.

Lemongrass stimulates digestion.
➡*Add 5 drops to 10ml almond oil and massage into the stomach. Or try the remedy, right, with eucalyptus oil.*

Oregano is highly antimicrobial.
➡*Add 3 drops to 5ml coconut oil and massage into the abdomen.*

Ravintsara is a powerful antimicrobial.
➡*Add 2–3 drops to a diffuser.*

SUPPLEMENTS

Supporting the diet can promote recovery.

Multi-vitamins keep nutrient levels high.
➡*Take a daily supplement.*

Probiotic supplements boost the gut.
➡*Look for a supplement with 10 billion live organisms per dose.*

LIFESTYLE

Take an oral rehydration solution. Buy or make your own with 1 litre (1¾ pints) water, 8 tsp sugar, and 1 tsp salt.

Rest at home for at least 48 hours.

REMEDY

Anti-viral room spray

*Combine 15 drops **lemongrass** essential oil with 10 drops **eucalyptus** essential oil in 2 tbsp each of **water** and **vodka**. Pour into a small, sterilized bottle and use as a room spray to clear the air.*

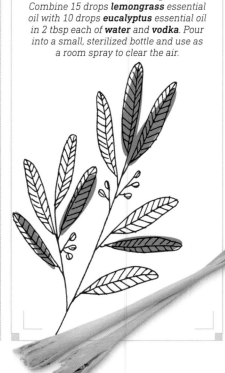

INFLAMMATORY BOWEL DISEASE (IBD)

This umbrella term describes two conditions: ulcerative colitis, which affects the colon – or the large intestine – only, and Crohn's disease, which can affect any part of the digestive system, including the mouth and the anus. Both conditions can cause symptoms of diarrhoea, abdominal pain, tiredness, and bloody stools.

HERBS

Anti-inflammatory and antispasmodic herbs ease discomfort, and mucilaginous herbs protect the mucous membranes, helping to heal gastrointestinal lesions. Herbs can also help to balance the immune response, and those that act as relaxants treat the underlying anxiety and stress that can accompany IBD.

Wild yam is antispasmodic and anti-inflammatory to promote healing.
➡ *Take 2–4ml tincture in a little water 3 times daily.*

Marshmallow root is mucilaginous, which means that it helps to soothe, protect, and heal the mucosal membranes. Take separately from other medications as it may impede their absorption.
➡ *Make a decoction: add 1 tsp dried marshmallow root per 250ml (9fl oz) boiling water; stand overnight. Take 130–250ml (4½–9fl oz) 3 times daily.*

Agrimony is an astringent herb that acts as a tonic to the gut lining, promoting rapid healing and reducing discomfort. It calms nervous tension. Avoid with constipation.
➡ *Infuse 1–2 tsp dried agrimony in 175ml (6fl oz) boiling water and drink 3 times daily.*

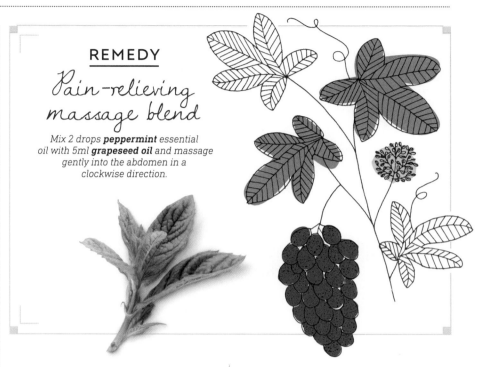

REMEDY

Pain-relieving massage blend

Mix 2 drops **peppermint** essential oil with 5ml **grapeseed oil** and massage gently into the abdomen in a clockwise direction.

Ashwagandha may help to calm and balance the auto-immune response and it eases anxiety and tension. Avoid in pregnancy or with hyperthyroidism.
➡ *Take 1–2ml tincture in a little water 3 times daily, or add 1 tsp of the powder to smoothies and cereals.*

ESSENTIAL OILS

Antispasmodic and analgesic oils relieve the pain and discomfort associated with IBD, and de-stressing oils can ease the emotional tension that can accompany IBD.

Peppermint helps to aid digestion.
➡ *See remedy with grapeseed oil, above.*

Sweet orange helps to settle the digestive system.
➡ *Mix 5 drops with 10ml sunflower oil and massage gently into the abdomen in a clockwise direction.*

FOOD

IBD can make it hard for your body to absorb the nutrients it needs from foods so a varied healthy diet is particularly important. While diet is a crucial factor in managing IBD, there is no one-size-fits-all approach, but certain nutrients are beneficial. It's also important to drink plenty of fluids to avoid dehydration. Aim to drink 1.5–2 litres (2¾–3½ pints) of water a day to aid digestion and avoid complications such as kidney dysfunction, joint pain, and gallstones.

Fibre-rich foods can increase the severity of IBD flare-ups so, while it's important to include fibre in the diet regularly, choose amounts and sources carefully according to what works for your digestion.
➡ *Include steamed or lightly cooked vegetables, canned or cooked fruits, and starches (such as porridges from oat, barley, or buckwheat) as well as wholewheat noodles and tortillas.*

Oily fish, such as salmon, mackerel, herring, and sardines, have an anti-inflammatory effect that can help to soothe and calm the digestive tract, and are also a good source of high-quality protein.
➡ *Include 2–3 portions weekly.*

➤ CONTINUED...

Liquid meals, such as smoothies or vegetable broths, provide the essential nutrients your body needs in an easy-to-digest form.

➨*Combine the foods that work for you into one liquid meal each day.*

WHAT TO AVOID

Excessive sugar and fat increase the risk of ulcerative colitis. Dairy products can sometimes trigger IBD so it may be worth investigating their effects on you.

SUPPLEMENTS

It is well worth consulting a qualified nutritionist who can help you identify and correct nutritional deficiencies to improve specific symptoms and your overall health.

Probiotic supplements can be as effective as conventional drugs in treating IBD. Mixed supplements containing a variety of *Lactobacilli* and *Bifidobacteria* will help to restore a healthy balance of bacteria in the gut.

➨*Look for a supplement with 10 billion live organisms per dose.*

Omega-3 marine oil can reduce inflammation in the digestive tract, lowering the need for anti-inflammatory drugs.

➨*Take 1–2g combined EPA and DHA 3 times daily.*

LIFESTYLE

Yoga and other gentle stretching exercises can improve energy levels and help to reduce constipation, gas, and abdominal bloating.

OTHER THERAPIES

Hypnotherapy can help to address emotional and psychological factors linked to IBD. Relief from stress may in turn relieve symptoms.

Acupuncture is successful in relieving symptoms in some sufferers.

DIVERTICULOSIS

This condition affects the colon, causing small bulges or pockets, known as diverticula, to develop in the intestinal wall. It is more common with age, thought to be due to a low-fibre diet, and often there are no symptoms. However, if the pockets become inflamed or infected, or if they rupture, they can cause pain and bleeding, known as diverticulitis, which needs urgent medical attention.

HERBS

Anti-inflammatory herbs help to reduce inflammation in the diverticula and ease spasms, while antimicrobial herbs help to fight infection. Herbs can also be used to improve and regulate overall bowel health.

Wild yam is anti-inflammatory and antispasmodic to help heal the bowel tissues and reduce pain.

➨*Take 2–4ml tincture in a little water 3 times daily.*

Chamomile is anti-inflammatory and antimicrobial. It also helps relieve spasms, and promotes healing of the gut lining. Avoid with *Asteraceae* sensitivity.

➨*Infuse 1–2 tsp dried chamomile in 175ml (6fl oz) boiling water and sip slowly throughout the day.*

Fenugreek seeds are anti-inflammatory and help to lubricate and soothe the colon. Avoid in pregnancy and with low thyroid activity. May impede the absorption of other drugs so take separately.

➨*Infuse 1 tsp crushed seeds in 175ml (6fl oz) boiling water and sip slowly throughout the day.*

FOOD

A low-fibre, high-fat diet significantly raises the risk of diverticulitis. A lack of essential nutrients can also weaken the colon wall, making it more likely for the small pouches to erupt.

Oily fish, such as salmon, mackerel, and sardines, are anti-inflammatory.

➨*Have 3–4 portions a week, grilled or lightly steamed.*

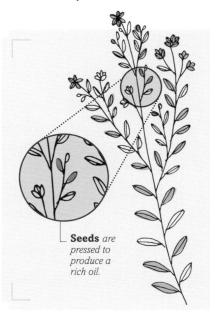

Seeds *are pressed to produce a rich oil.*

FOCUS ON

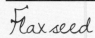
Flaxseed

PROFILE

The flaxseed plant is grown in cooler climes. It is grown primarily for its oil, which can dilute concentrated essential oils, and its seeds add valuable nutrients to the diet.

PROPERTIES

Flaxseed is anti-inflammatory and antioxidant. The seeds are fibre-rich and provide micronutrients such as manganese.

Flaxseed contains fibre and works as a bulk-forming laxative, softening stools and speeding transit time through the intestine. See box, opposite.
➤*Take 1 tbsp ground seeds a day. Try sprinkling over cereals, salads, soups, and vegetables.*

Leafy greens, such as spinach and lettuce, have fibre and important trace elements. A high consumption lowers the risk of diverticulitis.
➤*Include some in your diet each day.*

WHAT TO AVOID
Fresh garlic and horseradish.

SUPPLEMENTS

These can bolster the body against infection as well as strengthen the gut and help to balance intestinal flora.

Vitamin C supports tissue health and can help strengthen the wall of the colon, as well as fight infection.
➤*Take 1–3g daily in an "esterified" form, which is non-acidic and easily absorbed.*

Glutamine is an amino acid that helps the intestine to function properly.
➤*Take 400mg 4 times a day, between meals.*

Omega-3 fatty acids, such as those in fish oil, help fight inflammation.
➤*Take 1g twice daily.*

Probiotic supplements help maintain the health of the intestines.
➤*Look for a supplement that has up to 10 billion live organisms per dose.*

LIFESTYLE

Get regular exercise. Diverticulitis is more common with a sedentary lifestyle. Aerobic exercise has the greatest protective effect.

Avoid non-steroidal anti-inflammatory drugs (NSAIDs) and paracetamol, which raise the risk of diverticulitis. If you use these regularly for relief, consider a less damaging longer-term approach.

GALLSTONES

Gallstones form when cholesterol and bile pigments clump together to form stones in the gallbladder. It is easier to prevent gallstones than to treat them once formed. Preventative steps include avoiding aggravating foods and using supplements and herbs that increase the solubility of bile in the gallbladder.

HERBS

Herbs that increase the flow of bile can be beneficial. Combine these with ones that help to relax spasms, ease inflammation, and support digestive health.

Wild yam is relaxing and anti-inflammatory, relieving biliary colic – the term for the pain that occurs when a gallstone blocks the bile duct.
➤*Take 2–4ml tincture in a little water 3 times daily.*

Milk thistle is a liver and gallbladder tonic and boosts the flow of bile.
➤*Take 1 tsp to 1 tbsp ground seed 3 times daily. Or see recipe with oats, right.*

Barberry bark, a traditional remedy for gallbladder inflammation and gallstones, is a bitter herb that boosts bile secretion. Avoid in pregnancy.
➤*Take 1–5ml tincture in a little water 15 minutes before meals.*

WHAT TO AVOID
Ginger, turmeric, and peppermint.

ESSENTIAL OILS

Use essential oils that have a detoxifying action and anti-inflammatory properties.

Rosemary has cleansing properties and helps to reduce inflammation. Avoid with epilepsy.
➤*Add 3 drops to 5ml coconut oil and massage around the liver area.*

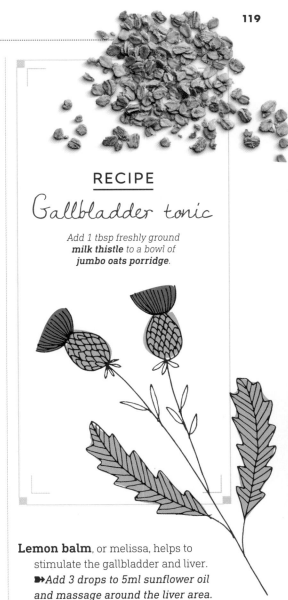

RECIPE
Gallbladder tonic

Add 1 tbsp freshly ground milk thistle to a bowl of jumbo oats porridge.

Lemon balm, or melissa, helps to stimulate the gallbladder and liver.
➤*Add 3 drops to 5ml sunflower oil and massage around the liver area.*

FOOD

Reduce your risk of gallstones by eating a diverse diet that is rich in vegetables, fruits, and dietary fibre. Drink 1.5–2 litres (2¾–3½ pints) water a day to keep the water content of the bile topped up.

Oats have a special mucilaginous fibre that helps to reduce the accumulation of damaging cholesterol.
➤*Replace wheat cereals with oats or oatmeal for a satisfying, energy-sustaining start to the day.*

➤ CONTINUED...

SKIN-ON BENEFITS

Eating almonds with their skin on delivers the most nutritional benefits. Flavonoids in the skin work with vitamin E in the nuts to reduce bad cholesterol.

Nuts and seeds, especially sunflower seeds, almonds, and hazelnuts, are rich in vitamin E, which helps prevent cholesterol build-up.
➧*Snack on a handful or sprinkle over cereals, porridge, and salads.*
WHAT TO AVOID
Saturated fats, cholesterol, animal proteins, sugar, and fried foods can lead to gallstones. Avoid, or limit, coffee, which can worsen symptoms.

SUPPLEMENTS

Deficiencies in certain vitamins have been linked to gallstones. Supplementing the diet ensures you get enough of these nutrients.

Vitamin C is essential for bile formation.
➧*Take at least 200mg and up to 1g daily.*
Calcium can help bind bile acids and decrease the risk of stone formation.
➧*Take at least 800mg daily.*
Vitamin E is necessary to prevent cholesterol build-up.
➧*Aim for 400iu daily.*

LIFESTYLE

Lose weight. Being overweight is a risk factor for gallstones. However, lose weight gradually as crash dieting also raises the risk.
Exercise regularly. Gallstones are more likely if you have a sedentary lifestyle.

APPETITE LOSS

Loss of appetite is common during convalescence, with some heart and liver conditions, and with cancer. It is also a symptom of emotional shock and grief. It is important to address appetite loss to avoid it impacting further on your health.

HERBS

Warming, aromatic, and stimulating herbs act as tonics for the digestive system, re-awakening appetite and revitalizing digestive organs and tissues.

Angelica root is a warming tonic that boosts appetite and digestion. Avoid therapeutic doses in pregnancy and high doses in strong sunlight and with anticoagulants.
➧*Take 2–5ml tincture in a little water 3 times daily.*
Cinnamon contains aromatic oils to help stimulate appetite. Avoid therapeutic doses in pregnancy.
➧*Sprinkle on toast, cereals, and desserts, try chai tea, or add a pinch to a mugwort infusion, below.*
Mugwort is mildly bitter, gently stimulating taste buds and digestion. Avoid therapeutic doses in pregnancy.
➧*Infuse 1–2 tsp dried mugwort in 175ml (6fl oz) boiling water and drink 3 times daily before meals.*

ESSENTIAL OILS

The aroma of certain oils stimulates the secretion of saliva and the digestive juices to prepare the body for eating.

Palmarosa acts as a tonic for the digestive system.
Ginger is an appetite stimulant.
Roman chamomile is a traditional remedy for appetite loss.

Cinnamon bark helps stimulate the secretion of gastric juices.
➧*Add 2 drops of any of the above oils to a tissue or diffuser and inhale.*

FOOD

It is important to stick to regular meal times, even if you consume only a small amount of food.

Broths and consommés are light and nutritious. Bone broth, made by slow cooking marrow bones, is rich in protein and trace elements.
➧*Make yourself or buy ready-made for a nourishing light meal.*
Bitter greens such as rocket, endive, radicchio, bitter lettuces, and kale stimulate the liver and gallbladder.
➧*Eat regularly with meals and in salads.*
Herbs and spices enhance the taste of food and help increase salivation and appetite. Chilli, turmeric, garlic, and cumin are good choices.
➧*Add to meals and dressings.*

LIFESTYLE

Address allergies that cause congestion. Try to keep your sinuses clear as loss of smell can lead to loss of appetite.

"Aromatherapy essential oils can stimulate the secretion of saliva and digestive juices to prepare for eating."

EATING DISORDERS

Anorexia and bulimia wreak havoc on mental wellbeing, emotional balance, personal relationships, and physical health. Physical recovery takes time, patience, and strategies.

HERBS

Herbs support the nervous system, easing anxiety, and help rebalance the emotions. Tonic herbs strengthen the mind and body.

Oatstraw is a tonic for exhaustion and helps reverse long-term debility. See box, right. Avoid with gluten sensitivity.
➽*Infuse 1–2 tsp dried oatstraw in 175ml (6fl oz) boiling water. Drink 3 times daily.*

Chamomile relaxes digestive action and calms nervous excitability and tension. Avoid with *Asteraceae* sensitivity.
➽*If eating is erratic, infuse 1 tsp each dried chamomile and oatstraw in 175ml (6fl oz) boiling water. Drink 1–3 times daily.*

Ashwagandha is calming, balancing, and strengthening, providing mental and physical support. Avoid during pregnancy or with hyperthyroidism.
➽*Take 1–2ml tincture in a little water 3 times daily, or add 1 tsp powder to smoothies and cereals.*

WHAT TO AVOID
Herbal laxatives such as cascara, senna, and rhubarb.

ESSENTIAL OILS

These can be calming and especially helpful for soothing emotions.

Rose is extremely nurturing.
Ylang ylang is an antidepressant.
Bergamot is emotionally uplifting.
➽*Add 5 drops of any of the above oils to 5ml base oil and add to a warm bath. Or add 2–3 drops to a diffuser.*

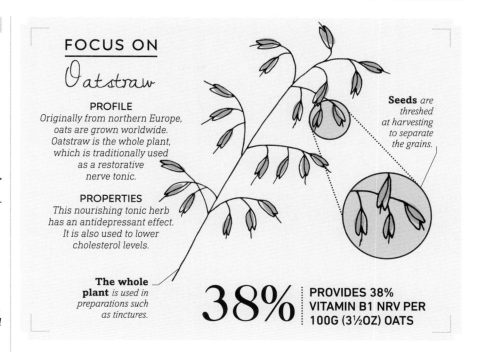

FOCUS ON
Oatstraw

PROFILE
Originally from northern Europe, oats are grown worldwide. Oatstraw is the whole plant, which is traditionally used as a restorative nerve tonic.

PROPERTIES
This nourishing tonic herb has an antidepressant effect. It is also used to lower cholesterol levels.

The whole plant *is used in preparations such as tinctures.*

Seeds *are threshed at harvesting to separate the grains.*

38% PROVIDES 38% VITAMIN B1 NRV PER 100G (3½OZ) OATS

FOOD

Restoring digestive health helps the body to absorb vital nutrients. Hydration is vital, too: chronic dehydration can affect both emotional and physical wellbeing.

Fermented foods such as yogurt, kimchi, sauerkraut, and kefir have beneficial bacteria for a healthy gut.
➽*Incorporate into the diet daily.*

Fibre is essential if there has been laxative abuse. Wholegrains, fresh vegetables, and pulses feed good gut bacteria.
➽*Include sources daily.*

Milk and dairy products help to restore phosphate and calcium levels.
➽*Include in your daily diet.*

Bananas, oranges, grapes, and peaches have digestion-boosting potassium.
➽*Have a fruit and yogurt smoothie.*

WHAT TO AVOID
In cases of bulimia, avoid processed and sugary foods. For anorexia sufferers, while these foods are not ideal, it is best not to discourage any food intake.

SUPPLEMENTS

Purging depletes the body of essential trace elements such as potassium and zinc.

Multi-vitamins, minerals, and omega-3 fatty acids aid immune and gut health.
➽*Take daily supplements.*

Potassium regulates the heart and blood pressure, and lowers the risk of stroke.
➽*Advised daily intake is 3500mg, which should also come from food. Talk to your doctor about dosage.*

Probiotic supplements add live cultures to the gut, while prebiotics feed already-present good bacteria.
➽*Look for capsules or powders with 10 billion live organisms per dose.*

LIFESTYLE

Gentle, non-competitive activities such as yoga can reconnect you to your body.

OTHER THERAPIES

Psychotherapy/counselling is advised.

OBESITY

There is an increasing awareness of the many factors at play behind excess calorie consumption. Emotional disorders, environmental chemicals, and lack of sleep can all contribute to obsessive eating.

HERBS

These boost digestion, balance blood sugar levels, support endocrine health, and enhance vitality in body and mind.

Nettle is a cleansing blood tonic. It also helps to balance blood sugars, detoxify, strengthen, and energize.
➽*Infuse 1–2 tsp dried nettle in 175ml (6fl oz) boiling water and drink 3 times daily. Or add to soups, stews, and salads.*
Fennel seed, a calming digestive tonic, may help reduce appetite cravings.
➽*Infuse 1 tsp dried fennel seed in 175ml (6fl oz) boiling water. Drink 3 times daily.*
Siberian ginseng (Eleuthero), a tonic, increases energy levels, stamina, and alertness. Avoid with acute infections.
➽*Take 3–5ml tincture in a little water 3 times daily.*
Schisandra, a liver tonic, stimulates the nervous system and energizes. Avoid with acute infections and barbiturates.
➽*Take 2–4ml tincture in a little water 3 times daily.*

ESSENTIAL OILS

These are supportive during weight loss, helping to control cravings and cleanse.

Cinnamon can be used to help regulate blood sugar.
Ginger can reduce sugar cravings.
➽*Add 5 drops of either oil to a bowl of hot water, lean over, cover your head with a towel, and inhale until the steam cools. Or add 2 drops of either to a diffuser.*
Grapefruit helps to detoxify and cleanse.
➽*See remedy with almond oil, below.*

FOOD

Eat plenty of fresh, plant-based, and whole foods. Drinking 300ml (10fl oz) of water before eating aids weight loss significantly.

Fermented foods such as miso, pickled cucumbers, and sauerkraut contain live cultures that help balance gut flora.
➽*Use as condiments with daily meals.*
Stone fruits such as apricots, prunes, cherries, and nectarines, are anti-inflammatory and have compounds that may fight metabolic syndrome due to obesity and insulin resistance.
➽*Try a stone-fruit skewer for dessert.*
Oily fish can lower levels of leptin – the hunger hormone – to help lose weight.
➽ *Eat daily to support weight loss.*
Baobab is a tropical fruit rich in fibre, which keeps you feeling full for longer.
➽*Add 15g (½oz) powder to a smoothie.*

REMEDY

Detox massage

*Add 5 drops **grapefruit** essential oil to 10ml **almond oil** and massage into the skin.*

WHAT TO AVOID

Diet or "lite" foods are often highly processed as well as being high in sugar and salt. Artificial sweeteners promote weight gain.

SUPPLEMENTS

Use to aid metabolism and reduce cravings.

Green tea extract has the polyphenol epigallocatechin-3-gallate (EGCG), which can increase metabolic rate.
➽*Take 300–800mg daily.*
Chromium helps reduce sugar cravings by regulating blood sugar levels.
➽*Take 600mcg chromium daily for 2 months to kick-start weight loss.*
CoQ10 is a vitamin-like substance important for creating energy in the cells, helping you avoid the tiredness that leads to snacking.
➽*Take 30–50mg daily with a fat-containing meal to aid absorption.*
Conjugated linoleic acid (CLA) is a healthy fat that is antioxidant and anti-inflammatory. It may help lower body fat around the abdomen as well as block the absorption of fat and sugar and increase insulin sensitivity.
➽*Take 1–3g daily.*

LIFESTYLE

Get sufficient sleep. Tiredness leads to poor food choices, and can alter key hormones that aid metabolism.
Remove obesogens. Heavy metals, as well as chemicals, found in plastics, fragrances, and flame retardants have been shown to promote weight gain.

OTHER THERAPIES

Acupuncture may aid weight loss.
Counselling can offer support.
Massage can raise body awareness.
Sauna can help to detoxify the body, aiding the elimination of environmental toxins.

GUT DYSBIOSIS

This commonly describes an imbalance in gut microflora, leading to poor absorption of nutrients and chronic fatigue. Poor gut health has also been linked to periodontal disease, inflammatory bowel disease, obesity, cancer, and colitis.

HERBS

Some herbs contain inulin, a prebiotic polysaccharide found in the roots, which boosts healthy gut bacteria. Bitter herbs are tonics and also support gut flora.

Dandelion root is a bitter digestive tonic that contains inulin, which improves digestive function and promotes healthy gut flora. Avoid with gallstones.
➡ *Take 2.5–5ml tincture in a little water 3 times daily.*

Burdock root contains inulin. It also stimulates digestive juices, promoting a healthy environment for gut flora.
➡ *Take 2–4ml tincture in a little water 3 times daily.*

Chicory root is bitter and beneficial for the liver, gallbladder, and pancreas. It contains inulin to support gut health.
➡ *Take 1–2ml tincture in a little water 3 times daily. Or try combining all three tinctures, see remedy, right.*

RAW OR COOKED?

Raw vegetables have enzymes that aid digestion. But the body absorbs more of substances such as carotenoids from cooked veg. Eat half raw, half cooked for gut health.

ESSENTIAL OILS

Dysbiosis can be exacerbated by stress. Choose oils that relax and strengthen.

Holy basil is uplifting and strengthening for mind and body. Avoid in pregnancy.
➡ *Add 3–4 drops to a diffuser.*

Lavender has deeply soothing and relaxing properties.
➡ *Sprinkle 2–4 drops on a tissue to inhale during the day, or sprinkle on your pillow to aid restful sleep.*

Mandarin is gentle, relaxing, and calming.
➡ *Add 5 drops to 5ml base oil for a massage blend or bath oil.*

FOOD

Bacteria in the gut have a direct effect on health and, in particular, immunity. Prebiotic foods support beneficial gut bacteria.

Buckwheat has prebiotic properties.
➡ *Breakfast on buckwheat flakes or porridge.*

Bananas contain small amounts of prebiotic inulin and are most effective as a prebiotic when slightly under-ripe.
➡ *Add to cereals or smoothies.*

Allium vegetables, such as garlic, onions, leeks, chives, and spring onions, are all prebiotic.
➡ *Eat raw or lightly cooked to maximize nutrients.*

"Long" pepper is a close relative of black pepper. In traditional Indian medicine, its tonic and digestive effects are used to treat dysbiosis.
➡ *Use in a spice grinder as a substitute for black pepper where a sweeter, spicier flavour is required.*

SUPPLEMENTS

Topping up nutrients can help to support the diet to optimize gut health.

Multi-vitamins help maintain gut health.
➡ *Take 1 daily.*

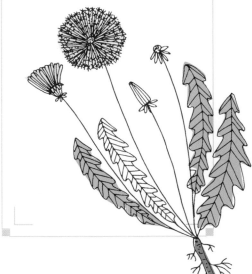

REMEDY

Gut-supporting decoction

*Make a decoction combining dried **dandelion root**, **burdock root**, and **chicory root**, using 30g (1oz) shredded dried roots to 500ml (16fl oz) water. Drink 90–175ml (3–6fl oz) 3 times daily.*

Probiotic supplements. Ones with *Lactobacilli* and *Bifidobacteria* help restore the bacterial gut population.
➡ *Look for ones with 10 billion live organisms per dose.*

Inulin, a prebiotic, improves absorption of nutrients and bowel regularity.
➡ *Take 1 daily.*

Aged garlic extract is odourless and higher in gut-healing antioxidants than regular garlic.
➡ *Take 400–600mg a day.*

LIFESTYLE

Avoid excessive use of antibiotics and non-steroidal anti-inflammatory drugs (NSAIDs), such as ibuprofen, as these can cause dysbiosis.

RECIPES FOR WELLNESS
SPREADS

These easy-to-rustle-up spreads make a delicious light lunch or quick snack to top up nutrients in the day. Simply blitz the ingredients – drizzling in any oil during blending – for 15–30 seconds, or until the desired consistency, then serve on toasted rye bread, oat cakes, or with crudités.

1

SPINACH AND CASHEW SPREAD

Pairing vitamin C-rich spinach with cashew nuts – high in protein and essential fats – gives this simple spread immune-boosting properties.

SERVES 1 • PREP TIME 10 MINS

85g (3oz) spinach leaves, steamed and squeezed to remove excess moisture

60g (2oz) cashew nuts

½ tsp grated nutmeg

salt and freshly ground black pepper

Nutritional info per serving:
Kcals 373 Fat 29g Saturated fat 6g Carbohydrates 10.5g Sugar 2.5g Sodium 34mg Fibre 3.5g Protein 15g Cholesterol 0mg

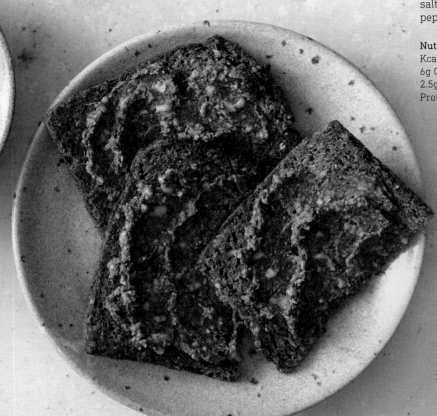

2

BUTTER BEAN AND MUSTARD SPREAD

Butter beans provide high-quality protein and digestive-supporting fibre, as well as a range of nutrients such as folate, potassium, phosphorus, magnesium, iron, and vitamin B6.

SERVES 2 • PREP TIME 5–10 MINS

200g can butter beans, rinsed and drained

1 tsp wholegrain or Dijon mustard

2 tbsp extra virgin olive oil

1 tbsp finely chopped flat-leaf parsley

freshly ground black pepper

Nutritional info per serving:
Kcals 159 Fat 11.5g Saturated fat 1.5g Carbohydrates 8g Sugar 0.8g Sodium 74mg Fibre 4g Protein 4g Cholesterol 0mg

3

AVOCADO AND FETA SPREAD

Avocado, a source of essential nutrients such as folate, potassium, and magnesium, is also high in monounsaturated fats, thought to play a role in reversing insulin resistance to regulate blood sugar levels, while tangy feta provides calcium for bone health.

SERVES 1–2 • PREP TIME 5–10 MINS

1 avocado, peeled and pitted

30g (1oz) feta

1½ tbsp coriander leaves

freshly ground black pepper

Nutritional info per serving:
Kcals 187 Fat 18g Saturated fat 5g Carbohydrates 1.5g Sugar 0.5g Sodium 154mg Fibre 3.5g Protein 4g Cholesterol 10.5mg

4

TOFU AND OLIVE SPREAD

Tofu contains all eight essential amino acids, which can only be obtained from the diet. Amino acids form the building blocks of protein, vital for cell renewal. Olives add antioxidant benefits as well as anti-inflammatory polyphenols.

SERVES 2–3 • PREP TIME 5–10 MINS

140g (5oz) tofu, broken into chunks

1 tbsp extra virgin olive oil

1 lemon, juice and rind

30g (1oz) olives, pitted and sliced

10g (¼oz) walnuts

30g (1oz) cherry tomatoes, halved

2 spring onions, sliced

¼ tsp dried chilli

¼ tsp turmeric

Nutritional info per serving:
Kcals 132 Fat 10.5g Saturated fat 1.5g Carbohydrates 2g Sugar 1.5g Sodium 140mg Fibre 1.7g Protein 7g Cholesterol 0mg

5

SPICY CHICKPEA SPREAD

Sustaining and high in protein, chickpeas provide manganese to support bone health, and folate, to boost heart health and help ease symptoms of depression.

SERVES 3–4 • PREP TIME 5–10 MINS

400g can chickpeas, drained and rinsed

2 tbsp extra virgin olive oil

1 tbsp ground cumin

1 tbsp turmeric

1 tsp dried chilli

3 tbsp lemon juice

freshly ground black pepper

Nutritional info per serving:
Kcals 130 Fat 7.5g Saturated fat 1g Carbohydrates 10g Sugar 0.5g Sodium 0mg Fibre 3.5g Protein 4.5g Cholesterol 0mg

URINARY SYSTEM

The kidneys and bladder perform the vital role of filtering and removing waste in the form of urine from the body, in the process maintaining a healthy balance of fluids and electrolytes, which is crucial to many bodily functions. Discover how hydrating, nutritious, cleansing, and protective nutrients, herbs, and essential oils can support urinary function, ensuring the smooth removal of waste, and how natural therapies and a tailored diet can help to resolve blockages and infections when these occur.

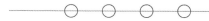

STAYING WELL
URINARY SYSTEM

A well-functioning urinary system that is able to remove waste efficiently is essential for overall health. Eating a diet that includes key micronutrients both supports and helps to optimize the health of the bladder, urethra, and kidneys. Healing herbs and therapeutic essential oils also provide extremely effective support, helping to cleanse and calm the urinary system to help it work smoothly and efficiently.

Foods

Being adequately hydrated and including key foods in your diet while avoiding dietary irritants can make a significant contribution to urinary health.

Hydration boost

Drinking plenty of healthy fluids – water is the best option for staying hydrated, but herbal teas are also beneficial and provide other benefits – is one of the simplest and most important measures to keep the urinary system working efficiently and help prevent infections. Hydration not only supports kidney function to help flush out toxins, but also boosts immunity – when your body is hydrated, it transports oxygen efficiently to ensure that cells, tissues, and organs perform optimally.

As well as drinking healthy fluids, eat foods with a high water content, such as watermelon, lettuce, celery, and cucumber.

Antibacterial foods

Eating foods with live bacterial cultures, such as natural yogurt, sauerkraut, kimchi, and kefir is a powerful way to repopulate the digestive tract with good bacteria after an infection and in turn strengthen the urinary tract's resistance to bacterial infections.

Vital fibre

Many aspects of modern diets can contribute to kidney and bladder problems. A diet high in fats and sugars and low in fibre raises the risk of kidney and bladder stones. High-fibre wholegrains such as wheat, corn, rye, millet, and barley help to remove stone-forming substances such as uric acid. Fibre-rich foods also prevent uncomfortable blockages in the intestines that can press on the bladder, so avoiding constipation has a knock-on benefit for bladder health.

As well as wholegrains, aim for a largely plant-based diet with limited meat to help lower levels of uric acid in your excretory system. Beans, dried peas, and lentils as well as nuts and

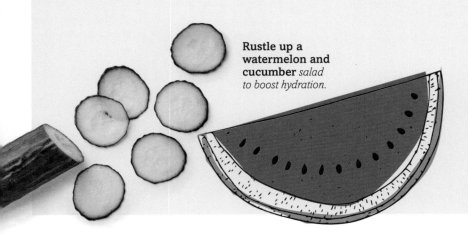

Rustle up a watermelon and cucumber *salad to boost hydration.*

> *"Being well hydrated is one of the most important ways to ensure that the urinary system is working efficiently."*

nut-based products are healthy high-protein alternatives to meat and are also low in substances called oxalates, which for some can lead to the formation of kidney and bladder stones.

ALKALINE FOODS

If you are prone to urinary tract infections, eating more alkaline-based foods may help to reduce recurrent infections and also make urination more comfortable when an infection does occur. Carrots, celery, black radish, barley grass, and cucumber as well as watermelon and bananas are all examples of alkaline foods that can promote health throughout the body. Where you can, try to buy organic produce to reduce your exposure to pesticide residues, which can affect immunity over the long term.

CALCIUM BENEFITS

Calcium-containing foods can bind to oxalates – substances that can lead to kidney stones – and stop these from being absorbed into the blood. If there is a tendency to kidney stones, getting enough calcium can be a helpful preventative measure. Dairy products such as yogurt, soft fish bones – ground down in tinned salmon – and greens such as kale and broccoli all provide calcium.

HERBS

Herbs contain several properties to support a healthy urinary system. Toning and calming herbs can help prevent inflammation, nerve sensitivity, and infection.

HERBS WITH A DIURETIC ACTION

Herbs with a diuretic effect are useful at the first sign of a urinary tract infection to reduce the symptoms and flush out bacteria. Stone root and corn silk help to increase urine flow, removing waste and excess water from the system. Buchu has a similar diuretic action and in addition contains volatile antibacterial oils that can help to both prevent and fight urinary tract infections.

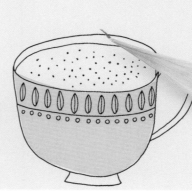

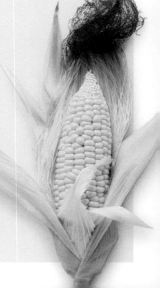

Infuse 1–2 tsp dried corn silk *in 175ml (6fl oz) boiling water for a detoxifying infusion.*

Soothing herbs

Mucilaginous herbs such as marshmallow and couch grass have a viscous or gelatinous quality that can help to soothe and calm any irritation in the urinary tract to prevent problems such as frequent urination. If there is inflammation in the mucous membranes of the urinary tract, the tissues become more vulnerable to infection, so these herbs can reduce the likelihood of an infection and are beneficial if you feel the initial symptoms of a urinary tract infection.

Marshmallow root is also diuretic, helping to encourage urine flow, and is an antioxidant herb, protecting the cells in the urinary tract from free radical damage.

Toning herbs

Certain herbs have a toning action on the bladder tissues. For example, horsetail is a toning herb that has a strengthening and calming effect on the lining of the bladder so can help to reduce the urgency and frequency of urination, which tends to increase naturally as we age as the bladder muscles become gradually weaker.

Essential oils

An essential oil massage can be an effective way to cleanse and boost the health of the urinary system.

Oils as antimicrobials

Antimicrobial and astringent essential oils promote and support urinary health. Uplifting cedarwood is antiseptic and astringent, so helps to keep infections at bay. Lavender, as well as being deeply calming, is also antiseptic, and thyme linalol has strong antiseptic properties to help manage urinary infections.

Citrus oils, such as lemon and bergamot, are cleansing and refreshing and also have antiseptic properties to help maintain urinary tract health. Add pre-diluted citrus oils or any of the above oils to a shallow sitz bath to help prevent infections taking hold.

Cleansing essential oils

Many essential oils have a detoxifying, cleansing effect that helps promote healthy bladder function and support the kidneys in expelling waste from the body to avoid an accumulation of toxins.

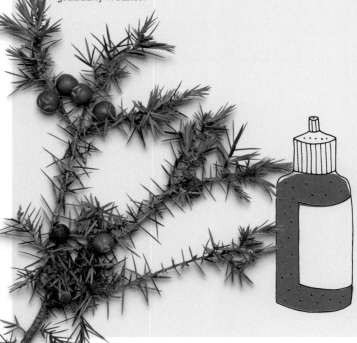

Add 4 drops juniper essential oil *to 10ml almond oil and massage over the kidney area to stimulate urine production.*

Pungent juniper berry and sweet and spicy fennel are effective detoxifying oils. Create a detoxifying, stimulating massage blend with either of these to massage gently over the kidney area. Dill and parsley also have a diuretic effect, reducing water retention and helping to flush out toxins. Juniper, a rejuvenating oil, also has a mild diuretic effect, as do grapefruit and mandarin.

SUPPLEMENTS

A healthy diet should provide vital nutrients, but if levels of key nutrients are low this can impact on urinary health so a supplement can be helpful.

BENEFICIAL BACTERIA

Probiotics help to populate the gut with beneficial bacteria to balance gut flora. Studies on probiotic supplements show that these can have specific benefits for urinary health. A daily dose of *Lactobacillus rhamnosus* and *L. fermentum* in particular can help prevent the overgrowth of harmful bacteria in the urinary tract, so reduce the risk of recurrent urinary tract infections.

MAGNESIUM BOOST

If you have suffered with kidney or bladder stones in the past you are more vulnerable to these forming again, so preventative measures are important. If you are susceptible, boosting your magnesium levels may help to inhibit crystal formation as low magnesium is an indicator for kidney and bladder stone risk. Dietary sources of magnesium are often high in the compound oxalate, which can contribute to the formation of stones, so a daily magnesium supplement can be a reliable way to top up levels. Magnesium also has a beneficial alkalizing effect on the body.

PROTECTIVE CRANBERRIES

Cranberries are a well-known remedy for urinary tract infections, and studies also suggest that they can help to prevent infection in the first place. Cranberries contain a substance called A-type proanthocyanidin (PAC-A), a naturally occurring antioxidant, and it's thought that PAC-A makes it harder for bacteria to adhere to the bladder. A cranberry extract supplement will deliver a standardized dose of PAC-A.

"Essential oils can be used in a massage to cleanse and boost urinary health."

TREATMENTS

URINARY SYSTEM

The kidneys, bladder, and urinary tract, which facilitate the removal of waste and toxins, can be affected by blockages and infections, which can cause discomfort and pain and compromise the efficient removal of waste from the body. A holistic approach to healing with gentle and stimulating herbs and essential oils and a tailored diet can be effective for relieving symptoms and treating ailments in the urinary system.

URINARY TRACT INFECTION (UTI)

Bladder infections are called cystitis, and infection in the urethra, urethritis. The kidneys can also be infected. Bacteria, especially *Escherichia coli*, often from the colon, is a major cause; non-specific urethritis can be caused by various bacteria. If a UTI is persistent, or there is blood in the urine or a fever, see a doctor urgently.

HERBS

Diuretic herbs promote urine flow, tonic and anti-inflammatory herbs support the urinary tract lining, and antimicrobials fight infection. Inflammation and irritation is eased by astringent or mucilaginous herbs.

Buchu contains volatile, antibacterial oils to fight infection and promote urinary flow. Avoid if breastfeeding.
➡ *Boil 175ml (6fl oz) water and let it stand for 1–2 minutes, then add 1 tsp dried buchu. Drink 2–3 times daily.*
Plantain is diuretic, antibacterial, astringent, and anti-inflammatory.
➡ *Infuse 1–2 tsp dried plantain in 175ml (6fl oz) boiling water. Take 3 times daily.*

Marshmallow leaf is a soothing mucilaginous herb that calms urinary tract irritation and promotes healing. Take separately from other medications as it may impede their absorption.
➡ *Infuse 1–2 tsp dried marshmallow in 175ml (6fl oz) boiling water per cup and leave overnight. Drink cold 3 times daily.*
Couchgrass is diuretic and contains mucilage to soothe and protect the mucosal lining and fight infection.
➡ *Make a decoction with 2–3 tsp dried couchgrass in 250ml (9fl oz) boiling water; take twice daily.*

ESSENTIAL OILS

Oils can act as diuretics to boost urine flow, can support the immune system, and are antimicrobial and anti-inflammatory.

Cedarwood is a gentle diuretic, recommended for treating cystitis.
Sandalwood is a traditional UTI remedy.
➡ *Take a 15-minute sitz bath: add 5 drops of either cedarwood or sandalwood essential oil to a warm hip-height bath.*
Bergamot has antiseptic properties.
Lavender has antimicrobial and analgesic actions.
➡ *Add 3 drops of bergamot or lavender oils to a warm bath and use a clean flannel to wash the affected area.*

FOOD

A nutritious wholefood diet will improve resistance to infection. Drink plenty of water every day to help flush out bacteria.

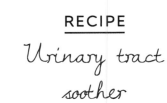

RECIPE

Urinary tract soother

*Blitz 2 **carrots** with either 1 **celery stick** or 1 **apple**, cored, until smooth. Drink daily.*

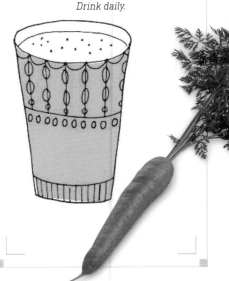

Carrot juice is high in anti-inflammatory beta-carotenes.
➥*See recipe, opposite.*

Live foods such as yogurt, kimchi, sauerkraut, tempeh, and kefir help to repopulate the gut with good bacteria, which in turn helps to strengthen resistance to infection.
➥*Eat a portion daily.*

Blueberries contain valuable antioxidants that prevent bacteria from sticking to the urinary tract wall.
➥*Snack on a handful regularly.*

SUPPLEMENTS

Antioxidant supplements can reduce inflammation, boost immunity, and repair the mucosal lining of the urinary tract.

Beta-carotene is an anti-inflammatory, helping to repair mucous membranes.
➥*Take up to 4mg daily.*

Cranberries contain antioxidant A-type proanthocyanidin (PAC-A), which makes it harder for bacteria to adhere to the bladder.
➥*Take as directed with plenty of water.*

D-mannose is a natural sugar in fruits, especially berries, which also prevents bacteria sticking to the bladder lining.
➥*Take 2g of powder dissolved in 200ml (7fl oz) water daily.*

Probiotic supplements help prevent the overgrowth of harmful bacteria and reduce the risk of recurrent UTIs.
➥*Look for a supplement with 10 billion live organisms per dose.*

LIFESTYLE

Harsh products damage the mucosal lining. Avoid feminine deodorants, douches, bubble bath, and harsh soaps.

Cotton underwear and loose clothes keep the urethra area dry, helping to discourage bacteria. Also wipe front to back to stop bacteria from the anus entering the urethra.

Pass urine immediately after sex.

BLADDER CONTROL

Loss of bladder control is caused by muscles or nerves not working well. It is most common in the elderly, chronically ill, or overweight. Stress incontinence is where a little urine leaks during physical activity; urge incontinence is an uncontrollable, urgent need to pass urine; nocturia is a need to urinate in the night.

HERBS

Depending on the cause, herbal infusions can soothe inflammation and bladder lining irritation and calm nerve sensitivity. Diuretic and tonic herbs are also helpful.

Angelica leaf relaxes the bladder muscles and helps to reduce urgency and frequency. Avoid in pregnancy and therapeutic doses if diabetic.
➥*Infuse 1–2 tsp dried angelica in 175ml (6fl oz) boiling water. Drink 3 times daily.*

St John's wort calms nerve activity. Avoid in pregnancy and high doses in strong sunlight. Taken internally, interacts with many prescription medicines.
➥*Infuse 1–2 tsp dried St John's wort in 175ml (6fl oz) boiling water. Drink 3 times daily.*

Horsetail helps reduce urgency, see below. Avoid with diabetes, gout, or kidney or heart disease. Seek medical advice if there is blood in the urine.
➥*Infuse 1–2 tsp dried horsetail in 175ml (6fl oz) water, 3 times daily, up to 4 weeks.*

LIFESTYLE

Pelvic muscle (Kegel) exercises strengthen the bladder muscles.

Avoid caffeinated and fizzy drinks, milk, sugar, sweeteners, honey, chocolate, citrus juices, and tomatoes.

OTHER THERAPIES

Biofeedback behavioural therapy can be as successful as conventional drugs.

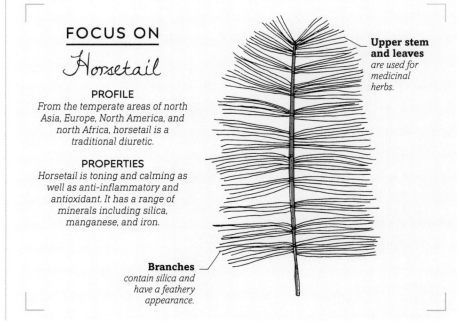

FOCUS ON
Horsetail

PROFILE
From the temperate areas of north Asia, Europe, North America, and north Africa, horsetail is a traditional diuretic.

PROPERTIES
Horsetail is toning and calming as well as anti-inflammatory and antioxidant. It has a range of minerals including silica, manganese, and iron.

Upper stem and leaves *are used for medicinal herbs.*

Branches *contain silica and have a feathery appearance.*

BLADDER STONES

If urine stays in the bladder too long and becomes very concentrated, substances in it react with each other to form crystals made up of oxalates, phosphorous, and uric acid, which enlarge over time. Passing them can be painful, but left in situ they can cause irritation and infection. Most cases affect men aged over 50 because prostate enlargement can obstruct the flow of urine, so it's important to get a prostate check.

HERBS

Diuretic herbs are beneficial, helping to increase urine flow and in turn dilute and promote the excretion of waste particles such as calcium. Anti-inflammatory and soothing herbs help reduce discomfort, and muscle-relaxing herbs may be helpful.

Stone root is a strong diuretic that is traditionally used for the dissolution of bladder stones.
➻*Make a decoction with 1–2 tsp dried stone root per 250ml (9fl oz) boiling water, and drink 3 times daily.*

FOOD

A diet high in fat, sugar, or salt with a low water intake can alter urine composition, increasing the risk of bladder stones. Eat a high-fibre, nutrient-dense diet and stay hydrated to lower the concentration of stone-forming minerals in the urine.

Wholegrain foods such as wheat, corn, rye, millet, and barley contain fibre that helps remove stone-forming substances from the body.
➻*Swap white, highly processed bread and cereals for wholewheat or wholegrain varieties.*

READY TO COOK

Dried lentils provide more nutrients than tinned ones and don't require any time-consuming soaking prior to cooking.

Plant-based protein is preferable to animal protein, which can raise the risk of uric acid-based stones. Beans, dried peas, and lentils are high in protein and low in oxalate.
➻*Make a three-bean salad, or try a vegetarian chilli rather than a meat-based one.*

Fresh fruit and vegetables provide digestion-boosting fibre, a range of antioxidant and essential nutrients, and also have a high water content that helps to keep you well hydrated.
➻*Eat at least two portions of both fruits and vegetables each day, ensuring that these form the basis of your daily diet.*

WHAT TO AVOID
High-fat meals. Try baking, grilling, or steaming your food instead of frying food or cooking with oil.

SUPPLEMENTS

If your diet is sub-optimal, a deficiency of certain important nutrients can contribute to the formation of bladder stones. Supplementation can help to support your diet to reduce the risk.

Magnesium can inhibit crystal formation. Taking a supplement can help ensure that you get sufficient amounts of this trace element.
➻*Take a recommended dose of 300–400mg daily.*

KIDNEY STONES

Painful kidney stones form when substances in the urine crystallize and grow into larger masses. Most of these stones are formed from oxalate or phosphorous, though some also form from uric acid, produced as the body metabolizes protein. Determining the kind of stone that has formed can help guide your choice of remedy.

HERBS

As with bladder stones, diuretic herbs help to boost urine flow to avoid the buildup of waste products such as calcium, while soothing anti-inflammatory herbs and muscle-relaxing herbs can ease pain and discomfort.

Stone root is used as a strong diuretic herb and is thought to help dissolve both bladder and kidney stones.
➻*Make a decoction with 1–2 tsp dried stone root per 250ml (9fl oz) boiling water, and drink 3 times daily.*

Gravel root helps prevent stones forming and may decrease the size of existing stones by promoting the excretion of waste products in urine. Avoid during pregnancy.
➻*Take 2ml tincture in a little water 3 times daily.*

Pellitory-of-the-Wall is a soothing diuretic herb that calms inflammation in the urinary tract and is beneficial for helping to reduce kidney stones.
➻*Infuse 1–2 tsp dried Pellitory in 175ml (6fl oz) boiling water. Drink 3 times daily.*

Corn silk is diuretic, anti-inflammatory, and soothes spasms in the urinary tract to help ease discomfort and pain.
➻*Infuse 2–4 tsp dried corn silk in 175ml (6fl oz) boiling water. Drink 3–4 times daily.*

ESSENTIAL OILS

Diuretic essential oils stimulate the action of the kidneys and accelerate natural detoxification processes.

Juniper berry helps to clear toxins. Try pairing with sunflower oil.
➡*See remedy, below.*
Fennel can be used to help eliminate toxins efficiently.
➡*Add 5 drops to 10ml almond oil and massage over the kidney area.*
Lemon is deeply cleansing and helps to detoxify.
➡*Add 5 drops to 10ml jojoba oil and massage gently into the skin over the kidney area.*

FOOD

A diet that is high in fats and sugars, and low in fibre, can generate damaging free radicals and has therefore been linked to a higher risk of developing kidney stones. Make sure you eat a fibre-rich, nutrient-dense diet. Drinking plenty of water – 1.5–2 litres (2¾–3½ pints) daily – will lower the concentration of stone-forming minerals in the urine.

Watercress and kale have high levels of calcium, which can actively reduce the risk of kidney stones forming.
➡*Eat raw or lightly steamed.*
Wholegrain foods such as wheat, corn, rye, millet, and barley, contain beneficial fibre to help remove stone-forming substances.
➡*Choose wholewheat or wholegrain types of bread and pasta.*
Plant-based proteins should replace animal proteins in the diet as much as possible as these make uric acid-based stones more likely. Beans, dried peas, and lentils are high in protein and fibre, both of which help to prevent kidney stones.
➡*Include pulses in meals and try pasta made from beans and pulses.*

Cold-water oily fish such as salmon, mackerel, sardines, and herring are rich in omega-3 oils, which can help prevent the formation of kidney stones. Sardines in particular – with the soft bones left in – have the added value of being rich in calcium.
➡*Enjoy sardines on wholemeal toast or with wholewheat pasta.*
WHAT TO AVOID
Oxalate-forming foods, such as spinach, kale, chocolate, beetroot, rhubarb, parsley, sorrel, tea, and most types of nut, because the compound oxalate can contribute to kidney stones. Fizzy drinks, which contain phosphoric acid, as this can contribute to the formation of stones. A high-salt diet increases the risk of bladder and kidney stones forming.

SUPPLEMENTS

Although it is best to get the nutrients you need from your diet, some supplements can be helpful to reduce levels of stone-forming substances.

Vitamin B6 can help decrease the production of oxalate.
➡*Take 40mg daily.*
Magnesium inhibits crystal formation. Taking supplements ensures that your body is receiving sufficient amounts.
➡*Take 300–400mg daily.*
WHAT TO AVOID
Long-term use of high-dose vitamin C supplements.

"Certain supplements can help to reduce levels of stone-forming substances."

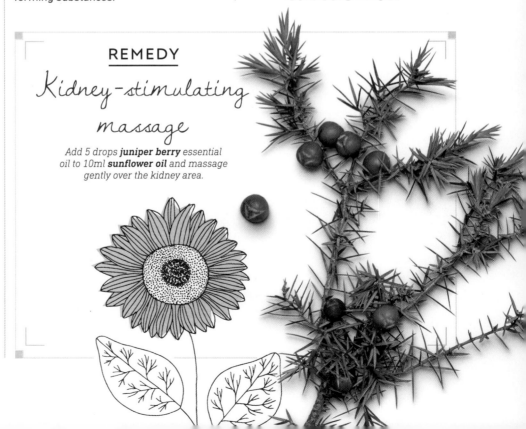

REMEDY
Kidney-stimulating massage

*Add 5 drops **juniper berry** essential oil to 10ml **sunflower oil** and massage gently over the kidney area.*

HOW TO MAKE
A SYRUP

A syrup is a traditional way of providing medicinal herbal remedies while softening the strong, bitter tastes of many herbs. This can make syrups especially appealing to children and a helpful way to introduce them to herbal remedies. The sugar or honey content also helps to preserve the water-based extract, avoiding the need to add alcohol or refrigerate the syrup.

Makes about 500ml (16fl oz)

YOU WILL NEED

500ml (16fl oz) herbal infusion or decoction (see p30 and p100)

500g (1lb 2oz) organic raw cane sugar or honey

large saucepan

wooden spoon

dark glass bottles

label

tincture (optional)

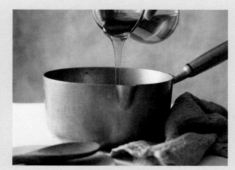

1 Sterilize all the equipment: wash thoroughly then dry in an oven at 140°C (275°F) or in a microwave for 30–45 seconds. Place the infusion or decoction in the saucepan and add the sugar or honey. To maximize potency, use a strong infusion or decoction.

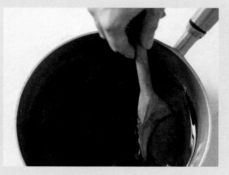

2 Gently heat the liquid, stirring continuously with a wooden spoon, until the sugar or honey has dissolved into the liquid.

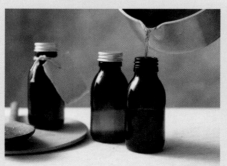

3 Leave the syrup to cool then decant into dark glass bottles and label with the herb and date. If you wish, add 1½–3½ tablespoons of a tincture before bottling for extra medicinal benefits. Take 3 teaspoons daily, or 1–2 teaspoons daily for children.

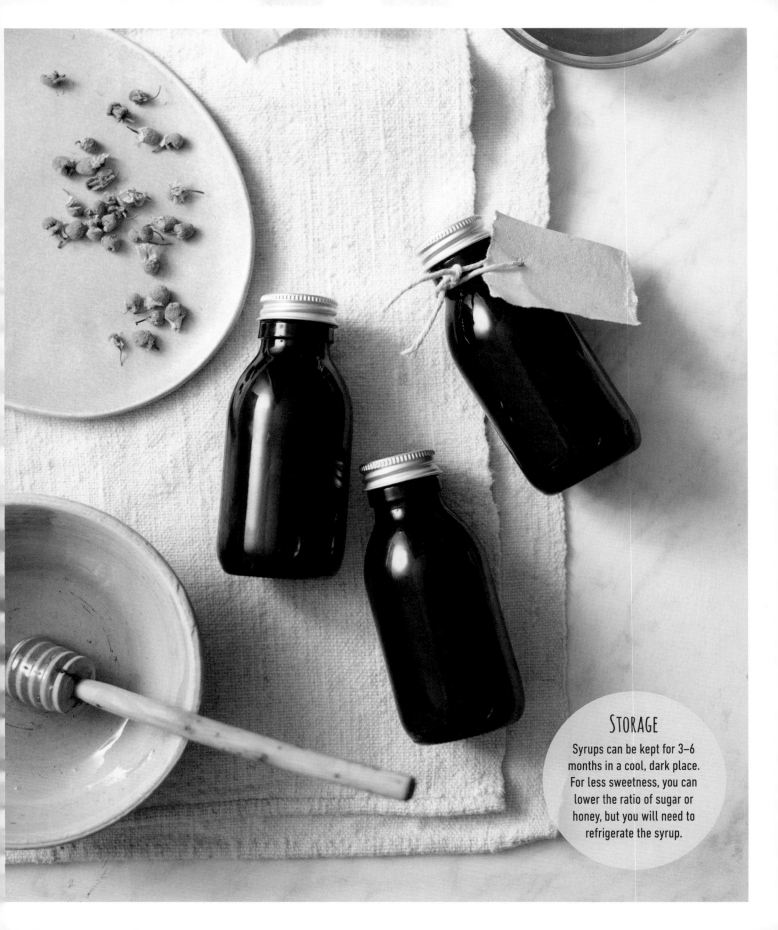

STORAGE

Syrups can be kept for 3–6 months in a cool, dark place. For less sweetness, you can lower the ratio of sugar or honey, but you will need to refrigerate the syrup.

HEART, CIRCULATION, AND BLOOD

All of our organs rely on a healthy circulatory system to pump blood effectively around the body and deliver oxygen and nutrients to each cell. Find out why the right nutrients are crucial for strong, healthy blood vessels and the efficient renewal of blood cells, and how holistic remedies can support diet by helping to tone blood vessels and boost circulation. When problems do occur, discover which nutrients, herbs, and essential oils can help to restore and boost circulatory health.

○ ─ ○ ─ ○ ─ ○

STAYING WELL

HEART, CIRCULATION, AND BLOOD

When working well, the cardiovascular system transports food, hormones, and oxygen efficiently to every cell in the body and removes metabolic waste. What we eat is crucial for heart health and the right nutrients can prevent a buildup of plaque in the arteries, as well as promote healthy blood cell renewal. Holistic remedies using herbs and essential oils can also help to strengthen the heart and blood and prevent conditions developing that can weaken circulation.

FOOD

What we eat can help to control blood pressure and cholesterol and keep blood vessels healthy.

BLOOD VESSEL BOOSTERS

Fibre-rich foods, such as wholegrains, pulses, and fruits and vegetables, promote heart health and strengthen blood vessels, reducing the risk of conditions such as varicose veins. Fibre-high foods can also supply other heart-healthy nutrients. For example, an anti-inflammatory antioxidant rutin, found in buckwheat seeds, unpeeled apples, and figs, is thought to strengthen blood vessels and reduce high blood pressure and cholesterol.

Chillies also help to strengthen blood vessels. Cayenne in chillies contains the compound capsaicin, which strengthens blood vessels and arteries, improving circulation to the extremities.

CHOLESTEROL BUSTERS

A diet based around vegetables and plant-based foods, naturally low in saturated fats and with soluble fibre, can lower cholesterol levels. Oats and barley contain a type of soluble fibre beta-glucan, which forms a gel-like substance that binds to cholesterol in the intestines and prevents it from being absorbed. Low-fat, protein-rich pulses are also a good source of beta-glucan.

Garlic also helps to balance cholesterol and is thought to help prevent platelets from clumping together, reducing the risk of clots and improving circulation. Garlic is most potent when eaten raw, so add raw garlic liberally to salad dressings and vegetables.

PROTECTIVE ANTIOXIDANTS

Deeply and brightly coloured vegetables and fruits are abundant in free radical fighting antioxidants, which help to prevent a dangerous buildup of plaque in the arteries. Grapes, for example, contain an antioxidant polyphenol called resveratrol, which boosts

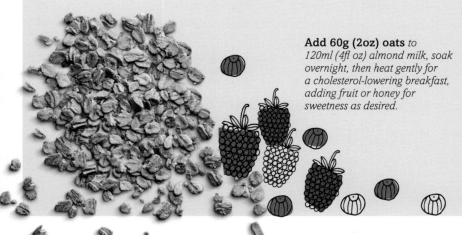

Add 60g (2oz) oats *to 120ml (4fl oz) almond milk, soak overnight, then heat gently for a cholesterol-lowering breakfast, adding fruit or honey for sweetness as desired.*

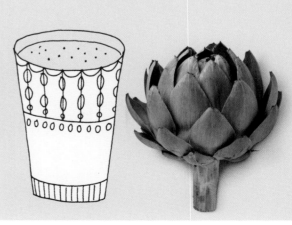

Make a cranberry compote: *simmer cranberries and orange zest for 5–10 minutes, add maple syrup, and enjoy with natural yogurt.*

> "Eating plenty of vegetables and plant-based foods can help to lower cholesterol levels."

circulation; orange and red produce contain beta-carotenes, which promote heart health; and cranberries and apples have anti-inflammatory flavonoids.

NUTTY BENEFITS

Nuts contain a mix of heart-boosting nutrients. Peanuts, walnuts, almonds, and cashews are high in vitamin E, which in food protects against heart disease, as well as fibre and plant sterols, hormone-like substances that help lower cholesterol. Pistachios are high in potassium, which can help to control blood pressure.

NUTRIENTS FOR HEALTHY BLOOD CELLS

Iron-rich foods, such as lean red meat, poultry, fish, pulses, dark leafy greens, and broccoli are essential for healthy red blood cells. The body also needs vitamin C and beta-carotenes to help it absorb iron. For beta-carotenes, try cantaloupe melon, carrots, sweet potatoes, and apricots, and for vitamin C, citrus fruits and peppers.

HERBS

Herbs can boost heart and circulatory health by supporting immunity, strengthening the blood, and increasing levels of energy and vitality.

STIMULATING HERBS

Stimulating herbs help to dilate blood vessels and increase blood flow in the body, oxygenating and nourishing tissues and boosting circulation to the extremities. Hawthorn, a stimulating heart remedy, is renowned for its ability to strengthen blood vessels and lower blood pressure. Ginkgo biloba, another popular circulatory herb, dilates the blood vessels to stimulate blood flow.

If there is a tendency to low blood pressure, panax ginseng, an adrenal stimulant, helps boost circulation. Rosemary has a tonic effect on the cardiovascular system to help boost the circulation.

Dilute juice from artichoke leaves and flower heads *with an equal amount of water and drink to support liver health. Or eat artichoke hearts regularly.*

Cholesterol-balancing herbs

Herbs can have a balancing effect on the body, helping to maintain healthy cholesterol levels in the blood by ensuring the efficient elimination of cholesterol through the liver, and also helping to balance and reduce unhealthy fats that are circulating in the blood stream. The high levels of antioxidants in fenugreek and globe artichoke also helps to protect the arteries from free radical damage.

Herbal blood tonics

Certain herbs work as nourishing, blood-building tonics. Nettles are a well-known traditional blood tonic. Iron-rich and with a high chlorophyll content, nettles help to boost red blood cell production to nourish cells around the body. Ashwagandha, a traditional Ayurvedic herb, also contains high levels of iron and is used to help strengthen the blood and increase vitality throughout the body.

Herbs to de-stress

The cardiovascular system is particularly sensitive to the effects of stress, which can lead to symptoms such as heart palpitations. Relaxing herbs, such as limeflowers, taken in a delicious infusion, can be extremely supportive during stressful periods, helping to control levels of anxiety and in turn reduce the risk of heart palpitations.

Circulatory toning herbs

Astringent herbs, such as horse chestnut and witch hazel, help to tighten and tone tissues, making them useful herbs for reducing the inflammation that is associated with varicose veins.

Essential oils

Soothing essential oils are used to help counter the stress and anxiety that can lead to circulatory problems, and also help to boost local circulation.

Blood pressure-balancing oils

Detoxifying and calming or sedative essential oils such as ylang ylang, yarrow, and lemon can be used in a massage to help control blood pressure during stressful periods. If you have a tendency to low blood pressure, a massage with circulatory stimulants such as rosemary and ginger can be beneficial.

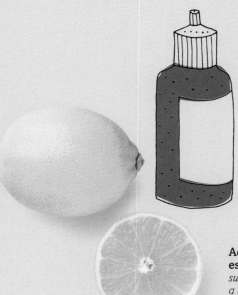

Add 4 drops lemon essential oil *to 10ml sunflower oil and enjoy a calming massage.*

"Essential oils can help to boost local circulation."

Oils to stimulate circulation

Essential oils are an effective way to improve local circulation if you have a tendency to cold hands and feet during chilly weather. Warming, luxurious oils, such as black pepper, ginger, and cypress, help to improve circulation and also have analgesic properties that can treat stiffness and pain.

Uplifting oils

For stressful days, uplifting essential oils such as lemon balm, neroli, and litsea soothe and calm, helping to reduce anxiety, avoid palpitations, and maintain emotional balance.

Supplements

A heart-healthy diet can be enhanced with well-chosen supplements, ensuring a reliable supply of nutrients to improve circulation and control cholesterol levels.

Getting the basics

A daily multi-vitamin and mineral supplement ensures levels of essential nutrients are maintained, supporting circulation.

Plaque-fighting garlic

Garlic, particularly "aged" garlic extract, is known for its cardiovascular benefits. When the bulbs are left to dry – for up to 20 months – not only is the odour removed, but levels of heart-healthy antioxidant phenols increase. Regular doses can help to prevent or even reverse the buildup of plaque in the arteries.

Omega-3 fatty acid supplements, derived from plants or marine sources, help to keep arteries in good condition and free from plaque. Taking these regularly helps to maintain healthy circulation and prevent blood clots.

Protective vitamin B

A daily B complex supplement boosts heart health. B vitamins, specifically folic acid, B6, and B12, help to break down a substance called homocysteine, high levels of which can damage blood vessel walls and lay the foundation for cholesterol deposits.

Circulation supporters

Antioxidant-rich rosehip powder and green tea supplements are fantastic choices for maintaining healthy circulation. Both of these contain compounds that protect cholesterol, preventing it from oxidizing and causing a buildup of plaque in the arteries.

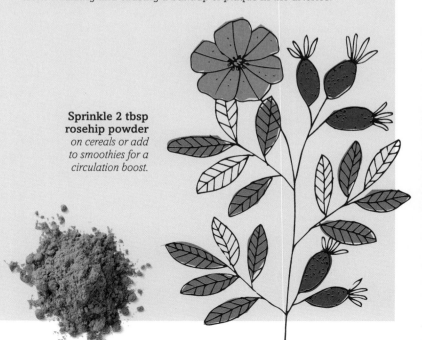

Sprinkle 2 tbsp rosehip powder *on cereals or add to smoothies for a circulation boost.*

TREATMENTS

HEART, CIRCULATION, AND BLOOD

When circulation is compromised so that oxygen and nutrients are not transported efficiently to tissues, or key nutrients are deficient in the diet, this can lead to a range of problems. Natural remedies stimulate blood flow and help keep blood healthy.

POOR CIRCULATION

A healthy circulation helps blood to move oxygen and nutrients around the body. If circulation in the arteries is slow, it can lead to Raynaud's and other problems such as chilblains, tinnitus, poor memory, and coronary heart disease. Poor blood flow in the veins causes varicose veins.

HERBS

Circulatory herbs help to dilate the blood vessels, increasing the blood flow and boosting the supply of oxygen and nutrients to the tissues and muscles around the body.

Ginkgo biloba relaxes blood vessels, boosting blood flow. Avoid in pregnancy, if breastfeeding, and with anticoagulant and antiplatelet medicines.
➡ *Take a 66mg leaf extract tablet, equal to 3300mg whole leaf, 1–3 times daily.*

Hawthorn is a strengthening tonic for the heart and is vasodilatory, improving peripheral circulation. Avoid with heart medication unless under medical supervision.
➡ *Infuse 1–2 tsp dried hawthorn in 175ml (6fl oz) boiling water and drink 3 times daily.*

Cayenne is a warming stimulant for the circulation taken internally and applied externally. Avoid with peptic ulcers, reflux, or on broken skin.
➡ *Take 1–2 drops tincture in water 3–4 times daily or add 10ml tincture to 3½ tbsp base cream for topical use.*

Ginger stimulates peripheral blood flow to help prevent problems such as chilblains, and also has pain-relieving properties. Avoid with peptic ulcers and gallstones.
➡ *Drink ginger root tea 3 times daily.*

ESSENTIAL OILS

Use oils that are rubefacient – causing the capillaries to dilate – to increase blood flow.

Ginger is a circulatory stimulant.
➡ *Add 5 drops to 10ml base oil and massage into the affected area.*

Rosemary acts as a stimulating tonic for the cardiovascular system. Avoid with epilepsy.
➡ *Mix 6 drops with a bath dispersant and add to a warm bath.*

Black pepper is warming so ideal for any conditions connected to the cold.
➡ *Add 5 drops to 10ml base oil and massage into the affected area.*

FOOD

Eat "warming" foods – experiment with hot spices and have warm drinks – and foods that support blood vessel health.

Oily fish, such as salmon and mackerel, contain omega-3, which aids circulation.
➡ *Have 2–3 portions a week.*

RECIPE

Blood vessel booster

Add a slice of chopped, fresh **chilli** to a cup of **blitzed vegetables** to kick-start circulation.

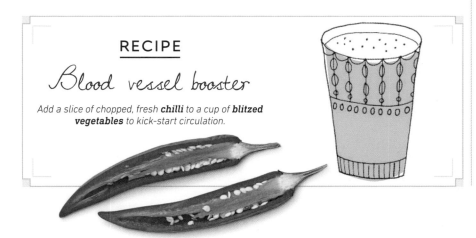

Oranges have bioflavonoids and vitamin C, which promote elasticity in vessels.
➽*Eat as a snack or freshly juiced.*

Cayenne, found in chilli peppers, strengthens blood vessels. Chillies are most potent raw or juiced.
➽*See recipe, opposite.*

Dark chocolate is rich in flavonoids, shown to boost circulation.
➽*Have 40g (1¼oz) 1–2 times a week.*

Apples and buckwheat contain rutin, a blood vessel strengthener.
➽*Eat buckwheat porridge and an organic apple a day.*

WHAT TO AVOID

Caffeine, because this constricts blood vessels, and salty and fatty foods.

SUPPLEMENTS

Supplements that thin blood and promote healthy veins can be supportive.

Garlic is a natural blood thinner and helps increase peripheral blood flow.
➽*Take 600mg daily.*

Vitamin C supports circulation by keeping veins and arteries healthy.
➽*Take 500mg to 1g daily.*

CoQ10 and vitamin E in combination aid peripheral circulation.
➽*Take 100mg CoQ10 and 500iu vitamin E daily.*

LIFESTYLE

Regular gentle exercise supports small blood vessels, avoiding blockages.

Wear appropriate outerwear: warm winter shoes, gloves and socks, and well-fitting shoes that aren't restricting.

Raise legs above heart level when you can to reduce the risk of varicose veins.

OTHER THERAPIES

Hydrotherapy with massage, or saunas with cold showers get blood flowing.

Acupuncture helps boost circulation.

Deep massage stimulates blood flow.

ANAEMIA

Insufficient haemoglobin – the oxygen-carrying pigment in red blood cells – or fewer red blood cells than normal can cause anaemia. Symptoms vary depending on the type and cause, but include tiredness, dizziness, shortness of breath, leg cramps, headache, and pallor.

HERBS

Herbs that act as blood tonics are strengthening and nutrient-rich, helping to support healthy blood cells and increase blood cell count. Herbs can also help to boost immunity and enhance energy levels to improve general health.

Nettle is an iron-rich strengthening blood tonic, high in chlorophyll, which helps to increase red blood cells.
➽*Eat fresh nettles in spring-time soups or infuse 1–2 tsp dried nettle in 175ml (6fl oz) boiling water. Drink 3 times daily.*

Yellow dock root is nutrient-rich, containing iron, potassium, and vitamin C; its cleansing action also boosts blood health. Avoid in pregnancy and if breastfeeding.
➽*Take 1–2ml tincture in a little water 3 times daily.*

Ashwagandha builds the blood cell count and is rich in iron to strengthen the blood. Avoid in pregnancy and with hyperthyroidism.
➽*Take 1 tsp powder in a warm milk drink with molasses for added iron and vitamins.*

WHAT TO AVOID

Astringent herbs, such as raspberry leaf, fenugreek, and yarrow, contain tannins and can interfere with iron absorption so take these separately from any iron medications, leaving three hours between the medication and the herb.

PITHY BENEFITS

If you don't mind its slightly bitter taste, avoid discarding the orange pith – this has as much vitamin C as the flesh and is also a good source of fibre.

FOOD

As well as iron-rich foods, include nutrients that aid the absorption of iron.

Liver is rich in iron and folate, which protects against some types of anaemia. Leafy greens, asparagus, and Brussels sprouts are also high in folate.
➽*Eat folate-rich foods daily; liver should be eaten only once a week.*

Cantaloupe melon has beta-carotene, which aids iron uptake. Also eat carrots, sweet potatoes, apricots, and squash.
➽*Start the day with ¼–½ melon.*

Citrus fruits are rich in vitamin C, which aids the absorption of iron.
➽*Have a citrus fruit or fresh juice daily.*

SUPPLEMENTS

These can aid efficient iron absorption.

Iron supplements may be advised.
➽*Take 40–200mg (dose determined by test results) ferrous sulphate 2–3 times daily, or an iron water supplement.*

Vitamin E deficiency is linked to anaemia.
➽*Take up to 400iu daily.*

Vitamin C is vital for iron absorption.
➽*Take 500mg to 1g daily.*

LIFESTYLE

Use cast-iron pans. There's evidence that these help raise blood iron levels.

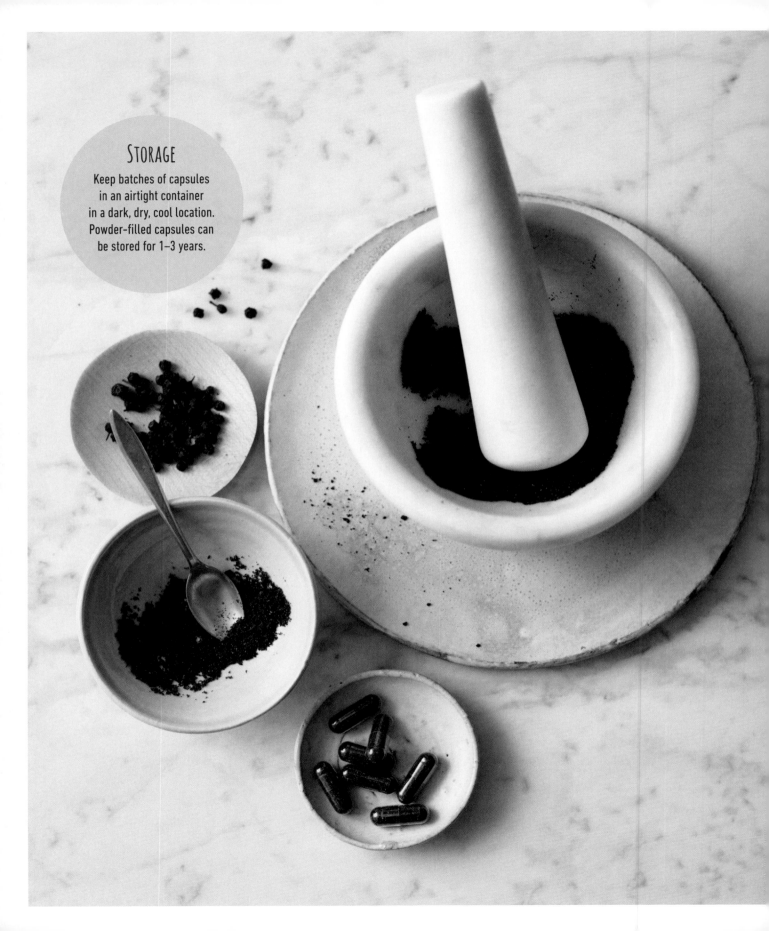

STORAGE

Keep batches of capsules
in an airtight container
in a dark, dry, cool location.
Powder-filled capsules can
be stored for 1–3 years.

HOW TO MAKE
HERBAL CAPSULES

With simple equipment, dried herbs can be ground down into powders and used to make your own herbal remedies in the form of easy-to-take capsules. Grinding down herbs into tiny particles gives the herb a larger surface area, which, in turn, allows the body to absorb more of its active constituents. Powders can also be used in poultices, or added to syrups, smoothies, and food.

Makes about 45 capsules

YOU WILL NEED

3 tbsp dried herbs

pestle and mortar, or coffee grinder

capsule-making machine, for either 735mg or 500mg capsules

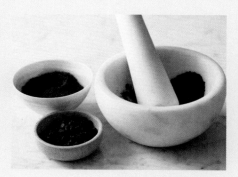

1 Grind the herbs in small batches with a pestle and mortar or coffee grinder. A pestle and mortar makes a finer powder with evenly sized particles that fill capsules more densely. If using a coffee grinder, grind in short bursts and use the grinder for herbal powders only.

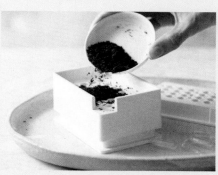

2 Before filling the capsules with the powdered herb, weigh an empty capsule and keep a note of its weight. After weighing, separate the two ends of each capsule and place in the capsule machine as instructed, ready for filling. Sprinkle the powder over the capsules and fill the capsules according to the manufacturer's instructions.

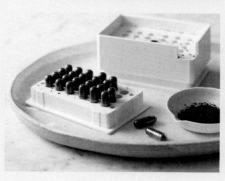

3 Once filled, remove the capsules from the machine. Weigh a filled capsule and subtract the weight of the empty capsule to ensure the dosage is correct. A full-capacity size "00" capsule is 735mg; a size "0" capsule is 500mg.

BLOOD PRESSURE

Hypertension, or high blood pressure, is a risk factor for heart disease and stroke. Hypotension, or low blood pressure, can restrict blood flow to the brain and other organs, causing dizziness if pressure is too low. The cause of blood pressure problems should be identified and treated.

HERBS

For high blood pressure, use herbs to help relax and dilate blood vessels and open up circulation, supported by relaxing heart tonics. Low blood pressure may benefit from circulatory or adrenal stimulants. Avoid stimulant herbs with hypertension.

FOR HIGH BLOOD PRESSURE

Hawthorn flowering tops and berries are heart tonics and nerve sedatives. Avoid with heart medication unless under medical supervision.
➥ *Take 3–5ml tincture in a little water 3 times daily, or make a fresh flower infusion in spring.*

Limeflowers relax the coronary arteries and nerves and open up circulation. Try combining with hawthorn, yarrow, and valerian.
➥ *See remedy, right.*

FOR LOW BLOOD PRESSURE

Rosemary stimulates circulation, especially to the head, and is a strengthening tonic herb. Avoid therapeutic doses in pregnancy.
➥ *Take 1–2ml tincture in a little water 3 times daily.*

Panax ginseng stimulates circulation and is a tonic for the adrenal glands to help strengthen circulation. Avoid with stimulants such as caffeine, asthma, nosebleeds, infections, or hypertension
➥ *Take powdered herb capsules, 400–500mg, 2–3 times daily.*

ESSENTIAL OILS

Oils that are detoxifying and calming or sedative can be used as hypotensives – lowering high blood pressure – while hypertensive oils help to raise blood pressure and are used for stimulating poor circulation.

FOR HIGH BLOOD PRESSURE

Ylang ylang is both hypotensive (lowering blood pressure) and sedative, helping to calm the mind.

Yarrow has hypotensive properties, helping to lower blood pressure.

Lemon is well known for its detoxifying effect and acts as a circulatory tonic.
➥ *Add 5 drops of any of the above oils to 10ml almond oil for a massage.*

FOR LOW BLOOD PRESSURE

Rosemary is a stimulant that can support low blood pressure. Avoid with epilepsy.

Ginger is a circulatory stimulant.
➥ *Add 5 drops of either of the above to 10ml grapeseed oil for a massage.*

FOOD

Numerous studies have shown that foods with a high antioxidant content, as well as those that are rich in potassium, can help to normalize blood pressure.

FOR HIGH BLOOD PRESSURE

Pomegranate juice, which is particularly high in heart-friendly antioxidants, has shown promise in lowering blood pressure.
➥ *Just 2 tbsp a day can be enough to make a difference to blood pressure.*

Walnuts are thought to be an effective way to lower high blood pressure associated with high cholesterol.
➥ *Include a generous handful – about 60g (2oz) – in your daily diet.*

Pistachios are a good source of potassium, which can help lower blood pressure. Dates are another reliable source of this essential mineral.
➥ *For a sweet treat, purée pistachios into a thick paste. Season with a pinch of Himalayan salt and stuff the mixture into whole de-seeded dates.*

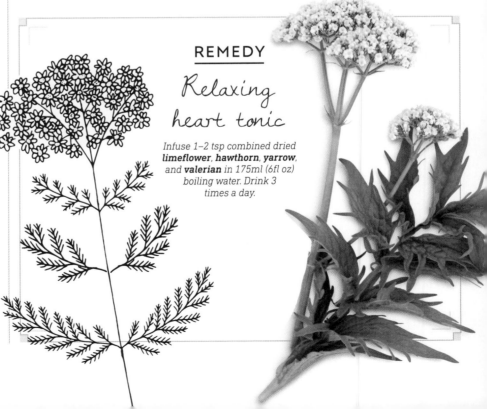

REMEDY

Relaxing heart tonic

*Infuse 1–2 tsp combined dried **limeflower**, **hawthorn**, **yarrow**, and **valerian** in 175ml (6fl oz) boiling water. Drink 3 times a day.*

> *"Studies show that a diet high in antioxidants and potassium helps to control blood pressure."*

Beetroot juice contains dietary nitrates, which can help to relax the blood vessel walls and therefore normalize blood flow in blood vessels – it is useful for both high and low blood pressure sufferers.
➼*Drink one glass a day on its own or in a mixed vegetable juice.*

FOR LOW BLOOD PRESSURE
Coffee and teas that contain caffeine can temporarily raise blood pressure in the event of an emergency – although this should not be used as a long-term strategy.

Salt can raise blood pressure, and those with hypotension are usually advised to add a little more – within reason – to their diets. People with high blood pressure may benefit from "Lo" or potassium salt as a substitute for sodium chloride.

WHAT TO AVOID
Alcohol should be limited or avoided.

SUPPLEMENTS

Supplements can boost dietary nutrients, supporting vascular health and circulation.

Probiotic supplements help lower systolic and diastolic blood pressure.
➼*Take a probiotic with 5–10 billion live organisms per dose daily.*

Garlic has been shown to reduce high blood pressure and is thought to be as effective as prescription drugs.
➼*Supplement with 600–900mg daily.*
Grapeseed extract contains antioxidant polyphenols, which are known to lower blood pressure.
➼*Take 25–150mg 1–3 times daily.*
Vitamin C, taken daily, helps to strengthen vascular tissue and has been shown to lower blood pressure to a similar extent as daily exercise.
➼*Take 500mg daily.*

LIFESTYLE

Eat smaller, more frequent low-carb meals throughout the day rather than fewer large meals to avoid the blood pressure drop that sometimes occurs after large meals.

Stay well hydrated. This is especially important for those with low blood pressure as dehydration can exacerbate the condition.

Sunlight is an important blood pressure "medication". Just 20 minutes of sunlight daily, without sun cream, alters levels of nitric oxide in the skin and blood, which in turn helps to lower blood pressure.

Compression stockings provide extra pressure to the feet, legs, and stomach, helping to stimulate circulation and increase blood pressure.

Yoga, both physical poses and breathing relaxation exercises, has been shown to reduce both systolic and diastolic blood pressure. Practise a yoga sequence daily at home and attend a regular class.

OTHER THERAPIES

Acupuncture has been shown to help lower chronic high blood pressure.
Mindfulness meditation is thought to be as effective as many drug interventions in bringing down high blood pressure.

HEART PALPITATIONS

Also known as arrhythmias, heart palpitations are a disturbance in the regular rhythm of the heart beat. Most types of palpitation are temporary, or due to stress, but regular palpitations with chest pain or shortness of breath should be treated by a doctor.

HERBS

Relaxing anti-anxiety and anti-stress herbs can be useful to help calm nervous palpitations. Cardiac tonics can also be used to strengthen the heart and to help regulate an erratic heartbeat.

Motherwort relaxes muscles and nerves and it is a strengthening tonic for the heart. Avoid during pregnancy, with heavy menstruation, or with palpitations.
➼*Take 1–4ml tincture in a little water 3 times daily.*
Limeflower is useful for relaxing spasms and relieving any nervous tension, in turn calming the heart and helping to lower high blood pressure.
➼*Infuse 1 tsp dried limeflower in 175ml (6fl oz) boiling water. Drink 3–4 times daily.*

BENEFITS BOTH WAYS
Beetroot juice holds on to nutrients such as vitamin C, depleted during cooking, though cooked beetroot is higher in dietary fibre.

➤ CONTINUED...

Hawthorn, a heart tonic, helps to strengthen the heart muscle. Avoid with heart medication unless under medical supervision.
➡️ *Take 3–5ml tincture in a little water 3 times daily.*

ESSENTIAL OILS

Therapeutic aromatherapy oils are useful in helping to control heart palpitations when these are linked to stress and feelings of anxiety.

Litsea cubeba has been used with success in clinical trials for cardiac arrhythmias.
Lemon balm has a calming effect on over-rapid breathing and also helps to soothe and calm a rapid heartbeat. See box, below.
Neroli helps to regulate the heart rhythm so can be beneficial for treating nervous heart conditions.
➡️ *Add 5 drops of any of the above essential oils to 10ml jojoba oil and use in a calming massage.*

SUPPLEMENTS

A few natural supplements may be helpful if you experience occasional palpitations.

Omega-3 marine oil stabilizes cardiac cell membranes to control palpitations.
➡️ *Take at least 1g daily.*
CoQ10 helps the muscles, including the heart muscle, to work properly.
➡️ *Take up to 30mg daily.*
Magnesium supports heart function.
➡️ *Aim for 200–400mg a day initially until symptoms resolve, then reduce your intake to 100–200mg daily.*

LIFESTYLE

Drink more water – at least 1.5–2 litres (2¾–3½ pints) daily. Dehydration can increase the risk of irregular rhythms.
Tackle insomnia. A lack of restful sleep raises the risk of an irregular heartbeat.
Avoid over-the-counter medicines that contain pseudoephedrine.
Lower stress. Chronic stress burdens the body and can lead to palpitations.

HIGH CHOLESTEROL

Cholesterol is a natural substance that the body needs to stay healthy. One type – high-density lipoprotein (HDL) is known as good cholesterol. The other type – low-density lipoprotein (LDL) – is unhealthy if there is too much, or it is damaged by free radical oxidation, increasing the risk of heart disease and stroke.

HERBS

These help reduce excessive cholesterol levels and balance blood fats, as well as reduce cholesterol production and increase its elimination via the liver.

Globe artichoke lowers blood fat and improves liver function to help reduce excess cholesterol. Avoid if sensitive to the *Asteraceae* plant family.
➡️ *Take a 250mg capsule of powdered leaf 3 times daily before meals.*
Fenugreek seed helps to lower cholesterol by slowing its absorption through the intestines. Avoid in pregnancy and with low thyroid activity. May impede the absorption of other drugs so take separately.
➡️ *Sprout seeds for salads, or infuse 1 tsp dried seeds in 175ml (6fl oz) boiling water and drink 3 times daily.*

FOOD

Switching to a plant-based diet that favours whole, fibre-rich foods over processed helps to control cholesterol.

Barley is a rich source of beta-glucan, a viscous soluble fibre, which has been shown to have similar cholesterol-lowering properties to oats.
➡️ *Use as a substitute for rice or on its own, using in a similar way to oatmeal.*

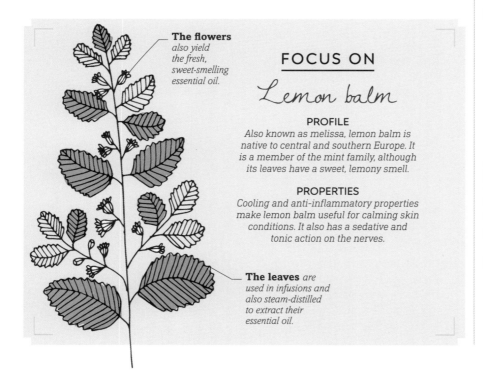

The flowers *also yield the fresh, sweet-smelling essential oil.*

FOCUS ON

Lemon balm

PROFILE
Also known as melissa, lemon balm is native to central and southern Europe. It is a member of the mint family, although its leaves have a sweet, lemony smell.

PROPERTIES
Cooling and anti-inflammatory properties make lemon balm useful for calming skin conditions. It also has a sedative and tonic action on the nerves.

The leaves *are used in infusions and also steam-distilled to extract their essential oil.*

Almonds increase levels of "good" HDL cholesterol, making this more active and helping reduce bad cholesterol.
➡️*Snack on a handful daily.*

Yogurt helps lower bad cholesterol and raise good cholesterol. *Lactobacillus acidophilus La5* and *Bifidobacterium lactis Bb12* cultures are beneficial.
➡️*Have 300g (10oz) daily, and unless on a diet use full-fat yogurt rather than low-fat artificially sweetened yogurt.*

Garlic has been shown to reduce high cholesterol and balance blood fats.
➡️*Add to food 3 times daily.*

WHAT TO AVOID
Limit red and processed meat.

SUPPLEMENTS

These enhance a healthy diet to help lower cholesterol levels and prevent oxidation.

Rosehip powder contains anti-inflammatory lycopene, which can protect LDL cholesterol from oxidation.
➡️*Add 40g (1¼oz) rosehip powder a day to apple juice, or take as a capsule.*

Probiotic supplements help lower cholesterol.
➡️*Take a daily broad-spectrum probiotic with 10 billion live cultures a dose.*

Green tea contains catechins, potent antioxidants that can lower cholesterol and protect against LDL oxidation.
➡️*Take a daily standard, caffeine-free supplement with 1300mg catechins.*

GARLIC PUNCH

Pulverizing garlic can increase its potency. Blitz 20g (¾oz) garlic with 1 tbsp anti-cholesterol lemon juice and drink as a shot or use as a dressing.

VARICOSE VEINS

Varicose veins are swollen and enlarged veins, usually blue or dark purple in colour. They may also be lumpy, bulging, or twisted in appearance and usually occur in the legs. Prolonged periods of standing, lack of exercise, and smoking are contributory factors.

HERBS

Tannins in astringent herbs tone and tighten the walls of veins and capillaries to reduce excessive dilation and leakages in blood vessels that can lead to varicose veins. Herbal circulatory stimulants are also used to help the rate that veins return blood to the heart.

Horse chestnut is astringent, anti-inflammatory, and also helps to tone the veins. Avoid with anticoagulants; if irritant to the stomach, take with limeflowers to soothe.
➡️*Take 1–4ml tincture in a little water 3 times daily.*

Witch hazel leaves are high in astringent tannins to help tone tissues and can be applied topically.
➡️*Make a cream, lotion, or gel using witch hazel water together with a horse chestnut infusion.*

Yarrow is an astringent blood vessel tonic and a stimulant for the circulation. Avoid during pregnancy and if you have a sensitivity to the *Asteraceae* plant family. Prolonged use can increase skin photosensitivity.
➡️*Infuse 1–2 tsp dried yarrow in 175ml (6fl oz) boiling water. Drink 3 times daily.*

ESSENTIAL OILS

Some essential oils are circulatory tonics, traditionally used to strengthen and support the circulatory system.

Cypress is known as a venous tonic, helping to strengthen veins.

Lemon is an excellent circulatory tonic, supporting healthy blood flow.
➡️*Add 5 drops of either of the above essential oils to 10ml calendula macerated oil and apply to the affected area with gentle upwards strokes, or use the blend in a small sitz bath. Alternatively, make a hot compress using 6 drops of either of the above essential oils in a bowl of hot water and apply to the affected area with a flannel or cloth.*

FOOD

Fresh wholefoods are packed with nutrients that can help to lower the risk of developing varicose veins.

Apples contain rutin, a flavonoid that strengthens capillaries.
➡️*Apples can be heavily treated with pesticides so have an organic apple each day.*

Watercress is a rich source of vitamin K.
➡️*Substitute watercress for lettuce as the base of your salads, or add to a green smoothie.*

Asparagus is rich in vitamins A, C, and K, which help strengthen the capillaries and veins.
➡️*Enjoy hot or cold as a side dish or salad ingredient.*

SUPPLEMENTS

B vitamins – in particular folic acid and vitamins B6 and B12 – help to break down a substance called homocysteine, which in excess can weaken the blood vessel walls.
➡️*Take a daily B complex that supplies 25–50mg of all the main B family vitamins.*

Vitamin C supports healthy circulation by keeping veins and arteries healthy and toned.
➡️*Take 500mg to 1g daily.*

➤ CONTINUED...

Vitamin E is an important vitamin for promoting vein health and therefore improving circulation.
➡*Take 1500iu daily.*

Vitamin K cream applied to varicose veins helps to strengthen capillaries.
➡*Apply daily to the affected area.*

LIFESTYLE

Wear compression stockings to support blood flow in the veins.

Avoid laxatives – both herbal, such as cascara and senna, and conventional.

Exercise regularly to boost circulation and aid weight loss if needed. Do 30 minutes exercise several times a week.

Avoid wearing high heels. Low-heeled shoes work the calf muscles more and so support the veins.

Elevate your legs. Take time each day to elevate the legs above heart level to stop blood pooling in them.

Avoid sitting or standing for long periods. Make a point of changing your position frequently to encourage blood flow and don't sit with crossed legs.

OTHER THERAPIES

Massage, especially vigorous types of massage such as Swedish, deep tissue massage, or lymphatic drainage, circulate the blood and lymph.

"Vigorous massage therapies help to move blood and lymph around the body to support the veins."

ATHEROSCLEROSIS

Atherosclerosis, a hardening of the arteries, is an early form of heart disease in which plaque builds up in arteries and limits blood flow to the major organs and extremities. Arterial plaque contains cholesterol, fat deposits, calcium, and fluid.

HERBS

Herbs can dilate blood vessels and improve blood flow. Herbs also balance and reduce fats in the blood and antioxidant herbs help to prevent arterial damage.

Hawthorn is antioxidant and opens up arteries to reduce atherosclerosis risk. Avoid with heart medication unless under medical supervision.
➡*Take 2–5ml tincture in a little water 3 times daily.*

Ginkgo biloba is antioxidant, helping to reduce arterial damage, and also stimulates circulation and dilates blood vessels. Avoid in pregnancy, if breastfeeding, and with anticoagulant and antiplatelet medicines.
➡*Take a 66mg leaf extract tablet providing the equivalent of 3300mg whole leaf, 1–3 times daily.*

FOOD

Eating a plant-based diet is one of the best ways to lower your risk of atherosclerosis. Base meals around vegetables, fruits, wholegrains, and legumes.

Pulses and beans supply fibre and protein and are low in fat.
➡*Eat more pulse-based dishes.*

Nuts and seeds are rich in vitamin E, fibre, plant sterols, and healthy fats.
➡*Eat a handful of walnuts or sprinkle 1 tbsp ground flaxseeds over salads, cereals, and soups daily.*

Sweet potatoes contain beta-carotene, which can help reduce the risk of arterial plaques. Other good sources include carrots, winter squash, cantaloupe melon, and apricots.
➡*Have a portion of one of these daily.*

Garlic reduces and balances cholesterol blood levels and prevents platelets sticking to promote healthy blood flow.
➡*Crush and add to dressings, soups, and meals 3 times daily.*

WHAT TO AVOID
Refined grains, added salt, and sweeteners. Salt intake should be no more than 1.5–2.4g a day.

SUPPLEMENTS

These can provide reliable amounts of nutrients to help reduce plaque formation and the tissue damage and inflammation caused by the oxidation of cholesterol.

Aged garlic extract has heart-healthy antioxidant phenols, which may help reverse the buildup of plaque.
➡*Take 2400mg every day.*

B vitamins help the body break down homocysteine, an amino acid that has been linked to an increased risk of heart disease and stroke.
➡ *Take 400mcg folic acid, up to 100mg vitamin B6, and up to 100mcg vitamin B12 a day.*

Omega-3 fatty acids can prevent the development of plaque and blood clots to protect against atherosclerosis.
➡*Take 1–4g daily.*

Beta-sitosterol, a plant sterol, prevents cholesterol absorption in the intestines.
➡*Take 800mg to 6g a day in separate doses, about 30 minutes before meals.*

OTHER THERAPIES

Acupuncture can help boost circulation, and address risk factors such as high blood pressure, smoking, and obesity.

Homeopathic remedies can be helpful for health throughout the body.

STROKE

A stroke is when circulation to the brain fails, depriving cells of oxygen, and can cause loss of vision and/or speech, paralysis, and confusion. Natural remedies can reduce risk factors and support recovery.

HERBS

These can help lower blood pressure, strengthen and dilate blood vessels, and reduce blood fats and inflammation.

Yarrow relaxes, dilates, and tones blood vessels and is anti-inflammatory. Avoid in pregnancy or with sensitivity to the *Asteraceae* plant family. Prolonged use can increase skin photosensitivity.
➤ *Infuse 1 tsp dried yarrow in 175ml (6fl oz) boiling water. Drink 3 times a day.*

Ginkgo biloba, an antioxidant, aids circulation. Avoid in pregnancy, if breastfeeding, and with anticoagulant and antiplatelet medicines.
➤ *Take a 66mg leaf extract tablet providing the equivalent of 3300mg whole leaf, 1–3 times daily.*

Feverfew reduces the risk of clotting. See box, right. Avoid in pregnancy or with anticoagulants.
➤ *Take 2ml tincture in a little water 3 times daily.*

FOOD

A plant-based diet with fresh produce provides vital antioxidants and nutrients.

Tomatoes have the antioxidant lycopene, linked to a lower risk of stroke in men.
➤ *Eat tomatoes regularly.*

Wholegrains significantly cut stroke risk.
➤ *Eat at least 2 portions a day.*

Chillies contain vitamin C and capsaicin to help support healthy blood vessels.
➤ *Add to soups, stews, and juices.*

Ginger has anti-clotting properties.
➤ *Add around 5g a day to fruit and vegetable juices, soups, and meals.*

WHAT TO AVOID
Research shows that sweet fizzy drinks and juice can impact artery health. High alcohol intake can affect heart rhythm.

SUPPLEMENTS

Target supplements to reduce stroke risk. A daily multi-vitamin provides key nutrients.

B vitamins help break down a substance called homocysteine, which in excess can damage blood vessel walls.
➤ *Take a daily B complex with 25–50mg of the main B vitamins.*

Garlic helps thin the blood.
➤ *Take 800mg of a high-quality garlic powder each day.*

Magnesium helps to lower blood pressure and reduce the risk of stroke.
➤ *Take 240–420mg daily.*

Potassium maintains fluid balance, and keeps organs and muscles functioning.
➤ *Take 3g daily if food sources are low.*

MAXIMIZING NUTRIENTS

Cooking tomatoes makes lycopene more available to the body, while ginger is most powerful when eaten fresh.

LIFESTYLE

Exercise regularly – a sedentary lifestyle almost doubles the risk of stroke, so aim to exercise at least 2–3 times a week and stay active generally.

Cut down, or give up, smoking.

Manage depression and anxiety as keeping these in check can help to lower the risk of stroke.

Yoga, practised regularly, can help improve balance, confidence, and mobility in long-term stroke survivors.

FOCUS ON

Feverfew
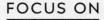

PROFILE
This is grown widely in northern temperate regions and was traditionally used to treat arthritis.

PROPERTIES
Feverfew is anti-inflammatory, dilating blood vessels and inhibiting platelet clumping. It can also be used to stimulate digestion.

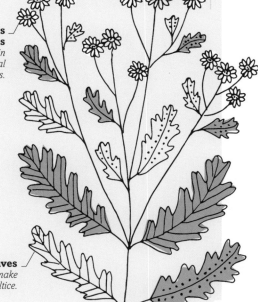

The flowers and stems *are used in medicinal infusions.*

The leaves *can be pulped to make a soothing poultice.*

BRAIN AND NERVOUS SYSTEM

Our brain and nervous system make up the body's control centre, sending messages via a complex network of nerves to govern our thoughts and actions and allow us to store information. Learn how to tailor your diet and use herbal and essential oil remedies to enhance memory and promote healthy nerve connections. If damage, inflammation, or disorders do occur, explore how holistic healing can help to remedy problems, cope with difficult symptoms, and support recovery.

STAYING WELL

BRAIN AND NERVOUS SYSTEM

This complex system benefits from care and attention to protect it from damage as we age and to help optimize its health. Key nutrients and targeted herbal and essential oil preparations support and strengthen neural health, keeping the mind and memory agile and maximizing brain function to keep you alert and focused throughout the day.

FOOD

Diet can be targeted to optimize the health of the brain and nerves. Key nutrients boost blood flow to the brain, help renew cells, and strengthen neural connections.

MEMORY BOOSTERS

Pungent herbs and spices, such as cinnamon, turmeric, and ginger, are not only rich in antioxidants, but also consuming these regularly is thought to help improve "working" memory – needed for everyday cognitive tasks such as decision-making, planning, and problem solving. The compound curcumin in turmeric, as well as boosting blood flow to the brain, is thought to help support memory by preventing plaque deposits forming in the brain.

Blueberries, and in fact berries of all kinds, are also thought to aid and improve memory. Berries are rich in antioxidant and anti-inflammatory plant pigments called anthocyanins, which studies suggest stimulate brain activity in the part of the brain that is connected to cognitive function, so helping to boost working memory.

BRAIN-CELL PROMOTERS

Certain foods are thought to support brain cell connections. Celery is rich in a substance called apigenin, which has been shown to build and strengthen connections between brain cells. Parsley, thyme, chamomile, and red pepper also contain this compound, so eat these foods regularly to boost brain health.

BRAIN-FUELLING FATS

The brain and nervous system needs a range of healthy fats to support brain cell renewal. Medium-chain triglycerides (MCTs), such as those found in coconut oil, are particularly beneficial because they are rapidly absorbed, providing an immediate source of fuel for the brain, so incorporate MCTs into your daily diet to support brain health.

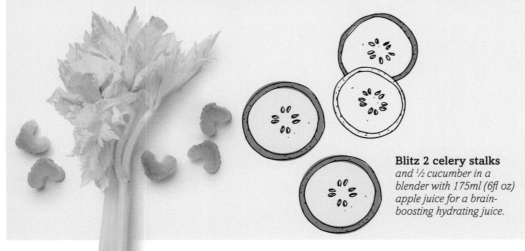

Blitz 2 celery stalks
and ½ cucumber in a blender with 175ml (6fl oz) apple juice for a brain-boosting hydrating juice.

> *"Essential nutrients can stimulate blood flow to the brain and strengthen neural connections."*

Take 1–2ml passionflower tincture *in a little water 3 times daily to strengthen and support the nerves.*

Foods to soothe

Almond skins contain a natural aspirin-like substance called salicin, which can help to ward off headaches, so if you find tension and stress are a headache trigger, try snacking on a handful of unpeeled almonds to stop pain building up when you are facing a stressful situation.

Apple cider vinegar may have an indirect effect that helps counter headaches. The acid in apple cider vinegar is thought to be milder than stomach acid, so when mixed with water, it can help neutralize excess stomach acid and ease headaches that are caused by digestive complaints.

Vital hydration

Staying well hydrated is crucial for optimizing brain function. Being dehydrated actually reduces brain volume and in turn impacts on brain function. Drinking plenty of healthy fluids throughout the day will help you stay alert and focused – aim to drink 1.5–2 litres (2¾–3½ pints) of water or herbal teas daily.

Herbs

Herbal preparations can both stimulate and relax the brain and protect it from the harmful effects of stress.

Anti-inflammatory herbs

As well as being used as a spice to flavour food, turmeric is also used in herbal preparations. Turmeric has neuro-protective properties that help to prevent inflammation and oxidative damage in the brain. In addition, turmeric provides a boost to the immune system, which helps to support neurological health throughout the body.

Tension-releasing herbs

Herbal preparations with ginger and chamomile have an anti-inflammatory effect that can help to ease tension in the body when you anticipate a stressful day or feel tension building.

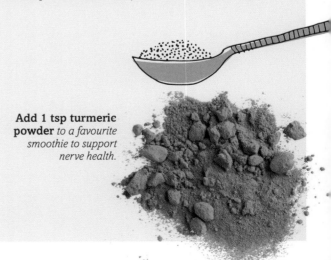

Add 1 tsp turmeric powder *to a favourite smoothie to support nerve health.*

Nerve-protecting herbs

Astragalus root is a popular Chinese medicine that is primarily used as an adaptogen – which is a type of herb that helps the body to function during periods of stress and therefore protects the body against the negative effects of physical, mental, or emotional stress. As well as its adaptogenic function, astragalus root also has protective properties that help to promote healthy nerve cell replication.

Nourishing nerve tonics

Popular sedative herbs, such as passionflower, vervain, and skullcap, act as nerve tonics to help strengthen and support nerve health and aid relaxation.

Herbs for memory

Stimulating herbs that help to boost circulation to the brain and therefore nourish and oxygenate tissues can be helpful for sharpening memory. Rosemary is a renowned herbal remedy for improving working memory. Or try uplifting lemon balm – actually a member of the mint plant family – which has been shown to improve cognitive function and memory, even in those with Alzheimer's.

Essential oils

Aromatherapy is a quick and effective way to calm the body and mind and counter the mental effects of stress, avoiding loss of focus and memory lapses.

Oils to release tension

Analgesic essential oils are beneficial where there is a tendency to tension headaches. Peppermint has a dual action, first cooling the mind, then warming to ease tension. Lemongrass is pain-relieving and its refreshing aroma stimulates the mind.

Mind-sharpening oils

Studies show that warming and anti-inflammatory rosemary can clear the mind rapidly and enhance mental clarity to refocus the mind and overcome mental fatigue.

Massage mind benefits

Chronic stress can exacerbate mental blocks, thwarting creative and mental processes, and also worsen existing nerve pain. Sedative oils, such as sweet marjoram, can warm and relax

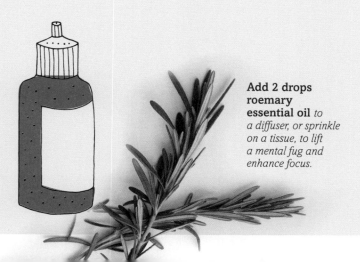

Add 2 drops roemary essential oil *to a diffuser, or sprinkle on a tissue, to lift a mental fug and enhance focus.*

Take resveratrol capsules – derived from grape skins – as directed to obtain the antioxidant benefits.

muscles and soothe nerves, while grounding and calming oils, such as vetiver, help to let go of held-in tension and promote relaxation, reviving spirits and re-energizing the mind.

SUPPLEMENTS

Nutrient deficiencies can hamper memory and brain function. Supplements can support the diet to sustain nutrient levels and promote healthy brain function.

ANTIOXIDANT PROTECTION

Antioxidant supplements may reduce or neutralize free radicals, protecting brain function in the short and long term. For example, resveratrol, derived from grape skins, is a polyphenol – an antioxidant plant compound – that has been shown to provide some protection against several neuro-degenerative disorders such as Parkinson's, Alzheimer's, and motor neurone disease.

CIRCULATION BOOSTER

Pycnogenol, derived from maritime pine bark, is believed to increase cerebral blood flow and improve brain function.

IRON CHECK

Iron deficiency, as well as causing fatigue, can lead to lower levels of dopamine in the part of the brain associated with movement, which in turn can damage the nerves and contribute to conditions such as restless leg syndrome. If tests show that iron levels are low, supplementing can be useful to protect and support the nerves.

BRAIN-ENHANCING B VITAMINS

The B vitamin family plays an important role in brain health, supporting the production of neurotransmitters such as serotonin, which affect mood and pain sensation. A daily B complex aids the production of neurotransmitters. Taking coenzyme Q10 (CoQ10), which acts like a vitamin, with a B complex may help to prevent migraines.

B vitamins also reduce levels of the amino acid homocysteine – high levels are toxic to the brain and linked to poor memory.

MAGNESIUM TOP UP

The nervous system requires adequate magnesium levels to function properly. A lack of magnesium may lead to migraines, so supplementing can be preventative.

"Therapeutic oils help to calm the mind and counter the negative effects of stress on the brain."

5

RECIPES FOR WELLNESS

SOUPS

Sustaining and delicious, these simple soups deliver a medley of nutrients, with vitamins and minerals from the vegetables retained in the liquid. Heat the oil in a pan, add the onion and garlic, and cook for 4 minutes. Add any spices and cook for a further 4–5 minutes, then add the remaining ingredients. Bring to the boil, simmer for 30–40 minutes, then serve, topping with any garnish.

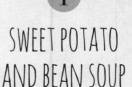

1

SWEET POTATO AND BEAN SOUP

This soup has heart-healthy credentials. Sweet potato is high in antioxidants to fight free-radical damage and prevent plaque build up in arteries, while antioxidant lycopene in tomatoes is linked to a reduced risk of heart disease.

SERVES 2–4 • **PREP TIME** 15 MINS • **COOK TIME** 40–50 MINS

1 tsp olive oil

1 red onion, diced

1 clove of garlic, diced

¼ tsp red chilli (or to taste), deseeded and diced

¼ tsp dried oregano

225g (8oz) sweet potato, peeled and diced

1 stick of celery, diced

1 small leek, sliced

400g can chopped tomatoes

400g can borlotti beans, drained and rinsed

500ml (16fl oz) vegetable stock

freshly ground black pepper

basil leaves, to garnish

Nutritional info per serving:
Kcals 165 Fat 1.5g Saturated fat 0.5g Carbohydrates 26g Sugar 10g Sodium 334mg Fibre 8g Protein 8g Cholesterol 0mg

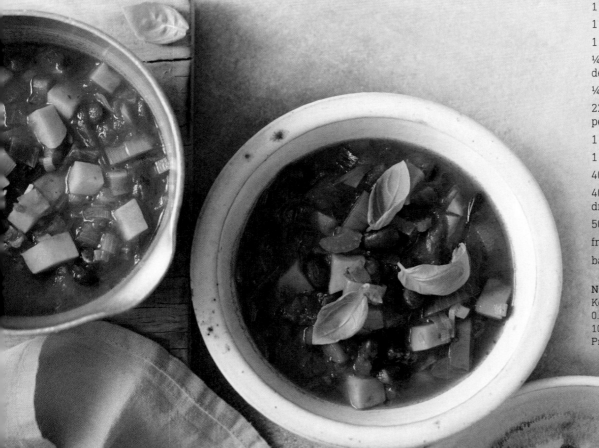

2
Fish Soup

Salmon provides cell-building protein and anti-inflammatory omega-3 fatty acids, while the main compound in ginger, gingerol, has potent anti-inflammatory and antioxidant properties.

**SERVES 4 • PREP TIME 15 MINS •
COOK TIME 40–50 MINS**

1 tbsp coconut oil

100g (3½oz) red onion, diced

1 clove of garlic, diced

¼ tsp chilli flakes

1 tsp lemon grass paste

1 tsp grated fresh ginger

300g (10oz) tomatoes, quartered

85g (3oz) green beans, chopped into 2.5cm (1 inch) slices

350g (12oz) fish-pie mix (salmon, cod, and haddock), cut into chunks

1 tbsp fish sauce

1½ tbsp lime juice

500ml (16fl oz) fish stock

400ml (14fl oz) coconut milk

2 kaffir leaves

Nutritional info per serving:
Kcals 346 Fat 26g Saturated fat 18g Carbohydrates 8g Sugar 6g Sodium 917mg Fibre 2.5g Protein 19g Cholesterol 52mg

3
Thai-style butternut soup

Squash is abundant in protective antioxidants, while sweetcorn and peas supply vitamin C to boost immunity and support collagen production.

**SERVES 2 • PREP TIME 30 MINS •
COOK TIME 40–50 MINS**

1 tsp coconut oil

1 small red onion, diced

1 clove of garlic, diced

1 tsp soy sauce

1 tsp red chilli, deseeded and diced

½ tsp turmeric

1 tsp lemon grass paste

2.5cm (1 inch) piece of fresh ginger, peeled and diced

225g (8oz) butternut squash, peeled, deseeded, diced, and roasted for 30 minutes at 200°C (400°F/Gas mark 6)

4 tbsp vegetable stock

60g (2oz) baby sweetcorn

60g (2oz) sugar snap peas

30g (1oz) rice noodles

175ml (6fl oz) coconut milk

grated zest of 1 lime

10 coriander leaves, to garnish

Nutritional info per serving:
Kcals 317 Fat 17g Saturated fat 14g Carbohydrates 31g Sugar 12g Sodium 561mg Fibre 5.5g Protein 7g Cholesterol 0mg

4
Tomato and Basil Soup

Lycopene in tomatoes has impressive disease-protecting properties, while red onion provides chromium to help regulate blood sugar levels.

**SERVES 4 • PREP TIME 10 MINS •
COOK TIME 40–50 MINS**

1 tbsp olive oil

200g (7oz) red onion, diced

2 cloves of garlic, diced

550g (1¼lb) tomatoes, halved

1 tbsp balsamic vinegar

750ml (1¼ pints) vegetable or chicken stock

2 tsp tomato purée

¾ tbsp basil, chopped

1 tsp freshly ground black pepper

Nutritional info per serving:
Kcals 54 Fat 0.5g Saturated fat 0g Carbohydrates 9g Sugar 8.5g Sodium 456mg Fibre 3g Protein 2g Cholesterol 0mg

5
Easy Vegetable soup

This medley of vegetables, packed with essential micronutrients, is coupled with fibre-rich lentils, which help to lower cholesterol and prevent blood sugar spikes. Adapt the vegetable mix to suit the season.

**SERVES 4 • PREP TIME 15 MINS •
COOK TIME 40–50 MINS**

1 tbsp olive oil

100g (3½oz) red onion, diced

1 clove of garlic, diced

1 tsp oregano

85g (3oz) carrots, peeled and sliced

100g (3½oz) green beans, chopped into 2.5cm (1 inch) slices

100g (3½oz) leeks, sliced

250g (9oz) new potatoes, sliced

390g can green lentils, drained and rinsed

1.5–2 litres (2¾–3½ pints) vegetable stock

Nutritional info per serving:
Kcals 190 Fat 4g Saturated fat 0.5g Carbohydrates 25g Sugar 6g Sodium 1211mg Fibre 7g Protein 10g Cholesterol 0mg

TREATMENTS

BRAIN AND NERVOUS SYSTEM

A healthy brain and nervous system depends on connections between billions of neurons, or nerve cells. Diet, lifestyle, mechanical damage, and ageing can all affect this complex system. Natural remedies and nutrients ease symptoms and support healing.

HEADACHES

Most headaches are linked to lifestyle rather than an underlying condition. Even so, headaches are the reason for more doctor visits than any other condition, and more drugs are prescribed, or bought, for headaches than for any other condition.

HERBS

Muscle-relaxing herbs help to ease pain. Migraines and cluster headaches – which strike intermittently over a period of time and may be hormone-linked – can benefit from liver tonics, which balance hormones.

Feverfew helps to prevent migraines. It also has bitter properties that support the liver. Avoid during pregnancy, or if taking anticoagulants.
➡ *Take a 50–200mg dried-leaf capsule daily.*

Ginger is anti-inflammatory and relaxes muscles, making it helpful for headaches and migraines, especially if accompanied by nausea. Avoid with peptic ulceration and gallstones.
➡ *Make a cup of freshly sliced ginger root tea and sip as required.*

Chamomile relaxes the central nervous system and has an anti-inflammatory action that helps to relieve headaches and migraines. Avoid with sensitivity to the *Asteraceae* plant family.
➡ *Infuse 1–2 tsp dried chamomile in 175ml (6fl oz) boiling water and drink 3 times daily.*

ESSENTIAL OILS

There are a number of therapeutic essential oils that can relieve both the causes and the symptoms of headaches. Identifying the underlying cause of a headache can help you to select the most appropriate essential oil and the best method of application.

Lavender is renowned for soothing and calming, making it especially helpful for headaches that are brought on by stress and anxiety.
➡ *Add 3 drops to a diffuser and inhale, or make a compress, as shown below.*

Peppermint has analgesic properties and is an effective traditional remedy for migraines.

Rosemary has a stimulating action and can ease headaches that are caused by concentrating for long periods of time. Avoid with epilepsy.
➡ *Add 3 drops of any of the above oils to a bowl of cold water and make a cold compress using a clean flannel or cloth to apply to the forehead or back of the neck.*

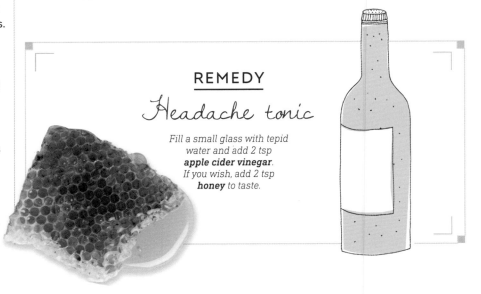

REMEDY

Headache tonic

Fill a small glass with tepid water and add 2 tsp **apple cider vinegar**. If you wish, add 2 tsp **honey** to taste.

FOOD

Foods can often cause headaches, but certain foods have soothing properties.

Almonds contain the natural "aspirin", salicin, in their skin.
➥*Eat a handful of unpeeled almonds when you feel a headache coming on.*
Apple cider vinegar works as a simple tonic for headaches that are linked to digestive distress.
➥*See remedy, opposite.*
WHAT TO AVOID
Foods that contain nitrates, such as processed and smoked meats, can trigger cluster headaches. Also, caffeine in coffee, tea, and chocolate constricts blood vessels and increases pressure in the head. Withdrawing caffeine can actually bring on headaches, so a gradual withdrawal may be needed.

SUPPLEMENTS

A tendency towards headaches may signal nutrient deficiencies.

Multi-vitamins can help make up for deficiencies in the diet that may contribute to headaches.
➥*Take a daily multi-vitamin.*
Magnesium deficiency is linked to migraines.
➥*Take 600mg daily for a few months, until brain levels of the mineral recover and symptoms resolve.*
CoQ10 may help prevent migraines.
➥*Take 150mg daily.*
B vitamins are vital for the production of neurotransmitters, such as serotonin, which mediate our perception of pain. B vitamins are also helpful for stress- and anxiety-related headaches.
➥*Take a B complex daily.*
Gamma-linolenic acid (GLA) from evening primrose, blackcurrant, or borage seed oil may reduce the likelihood of a headache.
➥*Take 500mg to 1g daily.*

> " *Nutrient deficiencies may explain a tendency towards headaches.* "

LIFESTYLE

Avoid indoor pollution. Dust, mould, cigarette smoke, cleaning products, and perfumes may trigger a sensitivity or allergic reaction, causing headaches.
Eye strain from being on a computer all day or working in poor lighting is a common cause of tension headaches.
Stay hydrated. Severe dehydration causes the brain to shrink away from the skull, causing head pain.
Weather changes, particularly in spring and autumn, are a common trigger for the type of migraine known as a cyclic headache.
Exercise regularly. Exercise can be as effective for treating headaches and migraines as conventional painkillers.
Avoid too many painkillers. Overuse of painkillers can cause a "rebound" or "overuse" headache. Try to find other ways to deal with the pain.

OTHER THERAPIES

Chiropractic and osteopathy can help relieve headache pain caused by poor or misaligned posture.
Reflexology stimulates pressure points in the feet to treat both the physical and emotional causes of headaches.
Acupuncture has been shown to be an effective treatment for headaches.

RESTLESS LEG SYNDROME

This is typified by an aching, pulling, itching, crawling sensation in the legs that makes it impossible to keep them still. Symptoms are generally worse during the night and while sedentary, and the condition is especially common during pregnancy.

HERBS

Antispasmodic and relaxing herbs help to relieve symptoms to enable you to rest and sleep. Nerve tonics can help to strengthen and support nerve health.

Passionflower is relaxing for muscles and nerves, relieving spasms and tension, and is a sedative, promoting sleep. May cause drowsiness.
➥*Infuse 1–2 tsp dried passionflower in 175ml (6fl oz) boiling water and drink 3 times daily.*
Vervain is a relaxing tonic for the nerves and eases tension. Avoid in pregnancy; excessive doses may cause vomiting.
➥*Take 2.5–5ml tincture in a little water 3 times daily.*
Skullcap is a nourishing nerve tonic and relaxes spasms and tremors.
➥*Take 3–5ml tincture in a little water 3 times daily.*

QUALITY CONTROL

High acid levels in apple cider vinegar mean it doesn't need chilling once opened as the acid guards against bacteria. To preserve quality, store in a cool, dark cupboard.

➤ CONTINUED...

ESSENTIAL OILS

Relaxing essential oils help to ease feelings of anxiety and stress.

Marjoram has analgesic, antispasmodic, and sedative activity.
➡ *Add 5 drops to 10ml base oil and massage into the legs.*
Vetiver is an effective sedative.
➡ *Add 6 drops to a bath dispersant.*

SUPPLEMENTS

A tendency towards restless legs may indicate some nutrient deficiencies.

Iron deficiency is linked to lower levels of dopamine in the area of the brain associated with movement. Before you supplement, have a blood test to check your levels. If you need a supplement, ferrous fumarate, ferrous sulphate, or ferrous gluconate are better absorbed than those containing ferric iron.
➡ *Doses up to 200mg 3 times daily may be effective.*
Folic acid can alleviate restless leg syndrome not linked to pregnancy.
➡ *Take up to 400mcg daily.*

LIFESTYLE

Disrupted sleep can worsen symptoms, so address irregular sleep routines.
Warm up, or cool down. Both heating pads or ice packs on the legs can relieve symptoms.
Gentle daytime exercise can help. Conversely, too much vigorous exercise may worsen symptoms.
Stress can exacerbate symptoms. Find ways to relieve anxiety.
Yoga helps balance sleep, mood, and blood pressure with restless leg syndrome.

OTHER THERAPIES

Acupuncture can be a useful longer-term treatment for the condition.

CARPAL TUNNEL SYNDROME

Carpal tunnel syndrome is pressure on the median nerve in the wrist, often due to repetitive movements. It causes tingling, numbness, and pain in the hand and fingers and reduces the ability to grip with or flex fingers.

HERBS

Anti-inflammatory herbs relieve swelling in the tissues around the median nerve to reduce pressure, while antispasmodic herbs can help to ease muscle tension.

Turmeric is antioxidant and reduces inflammation in the body to ease swelling and pain. Avoid therapeutic doses in pregnancy. May cause skin rashes or reactions in sunlight. Seek professional advice with gallstones.
➡ *Blend ½–1 tsp powder in warmed coconut milk and drink 3 times daily.*

St John's wort reduces nerve inflammation to heal and soothe pain locally. Avoid internally in pregnancy and high doses in strong sunlight. Taken internally, interacts with many prescription medicines.
➡ *Make a macerated flower oil and apply regularly to the affected area.*
White willow bark is anti-inflammatory and analgesic, easing nerve and muscle pain. Avoid in pregnancy, if breastfeeding, and with sensitivity to the salicylate plant family.
➡ *Take 1–5ml tincture in a little water 3 times daily.*

ESSENTIAL OILS

Analgesic and inflammatory oils can help to relieve some carpal tunnel symptoms. However, whichever therapeutic treatment you choose, it can often take months for the pain to resolve itself.

Sweet marjoram is a warming oil, which can relieve pain and discomfort.
Lemongrass is a soothing analgesic.

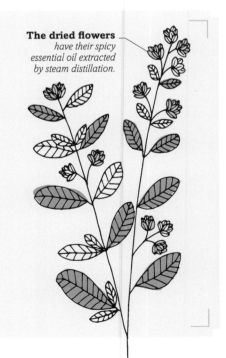

FOCUS ON

Sweet marjoram

PROFILE
Originating from the Mediterranean, this warming plant has a well-established history as a medicinal remedy.

PROPERTIES
Deeply relaxing, marjoram is renowned for its sedative properties and it has an analgesic action that relieves tension.

The dried flowers *have their spicy essential oil extracted by steam distillation.*

Peppermint has an effective anaesthetic action for pain relief.
➡*Add 5 drops of any of the above essential oils to 10ml almond oil and use in a massage, working from the hands to the neck.*

SUPPLEMENTS

Carpal tunnel syndrome is a mechanical problem of the wrist so supplements won't actually resolve the problem, but they may be supportive when taken alongside other approaches to tackling the condition, or be a preventative measure.

Vitamin B6 deficiency can increase vulnerability to carpal tunnel syndrome.
➡*Taking 50–200mg daily may help to relieve the symptoms.*

LIFESTYLE

Repetitive strain injury is a major cause of carpal tunnel syndrome. If you are making repeated movements that place a strain on your wrist you will need to stop these to allow time for healing to take place.
Wrist splints worn at night can help to relieve nerve pressure.
Diabetes and rheumatoid arthritis raise your risk of carpal tunnel syndrome so it's important to treat these conditions.

OTHER THERAPIES

Osteopathy and chiropractic both claim success in helping to treat carpal tunnel syndrome.
Acupuncture and electro-acupuncture, which uses small electric currents, can help reduce pain and swelling.
Yoga can help reduce pain and increase the strength of your grip.
Cold therapy can help. An ice pack applied to the wrist for 10–15 minutes, once or twice an hour can relieve pain.

MEMORY AND COGNITION

New brain cells may be generated at a slower rate as we age, but a decline in memory is not inevitable. Keeping an active brain and doing what you can to support brain health through diet and lifestyle supports the brain. If you notice a cognitive decline, seek medical advice as there may be a treatable cause.

HERBS

Stimulating herbs can be taken to boost brain circulation to nourish and oxygenate the tissues, while antioxidant herbs reduce cellular nerve damage. Herbs can also enhance nerve transmission to sharpen mental capacity.

Rosemary is a potent antioxidant and tonic herb that stimulates circulation to the brain. Avoid therapeutic doses during pregnancy.
➡*Take 1–2ml tincture in a little water 3 times daily.*
Ginkgo biloba is antioxidant and boosts oxygen delivery to the brain, improving cognition. Avoid in pregnancy, when breastfeeding, and with anticoagulant and antiplatelet medications.
➡*Take a 66mg leaf extract tablet providing the equivalent of 3300mg whole leaf, 1–3 times daily.*
Sage can improve memory and enhance feelings of alertness. In particular it has been shown to inhibit an enzyme called acetylcholinesterase (AChE), which breaks down acetylcholine, an important chemical messenger involved in information transmission in the brain. Avoid therapeutic doses during pregnancy and with epilepsy.
➡*Take a 300–600mg tablet daily, or take in a tincture or infusion. Can also be inhaled as an essential oil.*

FINE TO DRY

Rosemary retains its properties when dried. If you have an excess of the fresh herb, wash and dry the sprigs, tie them in a bundle, and hang in an airy room for about 2 weeks.

Lemon balm helps improve cognitive function and enhance accuracy of memory. Avoid with hypothyroidism.
➡*Infuse 1–2 tsp dried lemon balm in 175ml (6fl oz) boiling water and drink 3 times daily.*

ESSENTIAL OILS

Vaporizing, or diffusing, therapeutic oils into the environment can help to focus the mind and overcome mental fatigue.

Rosemary has a strong tradition as an aid for memory and concentration. Avoid with epilepsy.
Clove is relaxing and is used as a mental tonic, assuaging feelings of anxiety and enhancing focus.
Peppermint can help to clear the head and supports concentration.
➡*Add 3 drops of any of the above essential oils to a diffuser and inhale.*

FOOD

The most important foods for supporting memory and brain function are those that are rich in antioxidants.

Grape juice is high in antioxidants, including resveratrol, which enhances memory and brain performance.
➡*Enjoy a glass daily, or freeze fresh grapes and enjoy as a refreshing snack on a hot day.*

➤ CONTINUED...

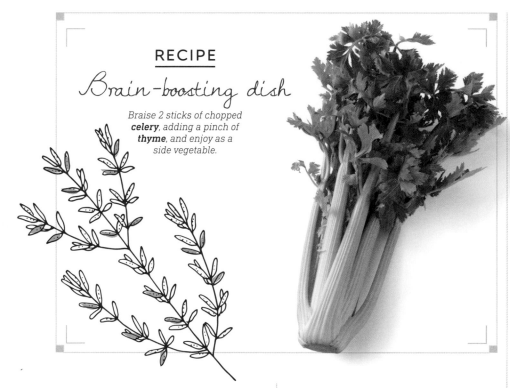

RECIPE

Brain-boosting dish

Braise 2 sticks of chopped **celery**, adding a pinch of **thyme**, and enjoy as a side vegetable.

Herbs and spices such as cinnamon, turmeric, and ginger, if eaten regularly, may improve "working" memory and cognition, needed for making decisions, planning, and problem solving.
➡ *Grind some cinnamon into your coffee or enjoy a chai tea.*

Blueberries are rich in antioxidants, in particular anti-inflammatory anthocyanidins, which can help to increase brain activity and support working memory.
➡ *Drink 500ml (16fl oz) blueberry juice daily.*

Celery contains a compound called apigenin, which helps to build and strengthen connections between brain cells. Other apigenin-rich foods include parsley, thyme, chamomile, and red pepper.
➡ *See recipe, above. Also snack on red pepper sticks and enjoy a cup of calming chamomile tea.*

WHAT TO AVOID
High-fat, high-sugar foods can take a heavy toll on brain function.

SUPPLEMENTS

Deficiencies in a wide range of nutrients can result in poor memory and reduced brain function. Vitamin B12 is the key nutrient for memory and cognition.

B vitamins, in particular B12, help to reduce levels of homocysteine, an amino acid that is toxic to the brain and linked to memory decline.
➡ *Take a B complex supplement daily.*

Pine bark extract can help to increase cerebral blood flow and improve brain function. Consult a medical practitioner if you have a bleeding disorder or diabetes before taking pine bark extract.
➡ *Take 100mg daily for 8 weeks.*

Vitamin D deficiency has been linked to rapid declines in memory and brain function. Many elderly people are low in this essential nutrient, which the body produces from sunlight and is hard to obtain from food alone.
➡ *Take 800–1000iu vitamin D3 daily.*

Selenium deficiency is linked to a fall in cognitive function and memory loss.
➡ *Take 100mcg daily.*

Docosahexaenoic acid (DHA) is a long-chain omega-3 fatty acid found in fish and marine plants. It can help to improve cognition in people with mild cognitive impairment, as well as boost the effects of B vitamins.
➡ *Take 200–300mg daily.*

Taurine is an amino acid that may help regenerate the hippocampus, the area of the brain associated with memory.
➡ *Take 500mg to 1g daily.*

LIFESTYLE

A daily nap can help to preserve memory and enhance the ability to think clearly.

Exercise regularly. Memory can deteriorate if physical fitness is poor.

Avoid smoking and alcohol. Smoking increases the risk of vascular dementia, while excess alcohol causes brain atrophy and depletes vitamin B.

Hydration is vital for memory and cognition. Dehydration affects brain efficiency and can cause memory loss and lack of concentration.

OTHER THERAPIES

Acupuncture can improve blood flow to the brain and subtle memory loss that precedes the onset of dementia.

FRESH OR DRIED?

Although sugar content is more concentrated in dried blueberries, they retain their antioxidant content and have plenty of fibre.

LIVING WITH NEURO-DEGENERATIVE DISEASE

Neuro-degenerative disease is an umbrella term for a range of conditions that primarily affect the way in which neurons function. These include Parkinson's disease, Alzheimer's disease, amyotrophic lateral sclerosis (ALS), motor neurone disease (MND), and Huntington's disease (HD). Some conditions, such as Huntington's, have no treatment. Others may be supported by diet and remedies to support nerve health.

HERBS

Herbs with "neuro-protective" activity can prevent neural inflammation and oxidative damage. They help to modulate the immune response, which may also help to prevent or treat some neuro-degenerative disease.

Turmeric protects against neural inflammation and has antioxidant and immune-modulating actions. Avoid therapeutic doses in pregnancy. May cause skin reactions in sunlight. Seek professional advice with gallstones.
➡ *Blend ½–1 tsp powder in warmed coconut milk and drink 3 times daily.*

Fleeceflower (He shou wu) is antioxidant and has neuro-protective properties. Avoid with diarrhoea and do not exceed the recommended dose.
➡ *Take 1–2ml tincture in a little water 3 times daily.*

Astragalus protects nerve cells and helps to modulate immune response. Avoid with acute infections such as influenza and colds and with immune-suppressant and blood-thinning drugs.
➡ *Take 2–4ml tincture in a little water 3 times daily.*

FOOD

Oxidative damage by free radicals may be a cause of neuro-degenerative disease. A diet of brightly coloured fresh foods high in antioxidants helps to fight free radicals.

Green tea contains theanine and antioxidant catechins, such as epigallocatechin-3-gallate, both of which protect the nervous system.
➡ *Have 2–3 cups a day, with a slice of lemon to increase antioxidant action. Also try incorporating matcha powder into green drinks or soups, or take a green tea supplement.*

Coconut oil is made up of medium-chain triglycerides (MCTs), which the brain can easily use as fuel. Avoid MCT supplements with diabetes or liver problems, during pregnancy, and when breastfeeding.
➡ *Use coconut oil for cooking.*

Acai has neuro-protective properties. See box, below.
➡ *Have a glass of acai juice daily.*

SUPPLEMENTS

These support deficiencies in the diet to boost brain function.

Lutein may help neutralize the free radicals that destroy nerve cells and lead to a decline in brain function.
➡ *Take 10mg daily.*

Resveratrol is a polyphenol that has been shown to protect against several neuro-degenerative disorders.
➡ *Take up to 1g twice daily.*

Zinc ensures healthy functioning of the central nervous system. A deficiency may contribute to neurological decline.
➡ *Lower-dose supplements of 8mg daily can be sufficient.*

LIFESTYLE

Go organic. Evidence increasingly shows that lifelong exposure to pesticides can make some individuals more vulnerable to developing neuro-degenerative diseases.

Drugs with anticholinergic effects – which are ones that inhibit some nerve impulses – can sometimes increase confusion. Talk to your doctor about medications and their possible side effects.

T'ai chi can deliver significant benefits for mild-to-moderate Parkinson's, including better posture, fewer falls, and improved walking ability.

FOCUS ON

Acai

PROFILE
Similar in appearance to a grape, this berry is a native of South America and has more antioxidants than any other berry.

PROPERTIES
Acai contains antioxidant apigenin, which has been shown to have anti-inflammatory and neuro-protective properties.

47% POWDER PROVIDES 47% VITAMIN A NRV PER 100G (3½OZ)

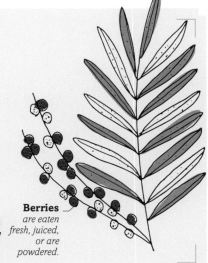

Berries *are eaten fresh, juiced, or are powdered.*

RESPIRATORY SYSTEM

The involuntary, continuous act of breathing provides us with life-giving oxygen and filters out carbon dioxide. When functioning well, this seamless process often goes unnoticed and acts as an effective frontline defence against germs and irritants. Discover how immune-boosting, clearing, and hydrating foods and natural remedies can help to keep our breathing apparatus in peak condition, and how natural approaches can soothe and unblock when inflammation and congestion occur.

○ ○ ○ ○

STAYING WELL
RESPIRATORY SYSTEM

The essential act of breathing, which brings oxygen into the body, removes waste and carbon dioxide from the lungs, and plays a role in the smooth functioning of the nervous system, can be hampered by viruses, bacteria, and allergens. Targeted nutrients and holistic remedies help to protect and strengthen the respiratory system, optimizing respiratory function and enabling the body to resist infection effectively.

FOOD

Key nutrients can help to strengthen the respiratory system – building resilience, preventing the respiratory tract from succumbing to infection, and reducing irritation from allergens.

IMMUNE-ENHANCING GARLIC

Garlic is potently antibacterial and antiviral, with decongestant and expectorant properties that can help to keep the lungs clear and ward off infection. Garlic also contains a substance called alliin, which when crushed turns into an unstable compound, allicin. In the body, allicin converts into the immune-boosting enzyme sulphur, which enhances the ability of white blood cells to fight viruses and germs. Raw garlic is most powerful as heat destroys some of the sulphur compounds, so add raw garlic liberally to salad dressings.

AIRWAY-CALMING CITRUS

Citrus fruits contain immune-enhancing vitamin C and phyto-nutrient bioflavonoids, both of which have anti-inflammatory and anti-allergenic properties to help calm the airways. During pollen season and when colds are circulating, eat plenty of citrus fruits to reduce irritation to the airways and boost immunity – and, if you do succumb to a cold, help speed your recovery.

NUTRIENT-DENSE MUSHROOMS

Mushrooms are a source of B vitamins, thought to boost disease-fighting white blood cells, as well as the antioxidant selenium, which studies show boosts the function of the immune system and also prevents free-radical damage to cells and tissues. Wild mushrooms, which are cultivated in the light, increase their levels of immune-enhancing vitamin D. Mushrooms also contain beta-glucans, a type of soluble fibre that supports disease-fighting white blood cells to boost immunity.

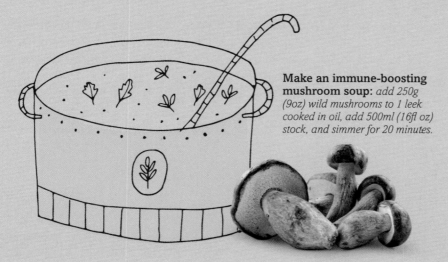

Make an immune-boosting mushroom soup: *add 250g (9oz) wild mushrooms to 1 leek cooked in oil, add 500ml (16fl oz) stock, and simmer for 20 minutes.*

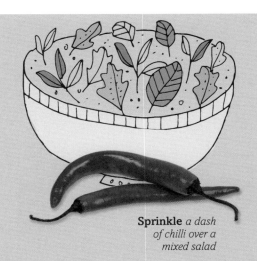

"Immune-boosting foods can prevent the respiratory tract from succumbing to infection."

Sprinkle *a dash of chilli over a mixed salad*

LUNG-SUPPORTING FATTY ACIDS

Ocean plants such as seaweed contain a type of fatty acid known as polyhydroxylated fatty alcohols, or PFAs. PFAs have excellent anti-inflammatory properties that help to strengthen the lungs. PFAs are also found in avocados, one of the few land plants to contain PFAs.

SINUS CLEARERS

Chilli peppers, hot mustard, curry, horseradish, and wasabi, used to add a flavourful punch to foods, have the added benefit of helping to open the nasal passages to keep sinuses clear.

HYDRATION BOOST

Staying well hydrated actually helps to prevent snoring. Drinking plenty of water and herbal teas not only maintains hydration levels to support bodily functions overall, but also thins out mucus, stopping secretions in the nose and soft palate becoming stickier and triggering snoring.

PROTECTIVE ANTIOXIDANTS

Matcha, finely powdered green tea leaves, is abundant in antioxidants to help reduce airway inflammation.

HERBS

Herbs with a healing or soothing effect on the respiratory system and ones that support a well-functioning immune system enhance breathing.

NATURAL ANTIHISTAMINES

Nettles, as well as being a rich source of chlorophyll and iron, both of which support immunity, are also natural antihistamines, helping to calm over-sensitive airways and soothe inflamed tissues. Try harvesting fresh nettles – which grow abundantly in the wild – in spring for a soothing nettle infusion to help protect the airways against the onslaught of pollen.

Add 1–2 tsp dried nettles, *or 2–4 tsp fresh nettles in spring, to 175ml (6fl oz) boiling water for a respiratory-calming infusion.*

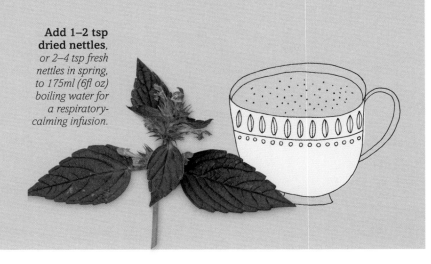

Protective berries

Elderberries provide excellent support during the cold and flu season. Anti-inflammatory flavonoids in the berries help to keep airways healthy and functioning optimally, and studies show that taking elderberry syrup regularly can ward off respiratory infection thanks to the berries' potent antiviral properties. If infection does take hold, a tea or tincture made from the flowers can soothe inflamed tissues and reduce catarrh and congestion. Do not eat raw elderberries as these can cause stomach upsets.

Tissue-toning herbs

If you're susceptible to snoring, toning herbs, such as raspberry leaf, sage, and agrimony, can help to tighten and tone the tissues around the mouth and soft palate to ease breathing.

Immune boosters

If you feel a cold coming on, echinacea can help to shorten its duration by enhancing the immune response. Echinacea has been shown to boost the response of white blood cells to infection and reduce inflammation in the airways. Similarly, golden seal has a powerful anti-infective action and reduces inflammation in the airways to support respiratory function.

Essential oils

Inhaling essential oils or diffusing them into the environment can calm and clear the respiratory tract.

Mucus-clearing oils

Essential oils can make effective decongestants. Cedarwood and sandalwood break up excessive catarrh and soothe the mucous membranes, and tea tree and bay laurel work as decongestants and are also highly antiseptic, helping to ward off germs.

Cooling peppermint

Peppermint has a cooling effect that can be useful for calming fever if infection does take hold. It also has an expectorant action and can help to keep the sinuses clear during the winter months, helping to build resilience to germs in the respiratory tract.

Throat-calming oils

Antispasmodic essential oils such as helichrysum and thyme have a calming action that can help to prevent the occasional tickle in the throat from developing into a chronic cough.

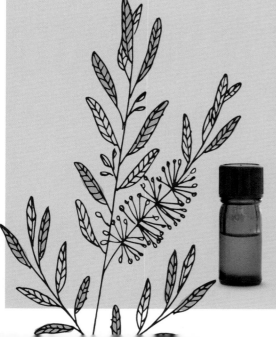

Add 4 drops tea tree essential oil *to a bowl of hot water, place a towel over the head to trap steam, and inhale for a decongesting inhalation.*

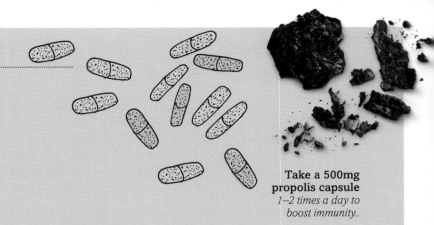

Take a 500mg propolis capsule *1–2 times a day to boost immunity..*

Lung-supporting oils

Ravintsara is a warming oil that is both antiviral and antiseptic, offering protection against germs, and it also has immuno-stimulant properties, which revive and support the immune system, boosting its resilience when defences may be lowered, for example, during times of stress.

Frankincense oil, with it spicy, resinous aroma, also supports respiratory function, soothing the mucous membranes and relaxing and deepening breathing when needed.

Supplements

Supplementing the diet can be an effective way to reduce sensitivity to allergens and boost respiratory health during the winter cold and flu season, especially if you succumb fairly easily to infections.

The essentials

A daily high-quality multi-vitamin and mineral supplement tops up nutrients and provides insurance against specific deficiencies that can leave the respiratory system vulnerable to infection.

Immune-supporting nutrients

Vitamin C supports immunity, and its role in collagen synthesis – the structural protein in body tissues – makes it instrumental for tissue health, in turn supporting and promoting lung health.

A zinc deficiency can increase susceptibility to germs. Studies show that zinc is anti-inflammatory and enhances immunity; taking a supplement at the start of a cold may reduce its severity and duration. Combine vitamin C and zinc for a immune-boosting punch to help to fight off colds and sinus infections.

Protective bioflavonoids

When viruses are circulating, propolis – a sticky, resinous mixture of beeswax, saps, and other substances that bees produce – is a source of antiviral and immune-protecting bioflavonoids. Do not give bee products to young children, or take if you have an allergy to honey or bee stings, or you are pregnant or breastfeeding.

Anti-inflammatory fats

Essential fatty acid supplements have significant anti-inflammatory effects that can help protect against chronic coughs. Try eicosapentaenoic acid (EPA) fish oils or gamma-linolenic acid (GLA) from borage oil to ward off a persistent cough.

"Targeted supplements can reduce sensitivity to allergens in the respiratory tract."

TREATMENTS

RESPIRATORY SYSTEM

Congestion and inflammation in the respiratory tract can lead to a range of conditions and complaints. Using natural remedies and eating key nutrients, as well as staying well hydrated, can help to relieve respiratory symptoms and reduce the duration of infections, as well as boost general immunity to lower the incidence of recurring infections. Reducing stress and getting plenty of rest are helpful for speedy recovery.

COLDS AND FLU

Catching a cold or flu is often inconvenient and unpleasant. It is also, to some extent, avoidable if you take preventative action. As well as boosting resistance, natural remedies can also help to shorten the duration of the illness if you do succumb to a virus.

HERBS

Antimicrobial herbs help to fight the infection and can be supported with herbs that boost immunity. Herbs that promote sweating and reduce fever can help to manage these illnesses.

THE RIGHT OIL

Ravintsara oil may be confused with ravensara. Therapeutic ravintsara is from the Madagascan camphor tree. Ravensara, from a different source, is used in perfumery.

Elderberry has proven antiviral activity to help fight infection.
➼*Make a fresh berry syrup in autumn or buy a syrup. Take 1–2 tsp daily.*

Echinacea is antimicrobial, anti-inflammatory, and boosts white blood cells. Avoid with immunosuppressants.
➼*Take 3–5ml tincture in a little water 3 times daily, or use with elderberry, see remedy right.*

Elderflower promotes sweating to lower fever and is a soothing anticatarrhal.
➼*Infuse 1–2 tsp dried elderflower in 175ml (6fl oz) boiling water. Drink 3–4 times daily.*

Yarrow induces sweating and is anti-infective. Avoid in pregnancy or if sensitive to *Asteraceae* plants. Over use can increase skin photosensitivity.
➼*Infuse 1–2 tsp dried yarrow in 175ml (6fl oz) boiling water. Drink 3–4 times daily.*

ESSENTIAL OILS

Oils can relieve a cough, sore throat, and congestion, and the fatigue or fever of flu.

Eucalyptus is a decongestant.
Ravintsara is an effective antimicrobial.
➼*Add 5 drops of either oil to a bowl of hot water to inhale (see Peppermint, below) or 2 drops to a diffuser. Or, add 3 drops to 5ml almond oil for a chest rub.*

Peppermint is cooling, helping to relieve fever and headache.
➼*Add 5 drops to a bowl of hot water, lean over, covering your head with a towel to trap the steam, and inhale until it cools. Or add 2 drops to a diffuser and inhale.*

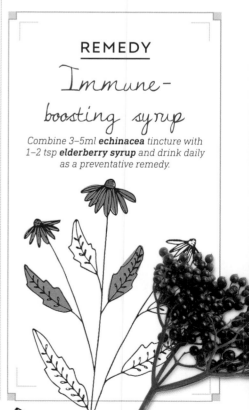

REMEDY

Immune-boosting syrup

Combine 3–5ml **echinacea** tincture with 1–2 tsp **elderberry syrup** and drink daily as a preventative remedy.

FOOD

When suffering with a cold or flu, eat light, nutrient-dense meals with complex carbohydrates and drink plenty of fluids.

Garlic and onions (preferably raw) are antibacterial and antiviral.
➡*Add a chopped garlic clove or a chopped raw onion to a soup or vegetables after cooking.*
Citrus fruits are rich in vitamin C, which can help to speed recovery.
➡*Have a glass of fresh orange or grapefruit juice daily.*
Shiitake, maitake, and reishi mushrooms have immune-boosting beta-glucans.
➡*Use instead of regular mushrooms.*
WHAT TO AVOID
Sugar, which rapidly depresses immune function.

SUPPLEMENTS

Supporting the diet when immunity is low can be beneficial.

Aged garlic extract can significantly reduce the severity and duration of colds and flu.
➡*Take 2.5g daily.*
Vitamin C and zinc lozenges can cut the duration of a cold.
➡*Look for ones with zinc acetate or zinc gluconate; take as directed.*
Propolis is rich in bioflavonoids, thought to give it antiviral properties.
➡*Take 500mg 1–2 times a day to relieve symptoms.*

LIFESTYLE

Stress is the main contributor to lowered immunity so take measures to relax.
Regular gentle exercise boosts circulation and immunity, but pushing past your limits may weaken immunity.
Cover your mouth when sneezing and wash hands to avoid reinfection and spreading germs to other people.

CATARRH

Catarrh is an overproduction and buildup of phlegm in the lungs, larynx, nose, and sinuses. It can be caused by a viral infection, such as a cold or flu, or by allergens.

HERBS

Astringent herbs can help to tone and calm inflammation to reduce catarrhal secretions, while clearing herbs help to expel excessive mucus. Herbs that are healing and soothing for your upper respiratory tract can ease symptoms.

Golden rod is anti-inflammatory, astringent, and an effective anticatarrhal. Avoid with sensitivity to the *Asteraceae* plant family.
➡*Take 2–4ml tincture in a little water 3 times daily.*
Elderflowers soothe and calm inflamed tissues and are anticatarrhal, helping to ease congestion.
➡*Infuse 1–2 tsp dried elderflower in 175ml (6fl oz) boiling water. Drink 3 times daily.*
Ground ivy is astringent and tones the mucous membranes, reducing secretions and calming irritation.
➡*Infuse 1–2 tsp dried ground ivy in 175ml (6fl oz) boiling water. Drink 3 times daily.*

ESSENTIAL OILS

A number of essential oils have expectorant and decongestant properties that help to clear the chest and lungs.

Thyme can be used as a strengthening respiratory tonic.
Fennel works as an antispasmodic and also as an expectorant, to help expel excess mucus.
Tea tree is strongly antimicrobial and expectorant.
➡*Add 5 drops of any of the above essential oils to a bowl of hot water, lean over, covering your head with a towel to trap the steam, and inhale until the steam cools. Or add 2 drops of any of the above to a diffuser and inhale. For tea tree, you can also try the remedy below, with almond oil.*

FOOD

Foods can help to reduce catarrh and can have an anti-inflammatory effect. Also drink plenty of water to thin out mucus.

Garlic has potent antimicrobial, decongestant, and expectorant properties.
➡*Add raw garlic to salads and dressings, or steep 3–4 peeled cloves in a bowl of boiling water to make an effective steam inhalation. Lean over, covering your head with a towel to trap steam, and inhale until it cools.*

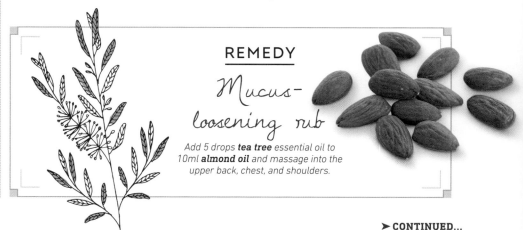

REMEDY

Mucus-loosening rub

Add 5 drops **tea tree** essential oil to 10ml **almond oil** and massage into the upper back, chest, and shoulders.

➤ CONTINUED...

"Supplements support respiratory health, breaking down mucus and fighting infection."

Apple cider vinegar actually has an alkalizing effect on the body that can help to reduce inflammation.
➠ *Take 1 tbsp in 250ml (9fl oz) of water each morning.*
WHAT TO AVOID
Dairy produce can be mucus-forming. Sugar and refined carbohydrates can also worsen symptoms.

SUPPLEMENTS

Top up a healthy diet with supplements that help to support respiratory health.

Vitamin C can help to combat an underlying infection.
➠ *Take 1–2g daily.*
N-acetylcysteine (NAC) is a modified amino acid that can break down mucus, making it easier to clear it away from the airways.
➠ *Take 250–500mg 1–2 times a day.*

LIFESTYLE

Allergies can be the root cause of chronic catarrh. Investigate your diet and environment for triggers.
Air conditioners and central heating can both make sinus inflammation worse by drying out the air. Turn them off and consider investing in a humidifier to moisten the air.

BRONCHITIS AND COUGHS

Coughing is a protective reflex to clear the lungs and airways of mucus and irritants. Bronchitis is an inflammation of the bronchial tubes, which bring air to the lungs, and often follows a cold or flu.

HERBS

Anti-inflammatory and expectorant herbs help to ease symptoms. Support these with antibacterial herbs to fight infection. Lung tonics help to strengthen the lungs and improve their resilience.

Elecampane is a powerful lung tonic. It soothes irritating coughs and helps expel excessive catarrh. See box, below. Avoid if sensitive to the *Asteraceae* plant family.
➠ *Take 1–2ml tincture in a little water 3 times daily.*

Thyme is an anti-inflammatory and antispasmodic herb, and has antibacterial and expectorant actions to help fight infections. Avoid therapeutic doses in pregnancy.
➠ *Infuse 1–2 tsp dried thyme in 175ml (6fl oz) boiling water. Drink 3 times daily.*
Mullein soothes the mucosal lining with its anti-inflammatory and relaxing action and is also antibacterial.
➠ *Take 2.5–5ml tincture in a little water 3 times daily.*

ESSENTIAL OILS

These can be used for their antispasmodic, expectorant, and antibacterial properties.

Bay laurel is antiseptic and can break down and expel mucus.
Cedarwood can help to break down excess mucus.
➠ *Add 5 drops of either of the above essential oils to a bowl of hot water, lean over, covering your head with a towel to trap the steam, and inhale until it cools.*

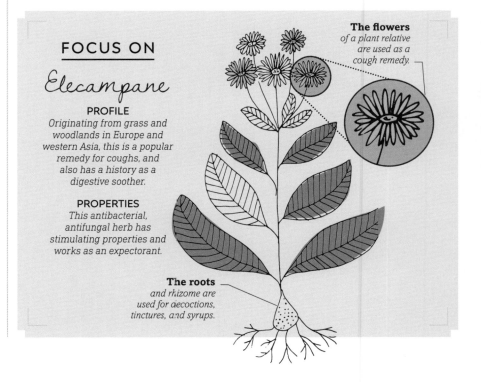

FOCUS ON

Elecampane

PROFILE
Originating from grass and woodlands in Europe and western Asia, this is a popular remedy for coughs, and also has a history as a digestive soother.

PROPERTIES
This antibacterial, antifungal herb has stimulating properties and works as an expectorant.

The flowers *of a plant relative are used as a cough remedy.*

The roots *and rhizome are used for decoctions, tinctures, and syrups.*

Sandalwood can soothe irritated mucous membranes.
➠*Add 2 drops to a diffuser and inhale.*

SUPPLEMENTS

Look for supplements that help to calm and heal inflamed, irritated airways.

N-acetylcysteine (NAC) may stimulate production of glutathione, a natural antioxidant, which is often depleted in bronchitis sufferers.
➠*Take 400mg daily.*

Beta-carotene has an antiviral action and can help to heal the mucous membranes.
➠*Take 6–15mg daily.*

Vitamin C with added bioflavonoids helps to calm inflamed airways.
➠*Take 500mg 3 times a day with food.*

Essential fatty acids such as GLA and EPA from borage oil and fish oils have significant anti-inflammatory effects on people with bronchitis.
➠*Take 500mg to 1g daily.*

OTHER THERAPIES

Homeopathy offers a number of remedies that can help to treat respiratory complaints.

Osteopathy and chiropractic may help to open up and relax the lungs.

Acupuncture can help to decongest, clearing the lungs of excess mucus.

SINUSITIS

The sinuses are air-filled pockets, or cavities, within the bones of the face. They have many functions, which include warming and cleaning the air we breathe and helping to resonate sounds. When they become inflamed, infected, or blocked by a buildup of mucus the result is sinusitis, which can cause tenderness and pain around the cheeks and forehead.

HERBS

Herbs help to calm and heal the lining of the sinuses, fight low-grade infections, and also help to clear congestion. These actions in turn promote the flow of fluids and reduce inflammation to ease pain and improve sinus health.

Plantain soothes and tones the sinus tissues, helping to balance secretions, and is antibacterial.
➠*Infuse 1–2 tsp dried plantain in 175ml (6fl oz) boiling water. Drink 3 times daily.*

Nettle is anti-allergenic and astringent, toning, soothing, and is decongesting for inflamed tissues.
➠*Infuse 1–2 tsp dried nettle in 175ml (6fl oz) boiling water. Drink 3 times daily.*

Golden seal is a tonic for the respiratory tract lining. It has a powerful anti-infective action and reduces inflammation. Do not take internally for prolonged periods. Avoid with hypertension, during pregnancy, and when breastfeeding.
➠*Take 1ml tincture in a little water 3 times daily.*

ESSENTIAL OILS

Essential oils can be used in combination with steam inhalation, and can help to support the immune system and remove and break down mucus.

RECIPE

Sinus clearer

*Chop a thumb-sized piece of **ginger** (see p178) into a cup and pour over 250ml (9fl oz) boiling water, then leave to steep for 5 minutes before drinking. Add a little **honey** to taste, if desired.*

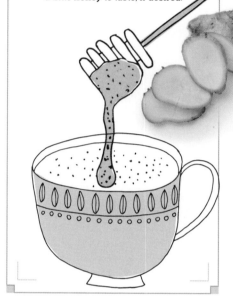

Niaouli is an excellent expectorant, and also has anti-allergenic properties.

Pine is soothing and healing and also acts as an antiseptic.

Helichrysum can help to break down mucus and is also antispasmodic.
➠*Add 5 drops of any of the above oils to a bowl of hot water, lean over, covering your head with a towel to trap the steam, and inhale until it cools. Or add 2 drops of any of the above oils to a diffuser and inhale.*

FOOD

Foods, or more specifically food allergies, may be a cause of chronic sinusitis so it can be worth testing for allergies. Some foods bring temporary relief to sinusitis.

➤ CONTINUED…

Chilli peppers, hot mustard, curry, horseradish, and wasabi may bring temporary relief for some sufferers by opening the nasal passages.
➡️*Add hot sauces and other spicy condiments to everyday foods.*

Peppermint is an effective decongestant.
➡️*Swap your coffee for 2–3 cups of peppermint tea daily.*

Ginger can help to loosen sinus congestion.
➡️*See remedy, p177.*

WHAT TO AVOID
Additives, including colourings and preservatives, can promote sinus inflammation. Dairy products can also be mucus-forming for some people, making the condition worse.

SUPPLEMENTS

Supplements can help to bolster your body's own natural immune response, so can help to support a nutrient-dense diet when immunity is low.

Vitamin C and zinc lozenges can help to support general immunity and fight sinus infections.
➡️*Look for ones with zinc acetate or zinc gluconate; take as directed.*

LIFESTYLE

Use an air purifier to remove dust, pollens, and other irritating particles from the air that may exacerbate sinusitis.

Check for allergens in your diet or environment.

Massage either side of the nose near the bottom of the nasal bones and at the outside of your nostrils as often as possible to help agitate mucus.

OTHER THERAPIES

Homeopathy offers several remedies that may help sinusitis symptoms.

ASTHMA

In this chronic lung disease, inflammation and spasm of smooth muscle in the bronchi narrow the airways and hamper breathing. If coughing, wheezing, chest tightness, and shortness of breath are severe seek urgent medical advice.

HERBS

Herbs support other treatments to relax and dilate airways, reduce inflammation, and act as expectorants to expel mucus.

Ginkgo biloba eases inflammation and hypersensitivity. Avoid in pregnancy, if breastfeeding, and with anticoagulant and antiplatelet medicines.
➡️*Take a 66mg leaf extract tablet equal to 3300mg whole leaf, 1–3 times daily.*

Liquorice soothes lung irritation, see box, right. Avoid with hypertension and in pregnancy, and large doses over prolonged periods.
➡️*Make a decoction with ½–1 tsp dried liquorice root per 250ml (9fl oz) boiling water and drink 3 times daily.*

Thyme, a lung tonic, is antispasmodic – relaxing and opening the airways – anti-inflammatory, and expectorant. Avoid therapeutic doses in pregnancy.
➡️*Infuse 1–2 tsp dried thyme in 175ml (6fl oz) boiling water. Drink 3 times daily.*

Hyssop, an expectorant, tones the lungs. Avoid in pregnancy.
➡️*Infuse 1–2 tsp dried hyssop in 175ml (6fl oz) boiling water. Drink 3 times daily.*

ESSENTIAL OILS

These fight infection, offer emotional support, and calm allergic responses.

Frankincense relaxes breathing.
Eucalyptus reduces congestion and expels mucus.

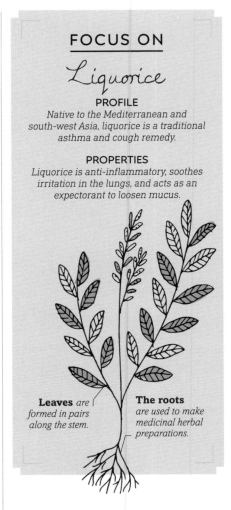

Pine has several properties that help ease pulmonary conditions.
➡️*Add 2 drops of any of the above essential oils to a tissue or diffuser and inhale.*

WHAT TO AVOID
Steam inhalation can worsen asthma in some people.

FOOD

Antioxidant and anti-inflammatory foods can help ease lung swelling and irritation.

Avocados have polyhydroxylated fatty alcohols (PFAs), which have excellent anti-inflammatory properties.
➡️*Enjoy a guacamole dip.*

Matcha, powdered green tea leaves, has anti-inflammatory antioxidants.
➡️*Enjoy a matcha latte.*

Sardines have omega-3 and vitamin D, both of which reduce inflammation.
➡️*Grill, adding lemon and garlic.*

Citrus has anti-inflammatory, anti-allergenic bioflavonoids and vitamin C.
➡️*Eat an orange a day or enjoy fresh orange juice for breakfast.*

WHAT TO AVOID
Saturated fats can increase inflammation, and sulphite, a preservative found in wine, dried fruits, pickles, and prawns, can trigger symptoms in some people.

SUPPLEMENTS

Certain nutrients can help reduce airway reactivity and severe attacks.

Magnesium – low intakes have been linked to asthma.
➡️*Tale 300–400mg a day.*

Vitamin C can support lung health.
➡️*Take 1g a day, or 1500mg a day for exercise-induced asthma.*

Vitamin D increases the effectiveness of medicines and reduces occurrence.
➡️*Take 800iu a day.*

Fructooligosaccharides (FOS) are a form of fermentable fibre that feeds good gut bacteria. Healthy gut flora can help control inflammation in the lungs.
➡️*Take 8g a day in drinks or on cereal.*

LIFESTYLE

Avoid air fresheners and cleaning products as well as allergens from dust, animal fur, mould, and pollens.

OTHER THERAPIES

Homeopathy can treat the whole body.
Acupuncture can fight allergens.
Flower remedies help calm panic.
Buteyko breathing involves breathing exercises aimed at relaxing the airways.

SNORING

There are two main types of snoring: palatal snoring is caused by vibration of the soft palate, while tongue snoring is caused by the base of the tongue restricting airflow at the back of the throat. Both types reduce sleep quality for the snorer and cause loss of sleep for partners.

HERBS

Herbs can tighten and tone the soft palate to help reduce snoring. Astringent and anti-inflammatory herbs can reduce swollen tissues and excessive saliva.

Raspberry leaf is astringent and tones the lining of the mouth and palate. Avoid in pregnancy until after the second trimester.
➡️*Infuse 1–2 tsp dried raspberry leaf in 175ml (6fl oz) boiling water. Drink 1–2 cups in the evening.*

Sage is astringent and is a traditional mouth and throat remedy. Avoid therapeutic doses in pregnancy and with epilepsy and avoid taking for prolonged periods of time.
➡️*Infuse 1–2 tsp dried sage in 175ml (6fl oz) boiling water. Gargle and drink 1–2 cups in the evening.*

Agrimony is astringent to the mouth and throat and toning, to relax tissues. Avoid with constipation.
➡️*Make an infusion as above or combine all three herbs in one infusion.*

ESSENTIAL OILS

Use essential oils to open the airways during sleep or to act as a decongestant.

Peppermint can relieve congestion.
➡️*Add 2 drops and 1 tsp glycerine to a glass of water. Gargle before going to bed, taking care not to swallow.*

Thyme works as a strengthening respiratory tonic.
➡️*Add 2 drops to a diffuser and inhale.*

Eucalyptus acts as a decongestant.
➡️*Add 5 drops of either of the above oils to a bowl of hot water, lean over, covering your head with a towel to trap the steam, and inhale until it cools. Or add 2 drops of either oil to a diffuser and inhale.*

LIFESTYLE

Stop smoking, reduce alcohol, and cut out allergens to reduce or even totally cure snoring problems.

Sleep on your side to reduce snoring and associated sleep apnoea (an interruption of normal breathing).

Weight loss can help to reduce snoring, so make an effort to lose weight if you think this might be a factor.

Keep nasal passages open with a hot shower before you go to bed, or try using nasal strips.

Try an anti-snoring mouthpiece, also known as a tongue-retaining device, which helps to reposition the jaw to make breathing both easier and quieter.

Allergens in bedrooms and in pillows can contribute to snoring. Wash and replace pillows regularly.

Keeping well hydrated can stop secretions in the nose and soft palate becoming stickier and therefore triggering snoring.

BEST STORAGE
Ripe avocados can be kept on a work surface if eating within a day or two. Otherwise, store them in the fridge because chilling halts the ripening process.

HOW TO MAKE
A POULTICE

A poultice is a traditional method of healing whereby moistened herbs are applied directly to the skin. The active plant constituents reach the deeper tissues and the bloodstream, producing a wider healing effect and making this an effective treatment for wounds, muscle and joint problems, and some internal conditions. Adding essential oils enhances the therapeutic benefits.

Makes 1 portion of paste

YOU WILL NEED

handful of dried herbs (or more if needed), finely chopped or powdered; or bunch of fresh herbs, bruised or crushed

freshly boiled water, enough to make a paste consistency

essential oils (optional)

gauze, or muslin cloth

bandage, plaster, or wound dressing

hot-water bottle (optional)

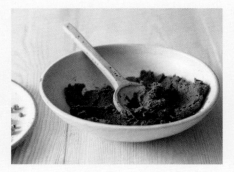

1 Mix the herbs with just enough water to moisten them thoroughly and form a paste. Stir until well combined, then add any essential oils, if using. Leave to cool slightly before applying to ensure the paste doesn't burn the skin.

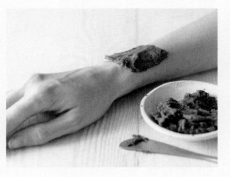

2 Apply the cooled paste directly to the skin, or spread over half a piece of gauze or muslin cloth, fold over the other half to cover the paste, and apply to the affected area.

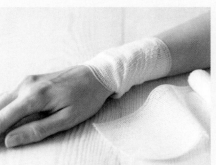

3 Bind the paste, or the filled gauze, with a separate piece of gauze, or a bandage, plaster, or wound dressing. Leave the poultice in place for 1–3 hours, using a hot-water bottle, warm clothing, or a blanket to keep it warm, if instructed. Reapply with a new batch of herbs if required.

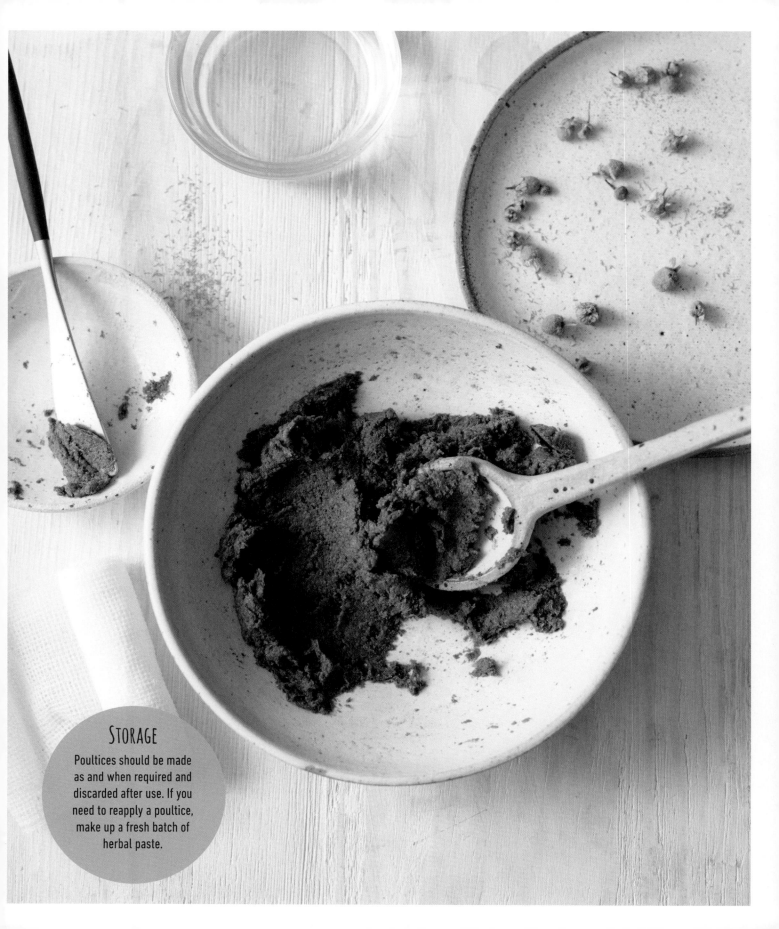

STORAGE

Poultices should be made as and when required and discarded after use. If you need to reapply a poultice, make up a fresh batch of herbal paste.

BONES, JOINTS, AND MUSCLES

A smoothly operating musculoskeletal system contributes significantly to quality of life, facilitating coordination, balance, and ease of movement so that we can carry out everyday activities with ease. Explore how key nutrients and holistic remedies help to nurture, strengthen, and protect these important parts of our bodies, and when damage and inflammation hamper the function of bones, joints, and muscles, learn how holistic approaches can offer support and promote healing.

STAYING WELL
BONES, JOINTS, AND MUSCLES

Giving constant care to our musculoskeletal system – the internal framework that supports and protects us and facilitates movement – helps to reduce the risk of injury and damage. Essential nutrients and holistic remedies can strengthen tissues, limit damage, and help maximize health in the bones, joints, and muscles.

FOOD

Eating a balanced diet with vital nutrients fuels the bones, joints, and muscles and regenerates tissues.

BONE-BUILDING NUTRIENTS

Calcium is essential for bone health. Ninety nine per cent of our calcium is stored in our bones, and it is vital for building and maintaining strong bones. Also, when levels of bone calcium are healthy, this ensures calcium reserves to help maintain levels in the blood, important for muscle function.

Calcium from food is the easiest to absorb and more likely to build strong bones than supplements, so eat calcium-rich foods daily. Good sources include yogurt, cottage cheese, and milk. Leafy greens, such as kale, collard, and mustard greens; watercress; nuts; tofu; raw cacao nibs; and tinned fish such as salmon, which contains soft, ground down calcium-rich bones, are also sources.

ESSENTIAL VITAMIN D

To absorb and utilize calcium, the body needs vitamin D. It is hard to obtain enough vitamin D from the diet and most vitamin D is made by the body in response to sunlight. However, foods such as eggs, oily fish, cheese, mushrooms, fortified cereals, and dairy do provide vitamin D, so include these in your diet regularly.

PROTECTIVE ANTIOXIDANTS AND ANTI-INFLAMMATORIES

Brightly coloured fruit and vegetables are rich in antioxidants, and a high consumption of vegetables is thought to support healthy bone density and musculoskeletal health. Antioxidant vitamins A and C, found in foods such as squash, dark leafy greens, and citrus fruits, help to combat the oxidative damage that can lead to damaging inflammation, helping to keep joints flexible.

Matcha – powdered green tea leaves – is rich in anti-inflammatory antioxidants (it has higher levels than standard green tea), which studies suggest can slow cartilage breakdown.

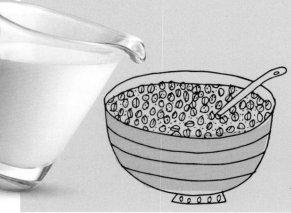

Milk or yogurt
with breakfast muesli provides a daily dose of essential calcium for bone health.

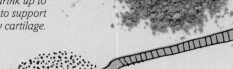

Add 1 tsp matcha powder *to 175ml (6fl oz) boiling water and drink up to 3 times daily to support healthy cartilage.*

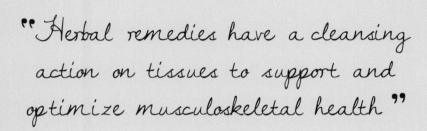

"Herbal remedies have a cleansing action on tissues to support and optimize musculoskeletal health"

Nutrients for bone tissue health

Zinc is an important micronutrient for bone tissue regeneration and a deficiency can impact on bone health. Sources include poultry, lean red meat, pulses, pumpkin seeds, and wholegrains.

Protein muscle fuel

Protein is vital for healthy muscles, helping to repair muscle cells and support the growth of new cells to ensure healthy muscle mass. Lean meat and fish, eggs, dairy, and nuts all provide protein. Try boiling marrow bones for a protein-rich broth that contains calcium and phosphorous for muscle and bone repair.

Joint lubricators

To reduce or prevent the inflammation that can lead to stiff and uncomfortable joints and limit movement, eat a diet that is rich in anti-inflammatory omega-3 fatty acids, namely eicosapentaenoic acid (EPA) and docosahexaenoic acid (DHA),

which help to lubricate the joints and ease movement. Good sources include oily fish such as salmon and mackerel, as well as flaxseeds, walnuts, and eggs.

Herbs

Herbal remedies can have significant benefits for the musculoskeletal system, reducing inflammation that can lead to stiffness, and cleansing tissues to support and optimize musculoskeletal health.

Detoxifying herbs

Diuretic herbs such as burdock root and celery seed have a cleansing action on body tissues, helping to remove waste products such as excess uric acid from the joints to promote healthy movement. Celery seed also has anti-inflammatory properties to help prevent joint stiffness and optimize movement.

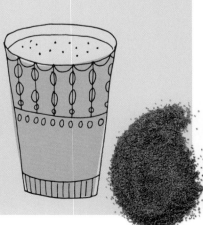

Add 1–4ml each celery seed and burdock root tincture *to a little water and take 3 times daily to help prevent stiffness.*

HERBS FOR CELL RENEWAL

Comfrey leaf contains a compound called allantoin, which speeds up cell regeneration, helping to promote musculoskeletal health and support healing where bone and tissue damage has occurred.

HERBS WITH PHYTOESTROGENS

A balance of hormones has a positive knock-on effect for bone health. During the menopause, a fall in oestrogen can impact on musculoskeletal health. Red clover contains plant oestrogens, or phytoestrogens, called isoflavones, which help to reduce bone density loss. Calendula also has an oestrogen-like action that increases calcium absorption to promote bone health.

ANTI-INFLAMMATORY HERBS

Repetitive actions or strenuous workouts increase the risk of nerve pain. Herbs such as St John's wort, known as an anti-depressant, can also reduce nerve inflammation to limit damage.

MUSCLE SOOTHERS

Antispasmodic herbs can help to calm muscles and release held-in tension and prevent aching. Valerian is both a powerful sedative and an antispasmodic, so can soothe muscles and promote deep, restful sleep so that muscle aches don't disturb sleep, which in turn enables the body to get the rest it needs to recuperate and revitalize muscles.

ESSENTIAL OILS

Aromatherapy offers a range of uplifting and warming oils that can be applied topically to revitalize joints and muscles and help optimize musculoskeletal health.

CIRCULATION BOOSTERS

Stimulating essential oils boost local blood circulation. Ginger is a comforting and warming oil that can be applied topically to help stimulate circulation to the tissues, reviving muscles and joints. Other warming oils include rosemary and sweet marjoram, which also have natural analgesic properties.

MUSCLE-SOOTHING OILS

Winding down after strenuous exercise or exertion is important to help muscles relax and avoid damage. Lavender has stress-busting properties that relax and soothe muscles after exertion.

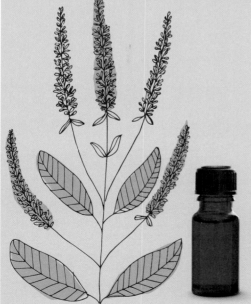

Add 4 drops peppermint essential oil *to a bowl of warm water and enjoy a reviving and energizing foot bath.*

Add 2 tbsp rosehip powder *to a bowl of creamy oats.*

Purifying oils

Cleansing essential oils aid natural detoxification processes to help prevent uric acid building up in the tissues and causing joint problems. A purifying massage with juniper and lemon oils helps to flush out toxins from tissues, supporting muscle health and reducing the risk of conditions such as gout and arthritis.

Oils to revive

Bones and muscles in the feet can feel the strain after an active day, making them vulnerable to long-term damage. A peppermint oil foot bath helps to revive feet – initially cooling them down, then promoting a feeling of warmth to revitalize tissues.

Supplements

Supplementing the diet protects the musculoskeletal system and boosts muscle, bone, and joint health.

Vitamin D top up

During the winter months or in colder climes it can be hard to obtain sufficient amounts of vitamin D – synthesized in response to sunlight – which the body needs to help it absorb calcium for healthy, strong bones. With dietary sources of vitamin D limited, supplements are a boost to bone health.

Nutrients for joint health

Omega-3 fatty acid supplements from oily fish or algae help to lubricate joints and are also thought to reduce the bone loss and inflammation that are linked to conditions such as osteoporosis.

Rosehip powder is rich in protective antioxidants to combat free radical damage, and contains a highly anti-inflammatory omega-6-like fatty acid, GOPO, to limit and prevent joint damage.

Vitamin B6 boost

If work involves repeated actions that increase the risk of strain, vitamin B6 intake, shown to relieve RSI, can be beneficial.

Protective nutrients

Vitamin C and quercetin help to eliminate excess uric acid to protect against conditions such as gout. A lack of vitamin C is also linked to reduced collagen formation, so keeping levels up promotes tissue growth and repair, while the flavonoid quercetin promotes bone cell growth to help bones cope with wear and tear.

"Uplifting and warming essential oils can help to revitalize joints and muscles."

TREATMENTS

BONES, JOINTS, AND MUSCLES

Well-functioning bones, joints, and muscles require strength and flexibility. Injuries, age, and lifestyle can impact on movement, leading to stiffness and debilitating pain. Natural remedies, diet, and supportive therapies can ease pain and restore movement.

BACK PAIN

Most adults experience back pain, particularly sciatica or lower back pain, at some point. The most common cause is work-related back injuries, but activities at home and at leisure are also a cause, as is stress. Back pain can be debilitating, stopping full participation in everyday activities and even preventing work.

HERBS

Relaxing herbs for nerves and antispasmodics for muscles can relieve tension and pain. Herbs that ease inflammation are beneficial and circulatory herbs can help revitalize stagnant tissues.

Valerian helps to relax the nerves and muscles and can also help to ease spasms. Avoid if taking sleep-inducing medication.
➨*Take 2.5–5ml tincture in a little water 3 times daily.*
Prickly ash is a circulatory stimulant, increasing blood flow into tense muscles. Avoid with anticoagulants.
➨*Take 2–4ml tincture in a little water 3 times daily.*

St John's wort reduces nerve inflammation to heal and soothe pain locally. Avoid taking internally during pregnancy and high doses in strong sunlight. Taken internally, it interacts with many prescription medications.
➨*Regularly apply a macerated flower oil to the affected area.*
Devil's claw is anti-inflammatory and analgesic, relieving pain, in turn easing movement in the back, and healing.
➨*Take 2–4ml tincture in a little water 3 times daily.*

ESSENTIAL OILS

Analgesic essential oils and those that increase local blood circulation, known as rubefacient oils, can be extremely beneficial in massage blends to relieve the pain of backache. To help relieve tension, take a bath using relaxing essential oils.

Rosemary is an effective analgesic and is very effective for releasing tension in stiff and overworked muscles. Avoid with epilepsy.
➨*Dilute 10 drops in 20ml (⅔fl oz) almond oil and use in a massage.*
Sweet marjoram boosts local blood flow to warm tissues and is analgesic, so is especially useful for muscular spasms.
➨*Dilute 10 drops in 20ml (⅔fl oz) almond oil and use in a massage.*

BEST STORAGE

Whether using St John's wort in liquid or capsule form, store it in an airtight container at room temperature in a dark, moisture-free place to stop active ingredients breaking down.

Lavender is an effective treatment for relieving muscular aches and pains and is also renowned for its relaxing properties, helping to ease tension.
➨*Dilute 6 drops in a bath dispersant and add to a bath of warm water.*

SUPPLEMENTS

These can be taken to help reduce inflammation and pain and accelerate tissue healing.

Vitamins B1, B6, and B12 taken together may help prevent a relapse of back pain linked to vertebral problems.
➨*Around 50–100mg each of vitamins B1 and B6, and 250–500mcg of vitamin B12, 3 times daily, is considered therapeutic.*

Proteolytic enzyme bromelain is anti-inflammatory, reducing pain and swelling and promoting faster healing of minor injuries in those with a variety of conditions, including back strain.
➡ *Take 100mg 3 times a day. Try taking for 12 weeks then have 4 weeks off.*

LIFESTYLE

Stay active. A sedentary lifestyle raises your risk of lower back pain. If your job involves a lot of sitting, make sure you balance that out with time for exercise and activities that keep you moving. Look for exercises specifically designed to improve back pain.

Lift carefully. Push rather than pull when you must move heavy objects. If you have to lift, let your legs do the work and avoid lifting and twisting simultaneously.

Replace your mattress. Sleeping on a medium-firm mattress supports the back and can reduce daytime pain.

Wear flat shoes or shoes with low heels (2.5cm/1 inch, or lower) to help prevent and ease lower back pain.

Quit, or cut down smoking. Evidence shows that nicotine increases lower back pain.

Consider losing weight. If you are overweight, you are more likely to have sciatica or lower back pain from a herniated disc or a pinched nerve.

Yoga keeps the spine flexible and less prone to injury – practise regularly.

OTHER THERAPIES

Acupuncture can relieve chronic lower back pain more effectively and for longer than many conventional treatments. Regular treatments may prevent relapses of back problems.

Visit a chiropractor or osteopath to relieve back pain caused by simple structural problems.

Alexander technique can correct poor posture, linked to chronic back pain.

NECK PAIN

Neck pain is a common problem, which tends to affect women more than men. It is rarely a sign of something serious. Usually it is caused by mechanical or postural strain or tension in the muscles or neck vertebrae.

HERBS

Herbs can relax the mind and body to relieve spasms and tension in the neck and ease movement. Use antispasmodic herbs for muscles and sedative herbs for nerves. Warming rubs also help with pain.

Passionflower helps to ease tension in the nervous system and relaxes the body. May cause drowsiness.
➡ *Infuse 1 tsp dried passionflower in 175ml (6fl oz) boiling water and drink 3 times daily.*

Valerian is a natural sedative and eases spasms in the body while relaxing nerve tension. Avoid if taking sleep-inducing medication.
➡ *Take 1–5ml tincture in a little water 3 times daily.*

White willow bark contains salicylic acid, which can ease pain and reduce inflammation. Avoid in pregnancy, if breastfeeding, and with sensitivity to the salicylate family of plants.
➡ *Take 2–4ml tincture in a little water 3 times daily.*

Cramp bark is antispasmodic and can be used to release tension that is held in the neck muscles. Cramp bark makes an effective remedy when combined with cayenne. Avoid cramp bark during pregnancy and when breastfeeding. Avoid cayenne internally with peptic ulcers and do not use on broken skin.
➡ *Make a topical cream: add 5ml cramp bark tincture to 50g (1¾oz) base cream, and add 5ml cayenne tincture. Apply to relieve pain.*

ESSENTIAL OILS

Many essential oils are both analgesic and also provide warmth to muscle tissues, releasing held-in tension and enhancing and supporting pain relief.

Eucalyptus works as an analgesic, providing effective relief for muscular aches and pains.
➡ *See remedy with jojoba oil, below.*

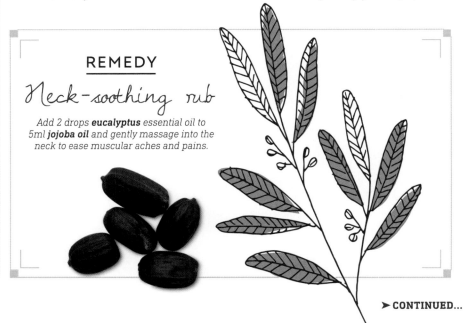

REMEDY
Neck-soothing rub

Add 2 drops **eucalyptus** essential oil to 5ml **jojoba oil** and gently massage into the neck to ease muscular aches and pains.

➤ CONTINUED...

" Therapies such as acupuncture can be effective treatments for relieving chronic pain."

Clove is mildly anaesthetic.
➡ *Add 5 drops to a bowl of hot water and apply a hot compress to the area using a clean cloth or flannel.*
Sweet marjoram is analgesic and warming.
➡ *Add 6 drops to 5ml bath dispersant and pour into a warm bath.*

LIFESTYLE

Heat can help to relieve pain. Try applying a hot compress or heating pad to provide some temporary relief.
T'ai chi, which combines deep breathing with slow and deliberate movements, can be beneficial for people suffering from chronic neck pain.
Daily stretching and strengthening neck exercises can help. Watch posture if sitting for long periods of time at a computer, and align the desk, chair, and screen at a comfortable height.

OTHER THERAPIES

Osteopathy and chiropractic can align vertebrae and ease muscle tension.
Alexander technique, which helps to improve posture, has shown more success at reducing chronic neck pain than standard medical treatments.
Acupuncture is a valuable treatment for relieving chronic pain.

KNEE PAIN

This can result from sports injuries, arthritis, or strain from overuse. The knee joint is vulnerable because it supports the full weight of the body and acts as a shock absorber when you run or jump. Seek medical help if the knee is acutely swollen or hot or you can't bear weight on it.

HERBS

Herbs can stimulate circulation to the joints, ease inflammation, and help repair tissues.

White willow bark is analgesic and has salicylic acid, which reduces inflammation. Avoid if pregnant or breastfeeding, or sensitive to salicylates.
➡ *Take 3–6ml tincture in a little water 3 times daily.*
Devil's claw is anti-inflammatory and analgesic, easing inflamed, stiff joints.
➡ *Take 2–8g daily in capsules.*
St John's wort reduces inflammation and heals damaged nerve tissue. Avoid in pregnancy and high doses in strong sunlight. If taken internally interacts with many prescription medicines.
➡ *Apply the macerated oil topically 2–3 times daily.*

ESSENTIAL OILS

Using analgesic, warming oils in massage helps to relieve local pain and stiffness.

Rosemary has analgesic properties. Avoid with epilepsy.
Sweet marjoram is warming and analgesic.
Ginger stimulates circulation.
➡ *Dilute 10 drops of any of the above essential oils in 20ml (¾fl oz) almond oil and use in a massage. Or dilute 6 drops of oil in a bath dispersant and add to a bath of warm water.*

SUPPLEMENTS

Natural supplements contain compounds that can help reduce joint inflammation.

Vitamin E can reduce inflammatory pain and help prevent joint damage.
➡ *Take 400iu vitamin E, containing d-alpha tocopherol and beta, delta, and gamma tocopherols.*
Rosehip contains an anti-inflammatory omega-6-like fatty acid called GOPO.
➡ *Take 2.5–5g daily in capsule form.*

LIFESTYLE

Wear well-cushioned shoes with a springy sole to prevent and lessen pain.
Rest – if you have injured your knee or it is very painful, keep it elevated and support with cold packs and bandages.
Warm up before exercise.
Losing weight can take pressure off knee joints and lessen pain.
Low-impact exercise carries less risk of knee injury. Yoga, swimming, and water aerobics are good choices.

OTHER THERAPIES

Acupuncture is effective for pain relief.
Homeopathy – injectable treatments have improved knee pain and stiffness in osteoarthritis sufferers.
Chiropractic and osteopathy help to increase mobility gently.

BANANA ROUNDS
If you have a glut of ripe bananas, try freezing peeled, sliced bananas on a baking tray, then transfer to a freezer bag. Defrost when required and add to cereals and porridge.

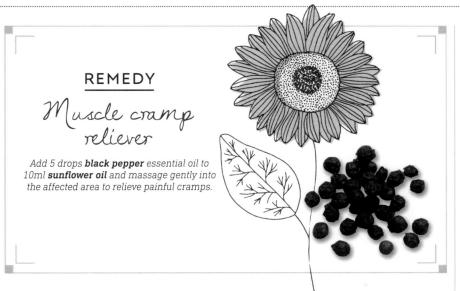

REMEDY

Muscle cramp reliever

Add 5 drops **black pepper** essential oil to 10ml **sunflower oil** and massage gently into the affected area to relieve painful cramps.

MUSCLE CRAMPS

Muscle cramps are not usually serious, but they can be incredibly painful. They can last minutes or hours and be debilitating. They are very common in the legs after heavy exercise, when you may be physically stressed and dehydrated.

HERBS

Antispasmodic herbs that reduce inflammation will relax muscles and help to ease stiffness. Circulatory stimulants will help to promote blood flow through the muscles to improve their function and general movement.

Cramp bark relaxes muscle tension to promote blood flow and movement. Avoid if pregnant or breastfeeding.
➡ *Take 4–8ml tincture in a little water 3 times daily.*
White willowbark is analgesic and anti-inflammatory, relieving pain and stiffness. Avoid if pregnant or breastfeeding, or sensitive to salicylates.
➡ *Take 3–6ml tincture in a little water 3 times daily.*

Ginkgo biloba increases blood supply to muscles and is anti-inflammatory to help relieve stiffness and cramping. Avoid in pregnancy, if breastfeeding, and with anticoagulant and antiplatelet medication.
➡ *Take a 66mg leaf extract tablet, providing the equivalent of 3300mg whole leaf, 1–3 times daily.*

ESSENTIAL OILS

Warming essential oils and rubefacient oils, which improve local circulation, can help to target pain relief, easing and reducing muscular stiffness and sudden pain from muscle cramping.

Lavender is extremely soothing, easing pain and cramping.
➡ *Add 5 drops to 10ml almond oil and massage into the affected area.*
Ginger is both warming and stimulating and acts as an effective analgesic, helping to ease the pain of cramps.
➡ *Add 5 drops to 10ml base oil and massage into the affected area.*
Black pepper has a warming action which is extremely effective for relieving muscular stiffness and aches and pains.
➡ *See remedy with sunflower oil, above.*

FOOD

Low levels of potassium, magnesium, and calcium have been linked to leg cramps.

Raw chocolate nibs are high in both calcium and magnesium.
➡ *Snack on chocolate nibs or sprinkle over yogurt or fruit salads.*
Tomato juice is rich in potassium.
➡ *Have a small glass daily to ward off leg cramps. Try spicing it up with a shot of chilli sauce to add pain-relieving curcumin.*
Bananas are potassium-rich.
➡ *Slice onto cereals or yogurts, add to fruit salads, or just keep one handy for a quick energy snack.*
Wholegrain foods supply magnesium.
➡ *Eat wholegrains daily.*
Apple cider vinegar provides potassium.
➡ *Combine 2 tsp apple cider vinegar with 1 tsp honey in a glass of warm water for a cramp-relieving drink.*
WHAT TO AVOID
Caffeine and alcohol can increase the risk of muscle cramping. Try cutting these out completely for a few weeks to see if symptoms resolve. If so either continue to avoid or reduce intake.

SUPPLEMENTS

If leg cramps are frequent, supplements may be needed to top up the diet.

Magnesium is taken for frequent cramps.
➡ *Take 350mg magnesium citrate daily.*

LIFESTYLE

Regular calf stretching exercises may help to prevent leg cramps reoccurring.
Adjust your bedding. Use pillows to prop up feet while sleeping on your back, or hang your feet over the end of the bed if you sleep on your stomach. Avoid tucking in blankets or bedding at the foot of the bed so you don't restrict the toes while asleep.

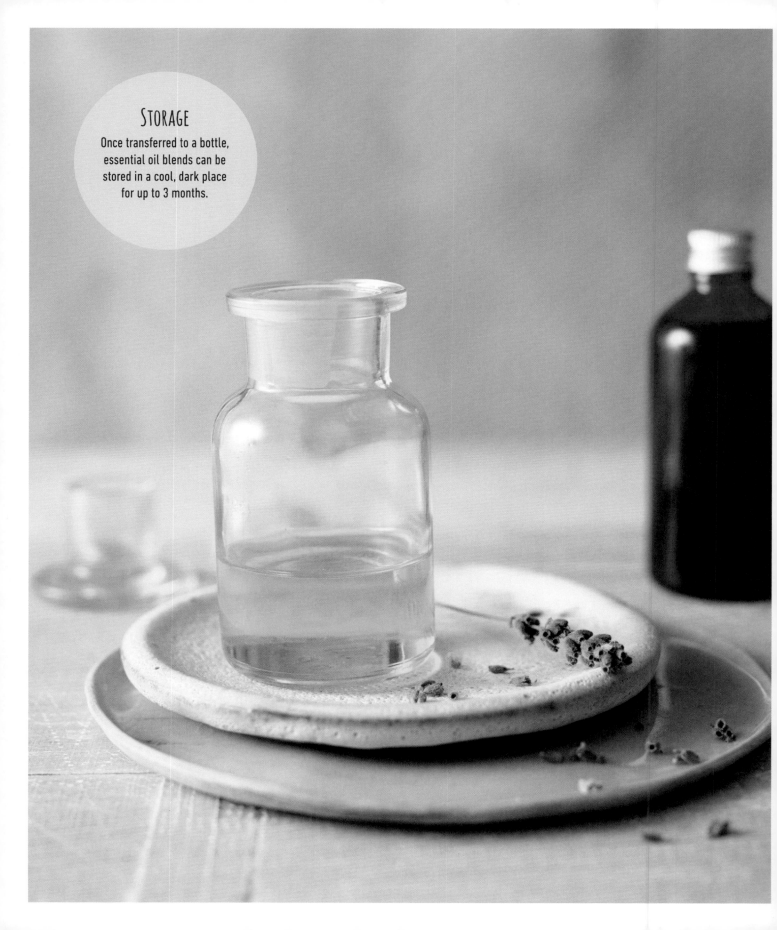

STORAGE

Once transferred to a bottle,
essential oil blends can be
stored in a cool, dark place
for up to 3 months.

HOW TO MAKE
AN ESSENTIAL OIL BLEND

Essential oils are highly concentrated substances so it is important that they are diluted in a base, or carrier, oil before use – only a few can be used neat. Medicinal bases, such as neem and St John's wort, add therapeutic benefits. Other base oils include almond, grapeseed, argan, olive, and jojoba. Dilutions can vary depending on whether a blend is being used on the face or on a wider area, as outlined below.

Makes 1½–2½ tbsp; multiply amounts for a larger batch

YOU WILL NEED

essential oil – a single oil or a blend – number of drops depends on use

1–2 tbsp base oil

small beaker or saucer

dark glass bottle

label

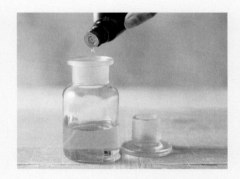

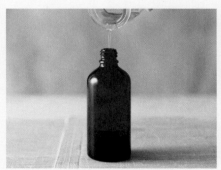

1 Add the essential oils to the base oil, in a beaker, saucer, or bottle. For a bath blend, add 4–6 drops essential oil to 1 tbsp base oil (or other bath dispersant such as whole milk) to disperse the oils in the water; for a body massage blend, add 7–15 drops essential oil to 1–2 tbsp base oil; and for a facial blend, add 3 drops essential oil to 1 tbsp base oil.

2 Either use the blend immediately in a bath or for a massage, or transfer to a sterilized dark glass bottle, seal, and label with the date and ingredients.

FROZEN SHOULDER

This common condition occurs when the ball and socket joint in the shoulder becomes inflamed, resulting in stiffness, pain, and a limited range of movement in the shoulder. It is more common in those who have a sedentary lifestyle, or who become sedentary for a period following an injury or an illness such as stroke.

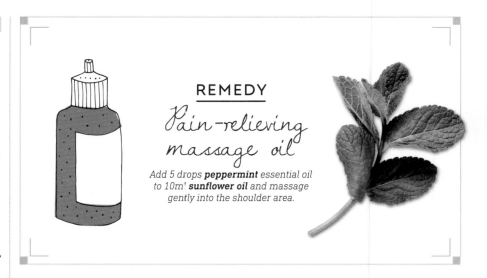

REMEDY

Pain-relieving massage oil

Add 5 drops **peppermint** essential oil to 10ml' **sunflower oil** and massage gently into the shoulder area.

HERBS

Herbs can help to reduce the pain and discomfort of frozen shoulder by stimulating the circulation to the shoulder joint, reducing inflammation and muscle stiffness, and supporting repair to damaged tissues.

White willow bark has analgesic properties and it contains salicylic acid, which helps to reduce inflammation. Avoid during pregnancy, when breastfeeding, or if you have a sensitivity to salicylates.
➡ *Take 3–6ml tincture in a little water 3 times daily.*

Devil's claw has an anti-inflammatory and analgesic action, making it useful for inflamed, stiff joints.
➡ *Take 2–8g daily in capsules.*

GRADUAL BENEFITS

Warming herbs such as prickly ash need a little time to take effect. Stick to the recommended dose and wait for the benefits.

Prickly ash is a warming stimulant for arterial and peripheral blood flow and eases muscular aches. Avoid with anticoagulant medication.
➡ *Take 2–4ml tincture in a little water 3 times daily.*

St John's wort reduces inflammation and heals damaged nerve tissue. Avoid internally in pregnancy and high doses in strong sunlight. Taken internally, it interacts with many prescription medicines.
➡ *Apply the macerated oil topically 2–3 times daily.*

Rosehip contains an omega-6-like fatty acid compound called GOPO. The powdered extract can relieve inflammation and help reduce pain.
➡ *Take 2.5–5g daily in capsules.*

ESSENTIAL OILS

Anti-inflammatory and analgesic essential oils can be used in massage blends or added to alternating hot and cold compresses to help relieve the symptoms of frozen shoulder.

Peppermint has stimulating properties that help to boost circulation and reduce pain.
➡ *See remedy with sunflower oil, above.*

Helichrysum has analgesic and anti-inflammatory properties.
➡ *Add 2 drops to 5ml base lotion and massage into the affected area.*

Lavender is an effective analgesic, easing discomfort.
➡ *Add 6 drops to a bowl of hot water and make a warm compress with a flannel. Apply to the shoulder for 7–10 minutes until the compress is at body temperature, then alternate with a cold compress. Repeat up to 5 times.*

LIFESTYLE

Exercise regularly to help prevent or improve frozen shoulder. Swimming gently exercises the upper body without putting undue strain on joints.

Heat may help to relieve ongoing pain and discomfort. Apply a hot compress or heating pad for temporary relief.

OTHER THERAPIES

Early physiotherapy is important to prevent the condition worsening and to maintain range of movement.

Chiropractic and osteopathy can help to increase mobility.

Acupuncture has been shown to provide effective relief for joint pain.

REPETITIVE STRAIN INJURY (RSI)

RSI is a musculoskeletal injury caused by repetitive movements, rigid posture, and other forms of chronic strain. It usually occurs in the wrist, but can affect other joints, such as the elbow. It can lead to the condition carpal tunnel syndrome (see p164). Symptoms include pain, stiffness, pins and needles, and loss of manual dexterity.

HERBS

Herbs reduce spasms and inflammation in the muscles, nerves, and connective tissues, easing pain and healing tissues.

Meadowsweet is anti-inflammatory. Avoid during pregnancy or with a sensitivity to salicylates.
➡ *Take 2–4ml tincture in a little water 3 times daily.*
Cramp bark is antispasmodic, relaxing muscles to relieve strain. See box, right. Avoid in pregnancy or if breastfeeding.
➡ *Add 5ml tincture to 50g (1¾oz) base cream and apply topically.*
Turmeric has a potent anti-inflammatory action to help reduce pain. Avoid therapeutic doses in pregnancy or with gallstones. May cause skin rashes.
➡ *Blend ½–1 tsp powder in warmed coconut milk and drink 3 times daily.*

ESSENTIAL OILS

Used in a massage blend or hot compress, essential oils can help to relieve inflammation and pain.

Eucalyptus has analgesic properties, offering relief from chronic pain.
➡ *Add 5 drops to 10ml arnica macerated oil and gently massage into the affected area.*

Peppermint is highly analgesic and used for pain relief.
Ginger is both analgesic and warming.
➡ *Add 6 drops to a bowl of hot water and make a compress using a flannel or cloth to apply to the affected area.*

SUPPLEMENTS

Anti-inflammatory supplements can help to manage pain.

Magnesium oil is effective for relieving pain and inflammation.
➡ *Apply topically. Look for one with easily absorbed magnesium chloride.*
Vitamin B6 eases carpal tunnel syndrome pain and may help other types of RSI.
➡ *Take 100mg daily for 3 months then switch to a B complex supplement.*

Vitamin C supports collagen production, helping to maintain the integrity of bones, muscles, skin, and tendons, as well as aid the absorption of B vitamins.
➡ *Take 1g daily.*

LIFESTYLE

Yoga, t'ai chi, and pilates strengthen muscles and flexibility and increase blood flow, reducing the risk of RSI and stimulating healing if RSI is present.

OTHER THERAPIES

Acupuncture can help to ease some of the pain and inflammation of RSI.
Homeopathy helps relieve RSI, carpal tunnel syndrome, and tendinitis – inflammation in a tendon.

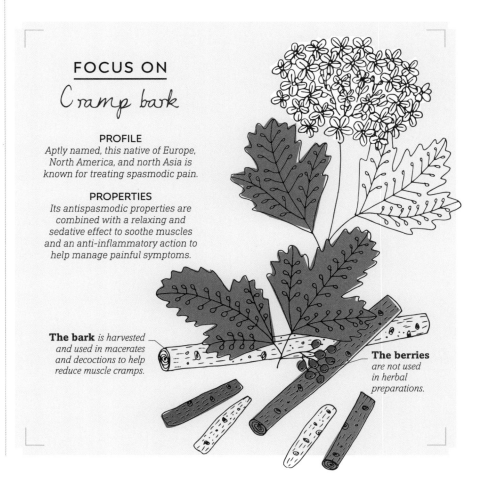

FOCUS ON

Cramp bark

PROFILE
Aptly named, this native of Europe, North America, and north Asia is known for treating spasmodic pain.

PROPERTIES
Its antispasmodic properties are combined with a relaxing and sedative effect to soothe muscles and an anti-inflammatory action to help manage painful symptoms.

The bark *is harvested and used in macerates and decoctions to help reduce muscle cramps.*

The berries *are not used in herbal preparations.*

SPORTS INJURIES

Being very physically active can make you more prone to bumps, tears, strains, and sprains, with pain ranging from annoying to debilitating. Most injuries heal with rest and support and natural approaches can help the healing process.

HERBS

Anti-inflammatory herbs can help to treat inflamed joints, muscles, or tendons, relieving discomfort and easing tension.

White willow bark is analgesic and anti-inflammatory. Avoid in pregnancy, if breastfeeding, and if sensitive to salicylates.
➡ *Take 3–6ml tincture in a little water 3 times daily.*
Devil's claw is analgesic and anti-inflammatory.
➡ *Take 2–8g daily in capsules.*
Arnica, an anti-inflammatory, stimulates blood supply for rapid healing. Do not use internally or on broken skin.
➡ *Make a cream with macerated arnica oil and arnica tincture.*

ESSENTIAL OILS

Essential oils can be used topically as "rubefacients", that is substances that improve the local circulation to promote tissue healing.

Lavender can ease pain and cramping.
➡ *See remedy with almond oil, below.*
Ginger increases circulation and is an effective topical analgesic.
➡ *Add 5 drops to 10ml base oil and massage into the affected area.*
Black pepper improves local circulation, providing effective relief for muscular stiffness and aches and pains
➡ *Add 5 drops to 10ml sunflower oil and massage into the affected area.*
Pine, a warming oil, is helpful for overexertion.
➡ *Add 6 drops to a bath dispersant.*

FOOD

Light, nutritious foods support the healing of tissues and bones.

Clear broth is protein-rich, in particular providing gelatine to support muscles, as well as bone-boosting minerals such as calcium and phosphorus.
➡ *Eat daily during recovery.*

LONGER LASTING

Lightly roasting pumpkin seeds then cooling them to lose excess moisture before storing them in an airtight container can extend their shelf life.

Fibre-rich vegetables, fruits, and legumes are also rich in vitamin C, magnesium, and zinc, all necessary for healing.
➡ *Consume daily.*
Pumpkin seeds have zinc for wound healing, tissue repair, and regrowth.
➡ *Snack on a handful or add to salads.*

SUPPLEMENTS

Supplements that reduce inflammation and pain support faster healing.

Vitamin C helps the body to make collagen, which maintains the integrity of bones, muscles, skin, and tendons.
➡ *Take 1g daily.*
Omega-3 fatty acids from fish or algal sources such as spirulina ease inflammation.
➡ *Take 1g daily.*
Proteolytic enzymes chymotrypsin, bromelain, papain, and trypsin reduce inflammation and pain and aid healing.
➡ *Take as directed.*

OTHER THERAPIES

Chiropractic and osteopathy rehabilitate by working on the spine.
Massage helps reduce muscle soreness.
Relaxation and stress-reducing practices such as meditation, muscle relaxation, and breathing can ease chronic pain and, with a strong link between stress and risk of injury, may prevent injury.

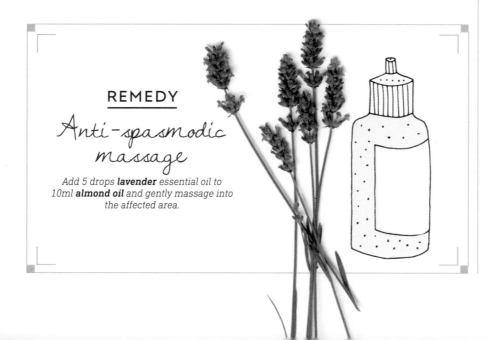

REMEDY

Anti-spasmodic massage

Add 5 drops **lavender** essential oil to 10ml **almond oil** and gently massage into the affected area.

BUNIONS AND HAMMER TOE

A bunion is an abnormal enlargement at the joint between the foot and the beginning of the big toe. Bunions develop over time, due to pressure, and while most don't affect walking, they can be painful. Another condition of the feet, which can be caused by pressure from a bunion or ill-fitting shoes, is called "hammer toe", where the middle joint of the second, third, fourth, or fifth toes becomes bent in the middle.

HERBS

Herbal remedies such as poultices, salves, or creams can be applied topically to help reduce any inflammation that is present and ease the pain caused by bunions and hammer toe.

St John's wort macerated oil can relieve nerve pain and reduce inflammation. Avoid internally in pregnancy and high doses in strong sunlight. Taken internally, it interacts with many prescription medicines.
➡️*Make a macerated oil and apply directly or use to make a salve or balm.*

" Herbal treatments can be applied topically to reduce inflammation and ease pain. "

Comfrey leaves are healing for bone and tissue damage and also relieve discomfort. Avoid on infected or deep skin lesions as it heals rapidly so could trap bacteria. Take professional advice before internal use.
➡️*Make a fresh poultice and apply directly to the bunion, or apply the macerated oil as with St John's wort.*

Castor oil is a traditional remedy for soothing inflammationn and in turn easing discomfort. Castor oil is rarely taken internally.
➡️*After bathing, smear onto the bunion directly, or soak a cotton wool pad and apply.*

ESSENTIAL OILS

Massaging with oils helps reduce the inflammation and pain that is associated with bunions and other foot problems.

German chamomile will help to reduce inflammation.
➡️*Add 2 drops to 5ml coconut oil and gently massage into the skin around the affected joint.*

Peppermint has a local anaesthetic effect that provides effective temporary pain relief.
➡️*Add 2 drops to 5ml coconut oil and gently massage into the skin around the affected joint.*

Rosemary has analgesic properties that can help to relieve pain effectively. Avoid with epilepsy.
➡️*Add 2 drops to 5ml base lotion and gently massage into the affected joint.*

LIFESTYLE

Properly-fitting shoes avoid putting unnecessary pressure on joints. Ideally, wear low-heeled shoes with a deep toe box. Adjustable shoes – with laces or straps – may provide comfort, and opt for those made from flexible materials such as leather. Avoid narrow or pointed shoes, which cramp the toes.

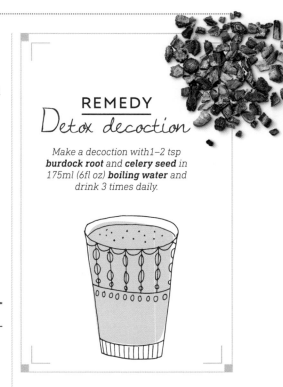

REMEDY
Detox decoction

*Make a decoction with1–2 tsp **burdock root** and **celery seed** in 175ml (6fl oz) **boiling water** and drink 3 times daily.*

GOUT

Gout is caused by a buildup of uric acid crystals – waste products from broken-down food – in the joints.

HERBS

Diuretic, cleansing, and anti-inflammatory herbs are beneficial.

Celery seed is anti-inflammatory and diuretic, helping remove uric acid from joints. Avoid the seeds in pregnancy.
➡️*Take 1ml tincture in a little water 3 times daily.*

Burdock root cleanses body tissues to remove toxins such as uric acid.
➡️*Combine with celery seed and/or nettle; see remedy, above.*

Nettle is diuretic and anti-inflammatory.
➡️*Infuse 1–2 tsp dried nettle in 175ml (6fl oz) boiling water and drink 3 times daily. Or apply topically as a compress.*

➤ CONTINUED...

ESSENTIAL OILS

Detoxifying essential oils help to reduce uric acid levels.

Juniper berry helps clear toxins.
➡*Add 5 drops to a warm foot bath and soak feet for 10 minutes.*
Lemon is a mild detoxifier.
➡*Add 5 drops to a bowl of hot water for a compress. Apply for 7–10 minutes, or until the compress is body temperature.*

FOOD

Staying hydrated and eating a plant-based diet helps decrease uric acid levels.

Montmorency cherries can reduce uric acid and ease the pain of gout.
➡*Take 30–60ml (1–2fl oz) of the liquid concentrate daily before bedtime.*
Coffee – moderate consumption may be associated with a reduced risk of gout.
➡*Drink daily in moderation.*
Low-fat dairy products may improve excretion of uric acid in the urine.
➡*Have low-fat milk or yogurt each day.*
Beans, pulses, and legumes are an excellent source of non-meat protein.
➡*Include regularly in meals.*
WHAT TO AVOID
Simple carbohydrates in white bread, cakes, sugary drinks, products with high-fructose corn syrup, marmite, yeast extract, alcohol, seafood, red meat.

SUPPLEMENTS

Anti-inflammatory supplements can ease symptoms and reduce frequency of attacks.

Vitamin C eases inflammation and lowers uric acid levels.
➡*Take 1g daily.*
Quercetin helps reduce uric acid and may provide relief from pain.
➡*Take 500mg daily with vitamin C.*
Omega-3 fatty acids ease inflammation.
➡*Take 1g daily with food.*

OSTEOARTHRITIS

This painful condition is caused by a gradual loss of cartilage and overgrowth of bone in the joints, especially the knees, hips, spine, and fingertips. Hard to prevent, it can be managed.

HERBS

Anti-inflammatory and detoxifying herbs help to heal joints and limit further damage; analgesic herbs ease pain; and circulatory herbs boost blood flow to the joints.

Meadowsweet has anti-inflammatory salicylic acid and is analgesic. Avoid in pregnancy or with salicylate sensitivity.
➡*Infuse 1–2 tsp dried meadowsweet in 175ml (6fl oz) boiling water and drink 3 times daily.*
Celery seed soothes nerves and is diuretic. Avoid the seeds in pregnancy.
➡*Take 1–5ml tincture in a little water 3 times daily.*

Bogbean, a traditional arthritis remedy, is anti-inflammatory and cleansing.
➡*Take 1–5ml tincture in a little water 3 times daily.*
Comfrey helps repair tissues (see box, below). Avoid on deep or infected skin lesions as it heals rapidly so could trap bacteria. Get advice before internal use.
➡*Make a macerate using 2 drops ginger essential oil and 10ml comfrey oil and apply regularly.*

ESSENTIAL OILS

Warming and analgesic oils are helpful. If arthritis is painful, don't massage the area.

Ginger is stimulating and analgesic.
➡*Add 6 drops to a bowl of hot water and make a hot compress. Apply for 7–10 minutes, or until the compress is at body temperature.*
Black pepper is analgesic and warming.
➡*Add 5 drops to 10ml coconut oil and massage into the affected area.*
Nutmeg will help to warm the joints.
➡*Add 6 drops to 5ml bath dispersant.*

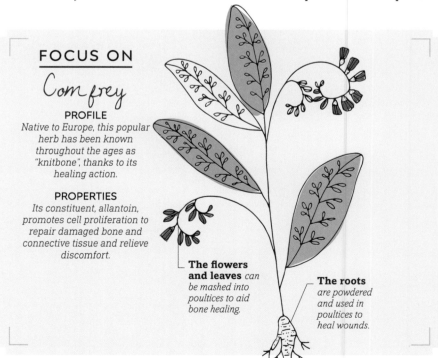

FOCUS ON

Comfrey

PROFILE
Native to Europe, this popular herb has been known throughout the ages as "knitbone", thanks to its healing action.

PROPERTIES
Its constituent, allantoin, promotes cell proliferation to repair damaged bone and connective tissue and relieve discomfort.

The flowers and leaves *can be mashed into poultices to aid bone healing.*

The roots *are powdered and used in poultices to heal wounds.*

FOOD

Foods with anti-inflammatory nutrients are supportive.

Cherries have anti-inflammatory anthocyanins to ease pain and stiffness.
➡ *Add to cereals, snacks, and yogurt.*
Matcha, powdered green tea leaves, is antioxidant-rich, slowing cartilage breakdown and reducing inflammation.
➡ *Have a daily matcha latte.*
A Mediterranean diet of fish, vegetables, fruit, cereals, beans, and olive oil can decrease swelling, tenderness, and pain and improve movement and vitality.
➡ *Base your daily diet on these foods.*
WHAT TO AVOID
Red meat, sugar, saturated fats, salt, and caffeine.

SUPPLEMENTS

Topping up key nutrients can delay the onset of osteoarthritis.

Vitamin C can prevent cartilage damage.
➡ *Take 1–2g daily.*
Vitamin E reduces inflammatory pain.
➡ *Take 400iu with d-alpha, beta, delta, and gamma tocopherols.*
Glucosamine sulphate eases symptoms.
➡ *Take up to 1500mg daily.*

LIFESTYLE

Regular moderate exercise that does not put stress on joints alleviates pain; losing weight reduces your risk.
High heels in later life increase risk as they shift weight, adding pressure to the knee joints. Wear well-cushioned shoes with a springy sole.
T'ai chi eases pain and stiffness.

OTHER THERAPIES

Acupuncture is helpful for pain relief.
Homeopathy is strengthening. Injected treatments have improved symptoms.

OSTEOPOROSIS

This means "porous bones" and describes any disease that reduces bone mass. Some bone loss is natural with age, but when bones become thin and brittle, symptoms such as loss of height, lower back pain, hip, wrist and spine fractures, and a bend in the spine, are more likely to occur.

HERBS

Osteoporosis due to oestrogen deficiency benefits from herbs that boost oestrogen levels. Herbs that improve gut health and nutrient absorption can be helpful.

Red clover has isoflavone compounds, which boost oestrogenic activity to limit bone density loss. Avoid high doses in pregnancy or with anticoagulants.
➡ *Infuse 2 tsp dried red clover in 175ml (6fl oz) boiling water and drink 3 times daily.*
Calendula has an oestrogen-like action, encouraging calcium absorption, and it supports liver function. Not suitable during pregnancy.
➡ *Infuse 1–2 tsp dried calendula in 175ml (6fl oz) boiling water and drink 3 times daily.*
Dandelion root, a digestive tonic, aids liver function and contains probiotic inulin to boost nutrient absorption. Avoid with gallstones.
➡ *Take 2–5ml tincture in a little water 3 times daily.*

FOOD

Calcium and other key micronutrients are vital to build bone strength and density.

Low-fat dairy such as yogurt and cottage cheese are calcium-rich, which is better absorbed from food than supplements.
➡ *Include 1–2 servings a day.*

Leafy greens such as kale, collard and mustard greens, watercress, and rocket supply magnesium, needed to balance calcium intake.
➡ *Make a pesto with kale, watercress or rocket, olive oil, lemon, and pine nuts.*
Legumes such as chickpeas and lentils have boron, which helps limit calcium and magnesium loss via urine.
➡ *Add to soups, stews, and salads or blitz into a hummus dip.*
WHAT TO AVOID
Caffeine increases urinary loss of calcium and magnesium. Heavy alcohol consumption increases risk.

SUPPLEMENTS

These can support the diet to improve bone mineral density and reduce fracture risk.

Omega-3 fatty acids from oily fish or algae (DHA and EPA) appear to reduce bone loss, as well as inflammation.
➡ *Take 1g daily.*
Vitamin D and calcium taken together promote strong bones.
➡ *Take 1g calcium and 400iu vitamin D3 daily.*
Green tea has polyphenols, which strengthen bones by improving collagen synthesis.
➡ *Take 100–750mg daily.*

LIFESTYLE

Losing weight takes pressure off bones. But after the age of 50, a little extra weight does protect bones in women and muscle mass protects men.
Quit smoking, a known risk factor for low bone mineral density (BMD).
Manage depression. Research shows a clear connection between this and BMD.
Weight-bearing exercise maintains bone strength. Walking and aerobics prevent bone loss and high-impact running and weight-training increase bone density.
Yoga boosts flexibility and bone strength.

SYSTEMIC DISORDERS

A complex interplay of hormones, metabolic processes, and body systems supports health, and imbalances can affect the whole body. Here we look at the crucial role diet and nutrients play in avoiding systemic problems and how holistic remedies can support the entire body, promoting balance and strengthening body systems. When imbalances and problems such as inflammation take hold, find out which nutrients and natural remedies can help to restore balance and support recovery.

○   ○   ○   ○

STAYING WELL
SYSTEMIC DISORDERS

Systemic disorders affect the entire body, rather than just a single organ or body part, and are often associated with chronic inflammation or with changes in immunity or metabolism. Preventative measures are key to avoiding systemic disorders taking hold. The nutrients your body receives, together with natural remedies, can support whole body health throughout life and ensure that body systems are working optimally.

FOOD

Eating a healthy, balanced diet has a profound and lifelong effect on health.

ANTI-INFLAMMATORY FOODS

The food we eat can have a considerable influence on levels of inflammation in the body. A diet based around fresh, organic whole foods, with fruits and vegetables, ensures a range of substances, such as antioxidant polyphenols, to fight the action of damaging free radicals and toxins to protect against inflammation.

HEALTHY FATS

Healthy oils help to optimize health throughout the body, preventing the inflammation associated with systemic disorders, providing fuel for the brain, lubricating joints, and maintaining skin health. Coconut oil is metabolized rapidly in the body, providing a quick source of energy. Although coconut oil contains saturated fat, this is made up of medium-chain fatty acids, which are easier to digest than long-chain fatty acids and less likely to lead to weight gain. Coconut oil also has an anti-inflammatory fatty acid, lauric acid, and antiviral properties to boost immunity.

Olive oil, particularly extra virgin olive oil, is a monounsaturated fat with well-documented health benefits. The phytonutrient oleocanthal in olive oil has an anti-inflammatory effect and olive oil also has protective antioxidants to boost immunity.

BERRY BENEFITS

Brightly coloured berries, such as strawberries, bilberries, and blackberries, contain antioxidant flavonoids to help fight disease. Flavonoids also help to lower insulin levels after eating, so consuming berries with a meal helps to control metabolism and avoid post-meal energy troughs. Bilberries also contain the antioxidant anthocyanin, shown to strengthen blood vessels by protecting them against the damaging effects of inflammation.

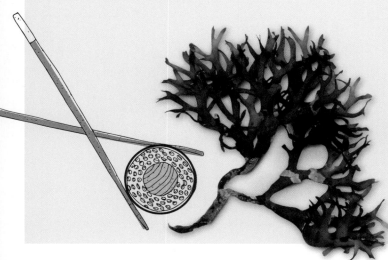

Add seaweed *to salads, eat as a side dish, or enjoy in a sushi roll.*

"Herbal remedies can help to manage stress and prevent it impacting on the body."

Nutrients for thyroid function

Seaweed contains iodine – a vital component of thyroid gland hormones, which play a role in metabolism and nerve function and which can only be obtained from the diet – as well as the micronutrients needed to metabolize iodine fully, such as selenium, zinc, iron, and vitamins A and E.

Balancing the gut

Fermented foods such as kimchi and live yogurt contain probiotics to top up good bacteria in the gut. A healthy gut flora boosts immunity, supporting health throughout the body.

Too many acid-forming foods can encourage inflammation, so alkaline foods such as green juices and nut milks are beneficial.

Fluid-balancing foods

Diuretic foods such as onion, aubergine, asparagus, watermelon, and green tea help to balance fluids, promoting healthy cell function and supporting the removal of waste and toxins.

Herbs

Herbal remedies help to strengthen immunity and balance hormone activity. Herbs also help to manage stress, preventing its effects from impacting on the body.

Tonic herbs to support the body

Tonic herbs help to strengthen body systems. For example, ashwagandha and skullcap promote healthy nerve function, while hawthorn acts as a tonic for the heart and vascular system, boosting circulation to the body tissues and ensuring that nutrients and oxygen are carried to cells around the body.

Liver tonics, such as milk thistle and dandelion root, support the liver's vital functions, including the elimination of toxins and regulation of hormones. Vervain is a tonic for digestion, in turn promoting immunity, while siberian ginseng (eleuthero) supports the adrenal glands, also boosting immunity.

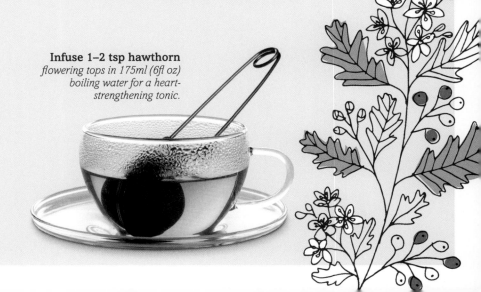

Infuse 1–2 tsp hawthorn
flowering tops in 175ml (6fl oz) boiling water for a heart-strengthening tonic.

Antibacterial effect

Herbs with an antibacterial action can be used to help improve skin health and balance bacteria naturally present on the skin, refreshing and helping to prevent problems such as body odour.

Supportive herbs

Many herbs have anti-inflammatory and antioxidant actions that can be supportive while undergoing treatments for conditions by reducing the side effects of medications, improving resilience, and strengthening immunity. Ginkgo biloba and gotu kola are effective antioxidant herbs, helping to prevent free radical damage in the body; while turmeric and white willow bark have anti-inflammatory properties that can support health.

The traditional Ayurvedic herb turmeric contains curcumin, which is powerfully antioxidant, as well as several active substances that can inhibit inflammation.

Diuretic herbs

Along with certain foods, herbs can also have a diuretic effect to help balance fluid levels in the body, promoting the removal of toxins and controlling inflammation. Dandelion leaf, hawthorn, juniper, and parsley are effective diuretics.

Essential oils

Therapeutic oils can have a range of actions to prevent chronic stress having a detrimental effect on the body.

Calming oils

Essential oils can have a reviving effect to help you cope with stress and in turn limit the potentially damaging impact of stress. Sweet orange is uplifting and also acts as a mild sedative to calm the mind and body. German chamomile has a calming effect on the mind and is anti-inflammatory to support tissue health.

Cleansing effects

Many oils have cleansing properties. Fennel, lemon, and juniper berry support eliminatory processes, helping to remove waste, stimulate lymphatic drainage, and ease congestion.

Anti-inflammatory oils

Essential oils can have effective anti-inflammatory effects throughout the body. Yarrow can be used in a targeted massage to reduce the aches and pains associated with inflammation, and

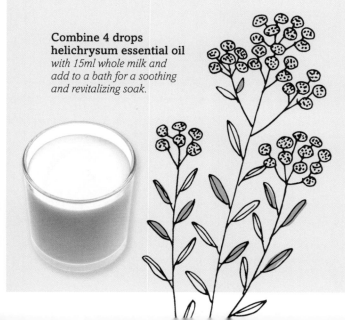

Combine 4 drops helichrysum essential oil *with 15ml whole milk and add to a bath for a soothing and revitalizing soak.*

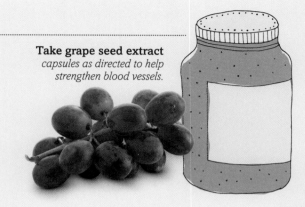

Take grape seed extract *capsules as directed to help strengthen blood vessels.*

also has a profound soothing action to help the body cope with stress. Helichrysum combines pain-relieving properties with an emotionally uplifting effect.

Supplements

Taking targeted supplements can support a healthy diet to boost health and immunity throughout the body.

The B Vitamin Family

A supplement that contains all of the B vitamins, including the related nutrient coenzyme Q10 (CoQ10), which acts in a similar way to a vitamin, can support cell metabolism and energy production and help to regulate the action of the thyroid gland.

Probiotics for Gut Health

A probiotic supplement can be especially useful after a course of antibiotics, when both good and bad bacteria are stripped from the gut. Probiotics help repopulate the gut with beneficial bacteria and restore a healthy balance of bacteria, which in turn promotes healthy immunity.

Magnesium Boost

A magnesium deficiency can lead us to feel more tired than usual and plays a role in chronic fatigue. Adequate magnesium also helps to improve insulin sensitivity and glucose control.

Energy-Boosting Nutrients

Spirulina, a naturally occurring algae, has potent antioxidant and anti-inflammatory effects and an impressive range of nutrients including protein, amino acids, and micronutrients to help prevent mental and physical fatigue during times of stress.

Rhodiola, a traditional eastern European folk medicine, is also used to enhance physical and mental performance.

Circulation Supporter

Resveratrol, a compound derived largely from the skins of red grapes, has powerful anti-inflammatory effects that can help to promote and support blood vessel health. Grape seed extract also has compounds to help boost circulation by strengthening blood vessels – antioxidant substances called oligomeric proanthocyanidins (OPCs) found in grape seed extract help to protect and strengthen blood vessels.

"Targeted supplements can support diet to boost health and immunity."

TREATMENTS

SYSTEMIC DISORDERS

Systemic disorders, which impact the whole body, can be caused by factors such as hormonal imbalances, inflammation, or problems with metabolism. Holistic remedies can support conventional treatments to promote recovery.

BODY ODOUR

We often associate body odour with sweat, but in fact sweat is almost odourless. However, acids in sweat are broken down by naturally occurring bacteria on skin, causing unpleasant body odour. How strong body odour is can vary from person to person and from day to day dependent on several factors. Rather than masking odour with perfumes, it is better to address the root cause.

HERBS

Herbs can be used to improve skin health and balance bacteria, refreshing the skin and reducing body odour. Improving liver and kidney function can also be supportive, promoting the effective cleansing of toxins from the body.

Sage has spicy camphor-like volatile oils, which have antibacterial properties and are toning, to help revitalize skin tissue. Avoid therapeutic doses during pregnancy and with epilepsy and avoid taking for prolonged periods of time.
➡*Infuse 2 tsp dried sage in 175ml (6fl oz) boiling water and blend into a body wash to use in the shower.*

Lavender is a refreshing herb with antimicrobial properties, helping to promote healthy skin.
➡*Infuse 2 tsp dried lavender in 175ml (6fl oz) boiling water. Add to your bath.*
Dandelion root is a strengthening tonic for the liver and the kidneys, improving digestive and excretory function. See box, right. Avoid with gallstones.
➡*Take 2–5ml tincture in a little water 3 times daily.*

ESSENTIAL OILS

Therapeutic essential oils can be used to prevent the bacteria that cause body odour from multiplying, leaving your skin feeling fresh and odour-free.

Bergamot is cooling and deodorizing.
Lemongrass works effectively as a deodorant.
Lavender works on the bacteria that cause body odour.
➡*Add 5 drops of any of the above essential oils to 5ml base lotion and apply to the affected area.*

FOOD

Eating a healthy, balanced diet that includes plenty of fresh vegetables and wholegrains, and limiting your sugar intake will help to promote skin health.

FOCUS ON

Dandelion

PROFILE
Several species of this traditional liver tonic are found in temperate regions in Europe, Asia, and South America.

PROPERTIES
Dandelion has diuretic properties and also acts as a strengthening tonic for the whole of the digestive system.

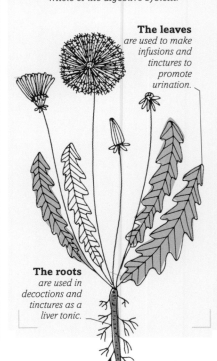

The leaves *are used to make infusions and tinctures to promote urination.*

The roots *are used in decoctions and tinctures as a liver tonic.*

Chlorophyll-rich foods, such as kale, spinach, and chard, and other dark green, leafy vegetables are beneficial. Chlorophyll is an antioxidant that gives vegetables their colour and acts as a natural deodorizer and cleanser in the body, neutralizing the bacteria that cause body odour.
➥*Try to include 2–3 servings with meals each week.*

Live foods such as kimchi – traditionally fermented vegetables – help to feed good bacteria already present in the gut. When there is an imbalance in gut bacteria, with low levels of beneficial bacteria, this can aggravate unpleasant body odour.
➥*Eat as a side dish or condiment.*

WHAT TO AVOID
Too much red meat, processed foods, foods low in fibre, and some strong spices, all of which may increase body odour. Excess sugar can trigger perspiration in some people, which when combined with bacteria on the skin can lead to unpleasant body odour.

LIFESTYLE

Wear cotton and other breathable fabrics. Some synthetic fabrics used in workout clothing are also breathable because they have fibres that wick sweat away from the skin.

Dry off thoroughly. Bacteria find it harder to take hold on dry skin so after a bath or shower, ensure that areas that sweat profusely are totally dry.

Avoid antibacterial soaps. Apart from contributing to global antibiotic resistance, they upset the natural bacterial balance on the skin. There's also little evidence they prevent body odour and they may dry out skin.

Check for diabetes. Without enough insulin, the body starts to break down fat for fuel, which causes a buildup of substances called ketones in the body, leading to diabetic ketoacidosis, which can produce a change in body odour.

> *"Vascular-strengthening tonic herbs help to improve circulation, while diuretic herbs remove excess fluid."*

FLUID RETENTION

The buildup of fluids in body tissues is known as oedema, which has a number of accompanying symptoms including bloating, muscle aches and other flu-like symptoms, fatigue, anxiety, and depression. Women tend to experience oedema more, often during menstrual cycles.

HERBS

Certain herbs can help to strengthen the capillaries. These herbs can be supported with vascular tonic herbs that improve the circulation, as well as and diuretic herbs, which assist the body in eliminating excess fluids.

Dandelion leaf acts as a diuretic to help expel excess fluids, and also contains potassium, which helps to balance mineral levels. Avoid with gallstones.
➥*Infuse 1–2 tsp dried dandelion leaf in 175ml (6fl oz) boiling water and drink 3 times daily.*

Horse chestnut strengthens capillaries and reduces local water retention. Avoid with anticoagulants. If irritant to the stomach, take with soothing limeflower.
➥*Take 1–4ml tincture in a little water 3 times daily.*

Hawthorn is a strengthening vascular and heart tonic, boosting blood flow. Avoid with heart medication unless under medical supervision.
➥*Take 2–5ml tincture in a little water 3 times daily.*

ESSENTIAL OILS

Detoxifying essential oils can be used to stimulate lymphatic drainage and help eliminate toxins.

Fennel is a detoxifying and diuretic oil.
Juniper berry is an effective detoxifier.
➥*Add 5 drops of either of the above oils to 10ml wheatgerm oil and use in a massage.*

Lemon, a cleansing oil, is recommended for detoxifying the body.
➥*Add 6 drops to a bath dispersant.*

FOOD

Some foods draw excess water from the tissues, relieving bloating. Dehydration exacerbates retention so drink plenty of healthy fluids throughout the day.

Protein deficiency can contribute to oedema. Plant-based proteins such as pulses and legumes are also rich in fibre, which may help reduce oedema.
➥*Eat plant-based proteins regularly.*

SUPER KALE
Kale delivers healthy nutrients whether raw or cooked. Raw kale has higher amounts of vitamin C and the B vitamins, while cooked kale releases more iron.

➤ CONTINUED...

Diuretic foods such as onions, celery, asparagus, and watermelon help to balance fluids.
➡️*Include regularly in your diet.*

Oranges and grapefruits contain a flavonoid, hesperidin, found abundantly in the pith, which strengthens capillaries to reduce leaking.
➡️*Eat the whole fruit, including the pith, in preference to the juice.*

WHAT TO AVOID
A high salt intake, which encourages oedema. Caffeine-containing drinks and alcohol are dehydrating, leading to fluid imbalances. Liquorice can also exacerbate oedema.

SUPPLEMENTS

These can help strengthen the capillaries to prevent fluid leakage into tissues.

Vitamin B6 helps to regulate oestrogen levels, which in turn can help to address fluid retention around the time of menstruation.
➡️*Take 25–50mg daily.*

Vitamin E can help boost capillary strength to reduce or stop leakage.
➡️*Take 600iu daily with food.*

Vitamin C boosts collagen production and strengthens tissues.
➡️*Take a daily 500mg to 1g supplement that includes rutin and bioflavonoids.*

LIFESTYLE

Consult your doctor about medications such as hormone drugs, painkillers, steroids, and blood pressure drugs, which can cause fluid retention.

Food allergies can lead to fluid retention. If concerned, get tested.

Gentle exercise, such as pilates, yoga, or swimming, can help combat oedema.

OTHER THERAPIES

Manual lymphatic drainage, a type of massage, can tackle fluid retention.

INFLAMMATION

The inflammatory process is a healthy protective mechanism linked to the immune system to aid healing. However, if inflammation is prolonged it can trigger serious diseases.

HERBS

Use antioxidant and restorative tonic herbs and ones that reduce inflammation and restore healthy metabolic processes.

Schisandra, an antioxidant, helps prevent cellular damage. It works particularly on the liver and brain. Avoid with acute infections and barbiturates.
➡️*Take 2–4ml tincture in a little water 3 times daily.*

Liquorice has steroid-like molecules, which can help to calm inflammation, especially if linked to auto-immune disorders. Avoid in pregnancy, with hypertension, and large doses over prolonged periods.
➡️*For a decoction, add ½–1 tsp dried liquorice root to 250ml (9fl oz) boiling water; drink 3 times daily.*

ESSENTIAL OILS

These can help to control the inflammatory response by boosting circulation and promoting tissue repair.

German chamomile has an anti-inflammatory action.

Yarrow is soothing and healing.

Helichrysum is anti-inflammatory and pain-relieving.
➡️*Add 6 drops of any of the above essential oils to a bath dispersant.*

FOOD

Foods that contain micronutrient polyphenols protect against inflammation.

Apples have the flavonol isorhamnetin, which helps to fight inflammation.
➡️*Keep an apple handy to snack on or have a baked apple for dessert.*

Turmeric has the anti-inflammatory compound curcumin.
➡️*Add a pinch to scrambled eggs, grate fresh root over roasted veg, or try the remedy with coconut milk, below.*

Red, purple, and black grapes provide resveratrol, a potent anti-inflammatory.
➡️*A daily glass is a therapeutic dose.*

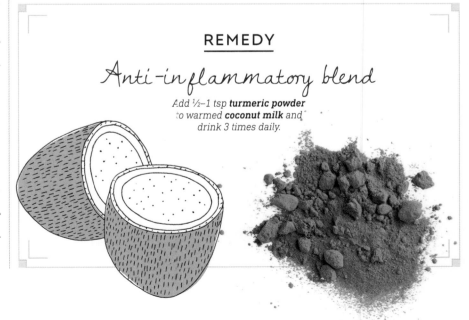

REMEDY

Anti-inflammatory blend

Add ½–1 tsp **turmeric powder** to warmed **coconut milk** and drink 3 times daily.

BEST UNPEELED

The skin of an apple houses over half its fibre and has a greater concentration of essential vitamins, so buy organic and don't discard the skin.

Legumes contain fermentable soluble fibre, which feeds good bacteria in the gut and reduces inflammation.
➥ *Use to make dips, or add to meals.*

WHAT TO AVOID
Overconsumption of refined sugars, saturated fats, and animal protein.

SUPPLEMENTS

Tackling chronic inflammation may require levels of nutrients that are hard to obtain from food alone.

Zinc deficiency triggers inflammation.
➥ *Take 8–11mg daily.*
Omega-3 supplements are calming.
➥ *Take 1–1.5g daily.*
Resveratrol reduces inflammation.
➥ *Take 150mg per day.*
Spirulina has antioxidant and calming anti-inflammatory effects.
➥ *Take up to 3g a day in a capsule.*

LIFESTYLE

Try meditation to relieve stress.
Chronic stress triggers the release of high levels of inflammatory hormones.
Get sufficient sleep. A deficit is linked to increased chronic inflammation.
Keep blood sugar under control.

OTHER THERAPIES

Massage reduces muscle inflammation.

VASCULITIS

This is an inflammation of the blood vessels. It causes a variety of changes in blood vessel walls, including thickening, weakening, narrowing, and scarring, which can restrict blood flow, resulting in organ and tissue damage. Vasculitis can range from a minor problem, with red patches on the skin, to a more serious systemic illness.

HERBS

Herbs can support the various tissues and organs affected by vasculitis. Anti-inflammatory herbs are foremost, supported by antibacterial and antiviral herbs where appropriate, as well as tonic herbs to improve immune function.

Holy basil is antibacterial, anti-inflammatory, and a strengthening tonic, used to help regulate immune function. Avoid in pregnancy.
➥ *Infuse ½–1 tsp dried holy basil in 175ml (6fl oz) boiling water and drink 3 times daily.*
Nettle is anti-allergenic, anti-inflammatory, and a strengthening blood tonic to support the kidneys.
➥ *Infuse 1–2 tsp dried nettle in 175ml (6fl oz) boiling water. Drink 3 times daily.*
Turmeric has a powerful and general anti-inflammatory action on the body. Avoid therapeutic doses during pregnancy and with gallstones. May cause skin rashes.
➥ *See remedy, opposite.*

FOOD

A diet that includes plenty of protective antioxidant-rich foods, such as fresh fruit and vegetables, is one of the best ways to support health and fight inflammation throughout the body.

Green tea has a range of antioxidant and anti-inflammatory compounds that can help to reduce inflammation.
➥ *Drink 2–3 cups daily, hot or cold.*
Bilberries are rich in anthocyanins, flavonoids that can help to protect and strengthen the blood vessels from the effects of inflammation.
➥ *The dried fruits can be brewed in a decoction, or try some bilberry jam.*
Buckwheat contains rutin, an antioxidant that helps to strengthen the blood vessels.
➥ *Buckwheat grains can be cooked like rice, or toasted and brewed as a delicious light tea. Buckwheat porridge makes a healthy breakfast.*

SUPPLEMENTS

These can support chronic inflammation by supplying a steady dose of antioxidants and strengthening the blood vessels.

Grape seed extract contains antioxidant compounds called oligomeric proanthocyanidins (OPCs), which protect and strengthen blood vessels.
➥ *Take 150–300mg daily.*
Vitamin C boosts circulation and tissue regeneration to keep veins healthy.
➥ *Take 500mg to 1g daily.*
Vitamin E improves vein health.
➥ *Take 750iu to 1g daily.*

" *Herbs that help reduce inflammation can treat body tissues affected by vasculitis.*"

CHRONIC FATIGUE (ME)

Chronic fatigue syndrome, also known as myalgic encephalomyelitis (ME), is a condition characterized by exhaustion that doesn't improve with rest. Its cause is unclear but it is thought that it may be a combination of genetics, viral infection, and inflammation from oxidative stress. For this reason it often requires more than one healing approach.

HERBS

Gentle tonic herbs that do not over-stimulate the body can be taken long term to help restore strength, while strengthening digestive tonics and immune-boosting herbs are supportive and also help to improve vitality.

Siberian ginseng helps to fight fatigue. It is also a strengthening tonic for the adrenal glands, which secrete hormones to help regulate the body's response to stress and are essential for vitality, as well as for the immune system. Avoid with acute infections.
➡*Take 2–4ml tincture in a little water 3 times daily.*

Astragalus, traditionally used for physical weakness, is an immune system tonic, which rebuilds strength and vitality. Avoid with acute infections and with immune-suppressant and blood-thinning drugs.
➡*Take 2–4ml tincture in a little water 3 times daily.*

Vervain acts as a digestive tonic, an antispasmodic herb, and also a strengthening tonic for the nervous system, helping to relax both mind and body. Avoid in pregnancy; excessive doses may cause vomiting.
➡*Take 2ml tincture in a little water 3 times daily.*

ESSENTIAL OILS

Aromatic essential oils can help to reduce the symptoms of ME.

Basil is refreshing, bringing strength and clarity to the mind. Avoid in pregnancy.
➡*Add 3 drops to a diffuser to inhale.*

Orange is gently sedative, helping to promote relaxation to restore strength, and is also emotionally uplifting.

Geranium can harmonize energy in both the mind and body.
➡*Add 5 drops of either orange or geranium to a bath dispersant to mix into a warm bath.*

SUPPLEMENTS

These can be helpful additions to a nutrient-dense diet to support immunity, fight fatigue, and lift low spirits.

Magnesium deficiency is known to play a role in ME.
➡*Look for a magnesium oil that contains magnesium citrate to use topically.*

Spirulina, a naturally occurring algae, is a rich source of protein, amino acids, and other essential nutrients and antioxidants. The supplement can be helpful in combating mental and physical fatigue.
➡*Take up to 3g a day in capsule form.*

Rhodiola is a traditional Eastern European folk medicine, used to enhance physical and mental performance and to fight depression.
➡*Take 400mg a day to help fight feelings of exhaustion.*

LIFESTYLE

Check your thyroid function and iron levels with your doctor to check low levels are not misdiagnosed as ME.

Relaxation techniques combined with gentle exercise can support body and mind. Try yoga, chi gung, and t'ai chi.

FIBROMYALGIA

This usually affects women and is characterized by chronic pain and fatigue. The cause is uncertain, but it may be linked to an excess of certain brain chemicals or a fault with the transmission of pain signals. Symptoms include muscle stiffness, sleep disturbances, gastrointestinal discomfort, anxiety, and depression.

HERBS

Tonic herbs are the main natural remedy for fibromyalgia, with the focus on herbs to improve circulation to the head and central nervous system. Herbs also help to relax muscles, calm the mind, and relieve pain. Start with low doses and build up gradually.

Gotu kola is a relaxing tonic for the brain and nerves. It enhances cognitive function and rebuilds connective tissues. See box, opposite. Avoid in pregnancy and with epilepsy. May cause skin sensitivity.
➡*Take 3–5ml of 1:2 tincture in a little water 3 times daily.*

Wild oats are restorative and a tonic for the nerves, making them useful for treating a state of debility.
➡*Take 2–5ml of the green milky seed tincture in a little water 3 times daily.*

FERMENTING FORMULA

Oxygen spoils the fermentation process so if making your own sauerkraut, make sure the cabbage stays submerged in its salty brine during the process.

FOCUS ON

Gotu kola

PROFILE
Native to south-east Asia, India, and Australia, this is used both as a salad ingredient and a medicinal remedy.

PROPERTIES
This tonic herb has antirheumatic and digestion-soothing properties. Its cleansing action makes it a healing topical treatment for skin complaints, and it is also used to enhance memory.

The leaves
are used in infusions, tinctures, and powders, or eaten to help restore digestion.

CoQ10, a vitamin-like compound, is necessary for the production of energy at a metabolic level and can help to reduce the pain and fatigue of fibromyalgia.
➡ *Take 300mg daily.*

Omega-3 fatty acids, from fish or algal sources, have an anti-inflammatory action that may help to reduce pain and stiffness.
➡ *Take up to 2g daily.*

Turmeric contains curcumin, well known for its antioxidant and anti-inflammatory effects.
➡ *Take up to 1g daily.*

Vitamin D deficiency has been linked to chronic pain.
➡ *Take a high-dose supplement of up to 1600iu vitamin D3 daily.*

LIFESTYLE

Insomnia can raise the risk of fibromyalgia, especially in women. A regular sleep routine is essential to combat pain and exhaustion.

Gentle regular exercise, especially swimming, can relieve pain and improve quality of life.

Yoga can be an effective way of managing fibromyalgia pain.

OTHER THERAPIES

Acupuncture can help to reduce pain and improve quality of life for those with chronic pain conditions.

Massage, with or without essentials oils, can aid relaxation, relieve pain, and reduce anxiety and depression. Weekly sessions are the most beneficial.

Liquorice interacts with the body's adrenal function, balancing hormones and restoring vitality, to help treat fibromyalgia. Avoid with hypertension and during pregnancy, and large doses over long periods.
➡ *Make a decoction with ½–1 tsp dried liquorice root per 250ml (9fl oz) boiling water, and drink 130–250ml (4½–9fl oz) 3 times daily.*

FOOD

A varied, nutrient-dense diet with whole foods is vital for supporting fibromyalgia, helping to manage discomfort and energize.

Goji berries and sour cherries contain natural melatonin, which promotes regular sleep cycles to help restore energy levels.
➡ *Snack on a handful of goji berries or have a glass of sour cherry juice before bedtime to aid sleep and reduce pain.*

Coconut oil, as well as being a source of quick fuel, is also anti-inflammatory and immune-supporting.
➡ *Use 3–4 tbsp each day in cooking, dressings, or just eaten on its own.*

Fermented foods such as sauerkraut and kimchi contain beneficial organisms that help balance gut flora.
➡ *Use as condiments for main meals several times a week.*

SUPPLEMENTS

Certain key nutrients can help to ease pain and fatigue so try to make these part of your daily regimen.

"A nutrient-dense diet with whole foods helps to manage discomfort and lift energy levels."

INSULIN RESISTANCE

Insulin is the hormone that helps our bodies metabolize, or burn, glucose from carbohydrates to use as energy or to store for later use. Insulin resistance is a precursor to type 2 diabetes (see opposite). It occurs when the body is unable to use the insulin it produces effectively. Being overweight is a risk factor.

HERBS

Herbal remedies can be used alongside lifestyle measures to help balance blood sugar levels and increase insulin sensitivity.

Milk thistle has hypoglycaemic properties, which means it helps to lower high blood glucose levels to restore balance. See box, below.
➡ *Take 175mg capsule daily of a standard milk thistle seed extract (made up of 80 per cent silymarin) or take as a powder, adding ¼–½ tsp to water or a smoothie.*
Cinnamon boosts the action of insulin in the body and helps to lower blood glucose levels. Avoid therapeutic doses in pregnancy.
➡ *Take 1–6g daily in capsules after meals.*
Holy basil has been shown to increase insulin sensitivity in cells and helps to lower high blood sugar levels. Avoid during pregnancy.
➡ *Take 2–3ml tincture in a little water 3 times daily.*

FOOD

Eat a low-sugar diet made up of foods that have a low glycaemic index. Certain foods help to balance insulin levels in the body.

Berries, such as strawberries, mulberries, cranberries, and blackberries, contain flavonoids, which can help lower insulin levels after a meal.
➡ *Purée a mix of berries and add to smoothies or make a berry compote to top porridge and yogurts.*
Broccoli is a rich source of the mineral chromium, which can help to balance blood sugar levels.
➡ *Steam and serve with olive oil, or purée with a little garlic and oil and use as a quick pasta sauce.*
Black seed oil, from the black cumin seed, can improve insulin resistance.
➡ *Use in dressings for salads or steamed vegetables.*

SUPPLEMENTS

You can support the diet with supplements that are anti-inflammatory and ones that improve insulin sensitivity.

Magnesium can boost insulin sensitivity and glucose control.
➡ *Take up to 420mg daily.*
Spirulina is a naturally occurring algae that has anti-inflammatory effects.
➡ *Take up to 3g daily in capsule form.*
Vitamin D can help improve the body's sensitivity to insulin.
➡ *Take 600iu vitamin D3 daily.*

LIFESTYLE

Lose weight if you are overweight.
Chronic stress is a risk factor for poor insulin sensitivity. Practise regular meditation to relieve stress.
Stop smoking as nicotine can hamper insulin sensitivity.
Exercise regularly to maintain a stable weight and improve insulin sensitivity.

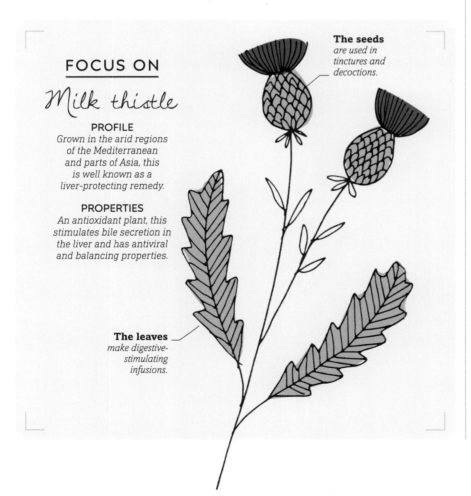

FOCUS ON

Milk thistle

PROFILE
Grown in the arid regions of the Mediterranean and parts of Asia, this is well known as a liver-protecting remedy.

PROPERTIES
An antioxidant plant, this stimulates bile secretion in the liver and has antiviral and balancing properties.

The seeds *are used in tinctures and decoctions.*

The leaves *make digestive-stimulating infusions.*

DIABETES

There are two main types of diabetes. Type 1, also known as insulin dependent diabetes, is rarer and comes on in childhood. This severe type of diabetes requires a lifetime on insulin. Type 2, or non-insulin dependent diabetes, is much more common, usually appearing in adulthood, and is caused by genetic inheritance and lifestyle.

HERBS

Herbs can support conventional medicines, helping to manage diabetes symptoms. Herbs with a hypoglycaemic effect – that help to lower high blood sugar levels – should only be used for early onset type 2 diabetes prior to orthodox medication as these can interact with medication.

Bilberries contain flavonoids, which can help to treat the vascular damage caused by diabetes.
➥*Add 20–50g (¾–1¾oz) bilberry powder daily to smoothies, cereals, or yogurt.*
Fenugreek seeds have a hypoglycaemic effect, helping to control blood sugar levels. Avoid in pregnancy and with low thyroid activity. Take separately from other drugs as it may impede their absorption.
➥*Infuse 1 tsp crushed dried fenugreek seeds in 175ml (6fl oz) boiling water and sip during the day.*
Ginkgo biloba boosts blood flow and can help to improve kidney function, which can suffer with diabetes. Monitor blood glucose levels carefully with ginkgo. Avoid in pregnancy, if breastfeeding, and with anticoagulants and antiplatelet medication.
➥*Take a 66mg leaf extract tablet equal to 3300mg of the whole leaf, 1–3 times daily.*

WHAT TO AVOID
Herbal diuretics. Take advice before using agrimony.

FOOD

Careful dietary control is essential. Foods with a low glycaemic index can help to control blood sugar levels. Generally, a high-fibre diet is helpful for lowering the glycaemic index.

Oily fish have omega-3 fatty acids, which, when abundant in the diet, reduce the likelihood of immune cells attacking insulin-secreting cells in the pancreas by 55 per cent.
➥*Aim to eat 2–3 times a week.*
Walnuts help to control blood glucose and blood lipids.
➥*Snacking on a handful 2–3 times a week offers protection against diabetes.*
Onion and garlic have been shown to lower blood sugar levels significantly.
➥*Use liberally in cooking, as the base to meals.*
WHAT TO AVOID
Hidden sugars, especially in low-fat foods and in fruit juices. Avoid sugary foods and drinks in general, artificial sweeteners, and all calorific foods.

SUPPLEMENTS

Key nutrients support glucose metabolism and insulin sensitivity. Supplementing the diet helps ensure that you are receiving the necessary levels of these nutrients.

Magnesium improves insulin sensitivity and glucose control.
➥*Take up to 420mg daily.*
Zinc has been shown to help control blood sugar levels in type 2 diabetes.
➥*Take 20–40mg daily.*
Chromium helps to regulate blood sugar levels and reduce sugar cravings, especially in overweight people.
➥*Take 500mcg daily.*

LIFESTYLE

If overweight, lose weight. Aim for a BMI score of less than 25.
Find ways to de-stress. Stress can deplete the body of magnesium, which helps to control blood glucose levels. This may explain why high levels of stress have been linked to poor glucose control.
Have a regular sleep routine and address insomnia – sleep deprivation can lead to poor glucose control.
Intermittent fasting – which involves restricted eating for some of the time – can help regulate blood glucose. Talk to a healthcare practitioner before trying this.
Exercise regularly. Aerobic exercise can prevent type 2 diabetes, while muscle-strengthening, on its own or in combination with aerobic exercise, improves diabetic control among diabetes sufferers.
Detox your home. Exposure to chemicals from perfumes, pesticides, flame retardants, and substances added to plastics such as phthalates has been linked to an increased risk of diabetes.

OTHER THERAPIES

Acupuncture may be helpful for regulating blood sugar.
Homeopathy strengthens and supports health in the whole body.

NO NEED TO CHILL

Onions don't need to be kept in the fridge – moisture in the fridge can cause onions to soften more quickly. Store onions in a cool, dry, well-ventilated place.

THYROID PROBLEMS

The thyroid gland produces hormones to regulate body temperature and energy. A hyperactive thyroid speeds metabolism, while an underactive thyroid slows down mental and physical functions. Seek a medical diagnosis before using remedies.

HERBS

Herbs help to rebalance the thyroid and treat symptoms such as constipation. Consult your doctor before using herbs with conventional thyroid treatments.

HYPERTHYROID REMEDIES

Lycopus (bugleweed) relaxes nerves to ease anxiety and slow a rapid pulse. Avoid in pregnancy, if breastfeeding, and with thyroid hormone treatment.
➡ *Take 1–2ml tincture in a little water 3 times daily.*

Motherwort is a relaxing nerve and heart tonic. Avoid in pregnancy, with heavy menstruation, or with palpitations.
➡ *Take 1–4ml tincture in a little water 3 times daily.*

HYPOTHYROID REMEDIES

Ashwagandha is a stimulant. Avoid if pregnant or with hyperthyroidism.
➡ *Take 1–2ml tincture in a little water 3 times daily.*

Kelp treats hypothyroidism caused by iodine deficiency. Do not give to children under 5. Be aware of heavy-metal toxicity in some sources.
➡ *Infuse ½ tsp dried kelp in 175ml (6fl oz) boiling water and drink 90–175ml (3–6fl oz) 3 times daily.*

WHAT TO AVOID

With hyperthyroid: bladderwrack, ephedra; caution with bacopa. With hypothyroid: caution with lemon balm, fenugreek, bugleweed.

FOOD

A wholefood, nutrient-dense diet helps to support thyroid treatments.

Seaweed, for hypothyroidism, provides iodine and the micronutrients needed for the proper metabolism of iodine.
➡ *Regularly add the powder to soups and dressings.*

Buckwheat is rich in selenium and B vitamins to calm hyperthyroidism.
➡ *Try buckwheat porridge.*

Brazil nuts provide selenium, which is essential for activating the main thyroid hormone, thyroxine.
➡ *Eat a handful daily.*

WHAT TO AVOID

Raw turnips, cabbage, mustard, pine nuts, cassava root, soybean, peanuts, and millet can affect absorption of iodine. Refined carbohydrates may feed an overactive thyroid. Iodized salt can lead to excess iodine.

LIFESTYLE

Avoid perfluorinated chemicals (PFCs), used to manufacture non-stick pans and stain-resistant fabrics, because these can raise the risk of hypothyroidism.

Medications such as steroids and some cough mixtures can affect thyroid function. Talk to your doctor before taking medicines.

Give up smoking. Smoking worsens symptoms that occur with an underactive thyroid.

De-stress. Severe grief or stress, for example from bereavement or divorce, can affect thyroid function.

Practise yoga. Several positions may support thyroid function.

OTHER THERAPIES

Acupuncture, combined with moxibustion (burning herbs), may help normalize thyroid function.

ADRENAL INSUFFICIENCY

Adrenal hormones, such as cortisol and aldosterone, play key roles in regulating blood pressure, digestion, metabolism, and the body's response to stress. Adrenal insufficiency occurs if adrenal glands do not produce enough of these hormones, causing conditions such as Addison's disease, with a range of symptoms.

HERBS

Tonic herbs work by protecting and strengthening the adrenal glands to help the glands manage excessive stress and regulate the release of stress-response hormones such as cortisol, which in turn prevents problems such as fatigue.

Liquorice supports the adrenal cortex – the part of the gland that produces hormones – helping to balance cortisol levels to manage the stress response. Avoid in pregnancy, with hypertension, and large doses over long periods.
➡ *Make a decoction: add ½–1 tsp dried liquorice root to 250ml (9fl oz) boiling water. Drink 130–250ml (4½–9fl oz) 3 times daily.*

Ashwagandha supports the adrenal glands and immune function. Avoid in pregnancy or with hyperthyroidism.
➡ *Take 1–2ml tincture in a little water 3 times daily.*

Skullcap has a relaxing, tonic effect on nerves affected by chronic stress, fatigue, and exhaustion.
➡ *Infuse 1–2 tsp dried skullcap in 175ml (6fl oz) boiling water. Drink 3 times daily.*

ESSENTIAL OILS

A number of essential oils support the nervous system and other factors associated with adrenal insufficiency.

Pine can help to relieve aches and pains and chronic tiredness.

Bergamot has uplifting properties that help to lift depression.

Vetiver is relaxing and beneficial for stress and anxiety.

➡️*Add 5 drops of any of the above essential oils to 10ml almond oil and massage over the kidney area.*

SUPPLEMENTS

Use supplements to support a healthy, wholefood diet, low in sugars, salts, additives, and refined carbohydrates.

B vitamins play an important role in cell metabolism and energy production.

➡️*Take a high-quality B complex daily.*

Vitamin C supports the production of cortisol in the adrenal glands.

➡️*Take 500mg to 1g daily.*

Probiotic supplements work via the gut to help the body cope with stress.

➡️*Look for a broad-spectrum supplement that contains at least 10 billion live organisms per dose.*

LIFESTYLE

Reduce stress levels with relaxation techniques such as meditation and spending time in nature.

Have a regular sleep routine and address causes of insomnia – sufficient sleep is vital for adrenal health.

SPICE IT UP

If using turmeric in cooking, freshly grated turmeric provides a punchier, more peppery flavour than dried.

CANCER SUPPORT

Natural remedies can be supportive during cancer treatment and during recovery, helping to boost immunity and energy levels. Discuss remedies with your doctor before using them.

HERBS

These can support the body during treatment by helping to manage side-effects, improve resilience, and strengthen immunity. The anti-inflammatory and antioxidant actions of herbs are beneficial.

Turmeric is anti-inflammatory, antioxidant, and has many beneficial actions to support treatment. Avoid therapeutic doses in pregnancy and with gallstones. May cause rashes.

➡️*Add ½-1 tsp powder to warmed coconut milk and drink 3 times daily.*

Astragalus can be taken during treatment to strengthen immunity and improve general health. Avoid with acute infections and with immune-suppressant and blood-thinning drugs.

➡️*Take 2–6g powder daily in smoothies or sprinkled on cereal.*

Milk thistle is antioxidant and strengthens and protects the liver.

➡️*Take 200–600mg concentrated extract daily.*

FOOD

The right nutrients can support you before, during, and after cancer treatment to help you maintain energy levels, better tolerate side effects, reduce the risk of infection, and support recovery.

Wholefoods are the most beneficial for supporting the body.

➡️*Eat whole fruit and vegetables rather than juicing, to get the most fibre and slow-release carbohydrates.*

> " *Herbal remedies can help to manage the side effects of treatments and boost immunity.* "

Protein from lean meat and dairy provide more of the important "buildup" nutrients that the body needs for repair, recovery, and energy.

➡️*Eat 500g (1lb 2oz) cooked meat each week.*

WHAT TO AVOID

Processed foods, especially salami, frankfurters, ham, bacon, and some sausages. Alcohol may be contraindicated. A very high-fibre or bulky diet is not ideal if appetite is poor or if experiencing bouts of diarrhoea.

LIFESTYLE

Try to eat organic. Regulations for organic foods and other products prohibit many cancer-causing substances.

Reduce stress. Cancer treatment can be particularly stressful and high levels of stress can hinder recovery. Find ways to relax such as spending time outdoors and practising meditation and yoga.

OTHER THERAPIES

Relaxing therapies such as music therapy can lessen anxiety and depression and improve quality of life.

Acupressure and acupuncture can help reduce chemotherapy-induced nausea and vomiting.

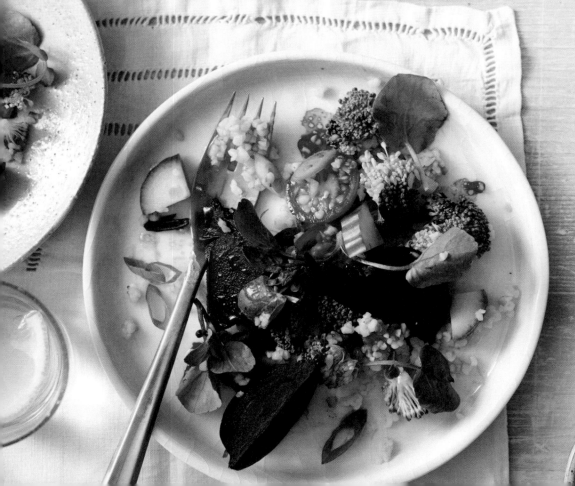

5

RECIPES FOR WELLNESS
SALADS

These satisfying salads are a meal in themselves – full of fibre, high-quality proteins, anti-inflammatory antioxidants, and essential micronutrients to boost health throughout the body. Simply place the salad ingredients in a large bowl. Prepare the dressing and either pour over the salad, or use as a marinade, as directed. Toss the dressing and salad ingredients together to combine well, and serve.

1

BULGUR, BEETROOT, AND BROCCOLI SALAD

This satisfying salad supports digestive and heart health. Low-fat bulgur wheat has essential minerals, protein, and fibre, vital for the digestion and circulation, and detoxifying compounds in beetroot support the liver.

SERVES 2 • PREP TIME 15 MINS •
COOK TIME 10 MINS

85g (3oz) bulgur wheat, cooked in 300ml (10fl oz) vegetable stock, as per packet instructions

115g (4oz) broccoli, chopped

250g (9oz) beetroot, cooked, peeled, and chopped

2 tbsp watercress

115g (4oz) cherry tomatoes, halved

2 spring onions, chopped

60g (2oz) cucumber, diced

For the dressing

2 tsp olive oil

2 tsp soy sauce

2 tsp lemon juice

Nutritional info per serving:
Kcals 310 Fat 5g Saturated fat 0.7g
Carbohydrates 49g Sugar 16g
Sodium 767mg Fibre 10g
Protein 12.5g Cholesterol 0mg

2 Rice Salad with spicy seeds

Nuts and seeds are high in anti-inflammatory omega-3 fatty acids. Pumpkin seeds also supply magnesium, which boosts muscle function, helps to balance fluids, and reduces fatigue.

SERVES 2 • **PREP TIME** 10 MINS • **COOK TIME** 25–30 MINS

200g (7oz) brown rice, cooked in 400ml (14fl oz) chicken or vegetable stock, as per packet instructions

2 spring onions, thinly sliced

¼ cucumber, sliced into matchsticks

60g (2oz) red pepper, deseeded and sliced into matchsticks

For the dressing
Cook ingredients in a wok for 3 minutes

1 tsp coconut oil

3 tbsp lemon juice

1 tbsp soy sauce

¼ tsp chilli flakes

1 tbsp pumpkin seeds

1 tbsp sunflower seeds

1 tbsp sesame seeds

Nutritional info per serving:
Kcals 587 Fat 16.5g Saturated fat 3.5g Carbohydrates 85.5g Sugar 5.5g Sodium 561mg Fibre 7g Protein 21g Cholesterol 0mg

3 Sprouted bean and alfalfa salad

Sprouted beans are densely packed with vitamins, minerals, enzymes, and fatty acids, and are the largest source of protein in the vegetable kingdom.

SERVES 2 • **PREP TIME** 5 MINS, PLUS COOLING • **COOK TIME** 10 MINS

125g (4½oz) quinoa, cooked as per packet instructions and cooled

200g (7oz) sprouted mixed beans

60g (2oz) alfalfa sprouts

For the dressing
Blitz ingredients for 30 seconds

1 tsp fresh ginger, peeled

¼ tsp red chilli, deseeded

60g (2oz) red pepper, deseeded and chopped

4 tbsp lemon juice

Nutritional info per serving:
Kcals 258 Fat 4g Saturated fat 0.5g Carbohydrates 39g Sugar 7.5g Sodium 45mg Fibre 8g Protein 13g Cholesterol 0mg

4 Courgettes with green beans and mint

Courgettes are high in immune-boosting vitamin C, as well as potassium, fibre, and vitamin K, while mint soothes indigestion and inflammation and stimulates digestion.

SERVES 2 • **PREP TIME** 5 MINS, PLUS COOLING • **COOK TIME** 25–30 MINS

150g (5½oz) brown rice, cooked as per packet instructions and cooled

125g (4½oz) courgettes, chopped and lightly steamed

125g (4½oz) greens beans, chopped and lightly steamed

For the dressing
Cook ingredients in a wok for 3 minutes

1 tsp olive oil

½ tsp red chilli, deseeded and diced

1 clove of garlic, diced

1 tbsp lemon juice (pips removed)

6 mint leaves

1 tsp fresh ginger, peeled and diced

Nutritional info per serving:
Kcals 322 Fat 4g Saturated fat 0.8g Carbohydrates 59g Sugar 3g Sodium 2mg Fibre 5.5g Protein 9.5g Cholesterol 0mg

5 Tofu, tomato, and watercress salad

Protein-rich tofu is also a great source of iron to support oxygen-carrying red blood cells, and calcium, vital for bone strength and density.

SERVES 2-3 • **PREP TIME** 5–8 MINS, PLUS COOLING AND CHILLING • **COOK TIME** 10–15 MINS

140g (5oz) basmati rice, cooked as per packet instructions and cooled

280g (9½oz) tofu, cut into cubes, marinated in the dressing, and chilled for 1 hour

100g (3½oz) cherry tomatoes, halved

75g (3oz) watercress

For the dressing

4 tbsp lemon juice

3 tbsp soy sauce

2 tbsp olive oil

1 tsp rosemary

1 tsp oregano

1 clove of garlic, diced

¼ tsp freshly ground black pepper

Nutritional info per serving:
Kcals 377 Fat 14.5g Saturated fat 2.5g Carbohydrates 42.5g Sugar 4.5g Sodium 850mg Fibre 3g Protein 17g Cholesterol 0mg

IMMUNITY AND INTOLERANCES

The immune system is vital for our survival. This intricate network of cells work together to identify, isolate, and attack invading pathogens to keep us healthy. A balanced gut flora plays a part in immunity and also helps to stop the body developing intolerances to foods. Find out how key nutrients and holistic remedies boost immunity and enhance the gut environment; and when the body is under attack, how natural healing can calm inflammation and help to rebuild a healthy immune response.

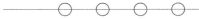

STAYING WELL

IMMUNITY AND INTOLERANCES

When working well, the immune system is our frontline defence against toxins, viruses, bacteria, and other harmful micro-organisms. Key nutrients and natural remedies can bolster defences to keep the immune system in peak form, and by promoting gut health, also reduce the risk of intolerances to certain foods.

FOOD

Ensuring your diet provides a variety of micronutrients helps to limit inflammation and optimize immunity.

PRO- AND PREBIOTICS

A healthy gut, as well as aiding digestion, also plays a vital role in supporting the immune system. The gut contains good and bad bacteria, but if bad bacteria outnumber beneficial bacteria, intolerances and disease-causing organisms can gain a foothold. A balanced diet high in antioxidant vitamins boosts immunity. "Live" foods, such as natural yogurt, kefir, and sauerkraut, contain probiotics – healthy bacteria – to support gut flora and reduce the risk of inflammation, intolerances, and disease.

Certain foods contain prebiotic substances, ones which feed the good bacteria already present in the gut. Asparagus, Jerusalem artichokes, onions, and garlic all provide prebiotics.

ANTIFUNGAL FOODS

Overuse of antibiotics, or a high-sugar, low-fibre diet can unbalance gut flora and lead to a fungal, or yeast, overgrowth and conditions such as thrush. Foods with antifungal properties can help to combat yeast infections. Coconut oil contains a natural antifungal compound, caprylic acid; and cruciferous vegetables such as kale, cabbage, broccoli, cauliflower, Brussels sprouts, rocket, cabbage, and radishes contain sulphur- and nitrogen-compounds called isothiocyanates, which fight fungal infection.

ANTIMICROBIAL FOODS

Some foods have broad antimicrobial properties that help to strengthen immunity. Mushrooms and grains such as barley, oats, and rye contain a soluble fibre known as beta-glucan. Beta-glucan enhances the action of bacteria-destroying white blood cells called macrophages, and so helps to boost immunity, speed wound healing, and may even increase the efficiency of

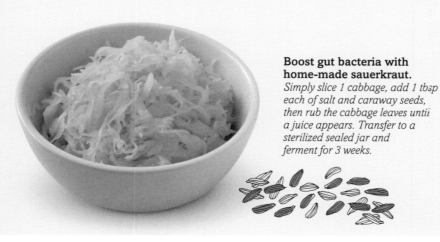

Boost gut bacteria with home-made sauerkraut.
Simply slice 1 cabbage, add 1 tbsp each of salt and caraway seeds, then rub the cabbage leaves until a juice appears. Transfer to a sterilized sealed jar and ferment for 3 weeks.

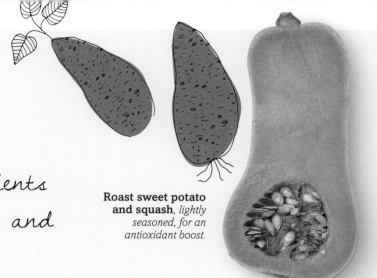

"A broad range of micronutrients helps to limit inflammation and boost immunity."

Roast sweet potato and squash, *lightly seasoned, for an antioxidant boost.*

antibiotics. Ginger also has an antimicrobial action. Compounds called shogaols and gingerols in ginger help to stimulate circulation and have an anti-infective effect. Garlic contains antiviral and antimicrobial allicin, which helps fight infection. Raw garlic is especially potent so add a clove of chopped garlic to soup or grate over vegetables to strengthen immune function.

ANTIOXIDANTS AND VITAMINS

Antioxidants, especially vitamins A and C, support disease-fighting cells. Squash, sweet potatoes, carrots, spinach, and cantaloupe melon are high in beta-carotene, which is converted into vitamin A in the body, while citrus and leafy greens provide vitamin C.

HYDRATING FOODS AND DRINKS

Dehydration affects cell function, making the body vulnerable to infection. Aim to drink 1.5–2 litres (2¾–3½ pints) of fluid a day in the form of water and herbal teas, and eat foods with a high water content, such as cucumber, melon, celery, and lettuce.

HERBS

Herbs have a range of actions that can help to strengthen the body's immune response and protect the body against harmful organisms.

IMMUNE-STRENGTHENING HERBS

Strengthening tonic herbs can help to maintain the health and vitality of the immune system, enabling the body to respond effectively to stress and debility. Siberian ginseng (eleuthero), a tonic herb with antioxidant properties that can help to restore and strengthen immune function, can be safely taken over long periods of time. Astragalus is a potent tonic herb that helps the body to manage short periods of mental or physical stress to help prevent stress impacting on the immune system; and myrrh is a revitalizing tonic known for its immune-stimulating and antimicrobial properties.

Take 3–5ml Siberian ginseng tincture *in a little water 3 times daily to strengthen immunity.*

ANTIBACTERIAL HERBS

Herbs can contain hundreds of active constituents that give them a complex antibacterial activity. The constituents work together to fight bacterial infections, internally and externally, and boost immunity. Echinacea enhances the immune response and is effective against bacteria such as *Staphylococcus* and *Streptococcus*. Golden seal is also active against a wide variety of bacterium including *Staphylococcus*, and boneset has potent immune–stimulating properties, similar to echinacea.

HERBS TO REGULATE THE BODY'S RESPONSE

Antihistamine and immune-regulating herbs can help to manage and reduce the response to foods that the body has an intolerance to. For example, thyme and nigella (black seed) have antihistamine and anti-inflammatory properties that can help to support healthy digestive function and restore and heal the gut lining when trigger foods that the body struggles to digest and process cause inflammation.

The common nettle, found throughout most of the world, is also able to reduce histamine and is thought to be particularly useful in offering protection during the pollen season.

ESSENTIAL OILS

Oils with antiseptic and antibacterial properties can assist the immune system in fighting off threats

ANTIMICROBIAL OILS

These oils guard against infection. Lemon is antimicrobial and boosts immunity, while eucalyptus and tea tree act as broad-spectrum antimicrobials against a range of bacteria. Eucalyptus also boosts immunity, and ravintsara is strongly antiviral.

CALMING OILS

Soothing oils can relieve tension, which when left unchecked can depress immunity. Sweet and spicy frankincense calms nerves and stimulates the immune response. Peppermint calms and is also a decongestant to tone the airways, while thyme is clearing.

OILS TO STIMULATE THE BODY

Ginger has a warming effect that helps to loosen inflamed joints and boost the appetite after illness or a period of stress.

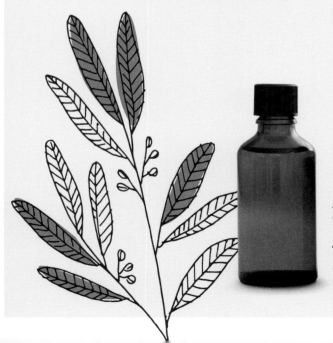

Add 20 drops of warming eucalyptus essential oil *to 75ml (2½fl oz) water and 1 tsp glycerine. Transfer to a bottle with an atomizer and use as a room-cleansing spray to eliminate germs.*

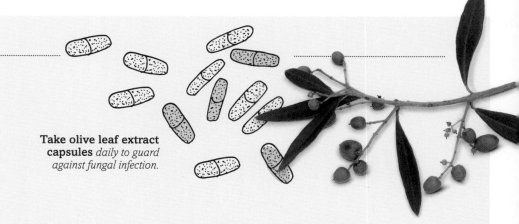

Take olive leaf extract capsules *daily to guard against fungal infection.*

Supplements

Certain supplements have immune-boosting properties that can support the diet.

Anti-inflammatory supplements

Vitamin D is anti-inflammatory. Studies show that when levels of this vitamin are low, we are more prone to colds, allergies, and infections. A daily supplement can help to boost immunity.

Allergic reactions can sometimes cause joint stiffness. Gamma-linolenic acid (GLA) in borage oil converts to a hormone-like substance called prostaglandin E1 (PGE1), an anti-inflammatory that reduces joint pain, inflammation, and stiffness.

Aloe vera juice has anti-inflammatory properties and also helps to heal the gut lining to promote healthy gut flora.

Antifungal properties

Olive leaf extract contains a substance called oleuropein, which is a powerful antifungal. Olive leaf is also rich in antioxidants, which help to prevent tissue damage from *Candida* overgrowth.

Gut-supporting supplements

Probiotic supplements deliver a guaranteed number of living organisms directly to the gut, which as well as supporting digestion, also ensures a more effective immune response. They can be especially beneficial after a course of antibiotics, which kill beneficial bacteria along with harmful species. Probiotics may also calm the body's overreaction to potential allergens.

Antihistamines

Histamine plays a key role in the inflammatory reaction to allergens, with high levels causing allergic symptoms. Bee pollen contains a range of antioxidants and vitamins that support general health and have an antihistamine effect. Note that bee pollen should not be given to young children, to those with an allergy to honey or bee stings, or taken during pregnancy or when breastfeeding.

A combination of vitamin C and the flavonoid antioxidant quercetin can have an antihistamine effect. Vitamin C also strengthens the walls of blood vessels to make them less permeable and aids the production of white blood cells – the frontline of the immune response.

"Antiseptic and antibacterial essential oils assist the immune system."

TREATMENTS
IMMUNITY AND INTOLERANCES

If the immune system is below par, or it overreacts to harmless substances or healthy tissues, infection and inflammation can occur. The body can also develop intolerances. Natural remedies bolster immunity and dietary strategies help to manage intolerances.

HAYFEVER

Hayfever, or allergic rhinitis, is an allergic reaction to pollen and this difficult condition has an increasing number of sufferers. Symptoms include a runny nose, itchy, watery eyes, and a sore throat.

HERBS

Some anti-inflammatory herbs act like natural antihistamines. Use together with soothing and anticatarrhal remedies.

Nettle reduces histamine and the inflammatory response to pollen.
Eyebright tones, calms inflammation in the lining of the nose and eyes, and is anticatarrhal.
Elderflower is anticatarrhal, soothes inflammation, and relaxes mucosal tissues to relieve discomfort.
➼*Infuse 1–2 tsp of any of the above dried herbs in 175ml (6fl oz) boiling water and drink 3 times daily; or combine, see remedy, right.*
Ginger is anti-inflammatory. Avoid with peptic ulcers and gallstones.
➼*Infuse a thumb-sized piece of fresh ginger in 175ml (6fl oz) boiling water and drink 3 times daily.*

ESSENTIAL OILS

Expectorant, anti-inflammatory, and immune-boosting essential oils offer relief from hayfever symptoms.

Thyme works as a respiratory tonic and expectorant.
Eucalyptus is an excellent decongestant.
Peppermint soothes and decongests.
➼*Add 4 drops of any of the above to a bowl of hot water, lean over, covering your head with a towel to trap the steam, and inhale until it cools. Or add 3 drops of an oil to a diffuser to inhale.*

FOOD

Key foods and nutrients can help to relieve allergenic symptoms.

Raw fruits and vegetables can reduce a tendency towards inflammation.
➼*Include in your diet daily.*
Rooibos, the caffeine-free tea, alleviates a runny nose and other symptoms.
➼*Drink daily during hayfever season.*
Oily fish, such as salmon and mackerel, are rich in anti-inflammatory omega-3.
➼*Aim to eat up to 3 portions of oily fish a week.*

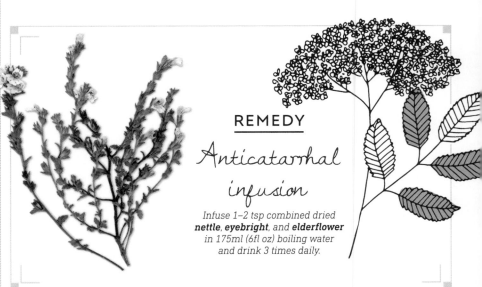

REMEDY

Anticatarrhal infusion

Infuse 1–2 tsp combined dried **nettle**, **eyebright**, and **elderflower** in 175ml (6fl oz) boiling water and drink 3 times daily.

WHAT TO AVOID

Caffeine and sugary snacks can trigger histamine release. Dairy can be mucus-forming so reduce your intake.

SUPPLEMENTS

Some supplements are anti-inflammatory, so calm an overreactive immune system.

Bee pollen has antioxidants and vitamins shown to reduce histamine levels. Do not give bee pollen to young children or take if allergic to honey or bee stings or if pregnant or breastfeeding.
➡️*Take 500mg daily.*

Probiotic supplements help to regulate the body's response to allergens.
➡️*Take a supplement with up to 10 billion live organisms per dose.*

Quercetin has antioxidant, antihistamine, and anti-inflammatory properties.
➡️*Take 500mg 2–3 times daily until symptoms are under control, then reduce to 500mg once a day.*

Vitamin C supports healthy immunity and protects the mucous membrane. It works well with quercetin (see above).
➡️*Take 500mg daily.*

LIFESTYLE

Being by the sea and in woodland can reduce symptoms.

Manage stress. Stress symptoms such as a raised heart rate and lowered breathing rate exacerbate hayfever.

Ionizers release negative ions into the atmosphere to counter histamine-triggering positive ions.

Check for food allergies or sensitivities.

Avoid smoky or polluted atmospheres.

Wear wrap-around sunglasses to keep pollen from getting into the eyes.

OTHER THERAPIES

Homeopathy treats the whole body to help calm hayfever.

Acupuncture helps reduce inflammation.

CANDIDA

Candida albicans **is a yeast that usually resides in the body, its levels kept in check by the immune system. If immunity is weakened, it can flourish, causing fatigue, headache, depression, joint pain, and poor focus. Thrush is an overgrowth of** *Candida* **in the vagina or the mouth. Get medical advice with recurrent episodes.**

HERBS

Use antifungal herbs and ones that boost immunity and promote gut flora. Cleansing herbs eliminate toxins and heal tissues.

Oregano is a key antimicrobial herb with specific activity against *Candida*. Not suitable during pregnancy.
➡️*Take 150mg capsules of oregano oil as directed.*

Pau d'arco is immune-stimulating and also antifungal to help expel *Candida*. Not suitable during pregnancy.
➡️*Make a decoction with 1–2 tsp dried Pau d'arco bark to 250ml (9fl oz) boiling water. Drink 3–6 times daily.*

Calendula is antifungal and anti-inflammatory to soothe infected tissues. Avoid internal use during pregnancy.
➡️*Take an infusion or tincture and also apply in creams or pessaries.*

Thyme is an antifungal and tonic herb. Avoid internal use during pregnancy.
➡️*Infuse 1–2 tsp dried thyme in 175ml (6fl oz) boiling water and drink 3 times daily; or for vaginal thrush, apply the infusion topically.*

Aloe vera juice heals the gut lining and supports gut flora. Avoid in pregnancy.
➡️*Take 15ml of juice 2 times daily.*

ESSENTIAL OILS

Oils can be antifungal and boost immunity. Use non-sensitizing oils for vaginal thrush.

Tea tree has antifungal properties that can be used to control *Candida*.
➡️*For oral thrush, add 2 drops to 1 tsp salt and dissolve in a glass of warm water, then gargle. For vaginal thrush, add 5 drops to a warm bath filled to hip height and take a 15-minute sitz bath.*

Lavender can help to improve the immune response and has analgesic and antimicrobial properties.
➡️*Add 5 drops to 10ml apricot oil and use in a full-body massage. For vaginal thrush, add 3 drops to a warm bath filled to hip height and take a 15-minute sitz bath.*

Thyme is helpful for infections and can strengthen the immune system.
➡️*Add 5 drops to 10ml almond oil and use in a full–body massage.*

FOOD

Foods with powerful antifungal effects can help control *Candida*. Also eat plenty of immune-boosting antioxidant foods.

Coconut oil contains a natural antifungal, caprylic acid.
➡️*Use for cooking, add to smoothies and dressings, or eat 1–2 tbsp daily on its own.*

Garlic is rich in sulphur compounds, specifically antifungal allicin.
➡️*It is especially powerful eaten raw; add to salads and dressings.*

Cruciferous vegetables, such as kale, cabbage, broccoli, cauliflower, Brussels sprouts, rocket, and radishes, have isothiocyanates, sulphur- and nitrogen-containing compounds that fight *Candida*.
➡️*Eat daily, raw or lightly steamed.*

Live foods such as yogurt can help balance gut flora.
➡️*Eat a portion daily – add to smoothies, cereals, or to cooked meals.*

WHAT TO AVOID

Sugar and cheese.

➤ CONTINUED...

SUPPLEMENTS

Candida overgrowth can affect the body's ability to absorb key nutrients efficiently so supplements can support diet.

Magnesium deficiency may make you more prone to *Candida* while adequate levels may help your body fight *Candida*.
➤*Take up to 300mg magnesium citrate – a highly bioavailable form – daily.*

B complex vitamins help strengthen immunity, protect cells from oxidative stress, and fight inflammation.
➤*Take a supplement with at least 25mg of all the main B vitamins.*

Olive leaf extract is rich in antioxidants and has oleuropein, a strong antifungal.
➤*Take up to 1500mg daily in capsule form in divided doses.*

Psyllium seeds provide soluble fibre to ensure regular bowel movements and remove the waste that *Candida* feeds on.
➤*Take the powder in a little water or capsules as directed before bedtime.*

Probiotic supplements are helpful after antibiotics as they repopulate the gut with healthy bacteria.
➤*Take a broad-spectrum supplement with up to 10 billion live organisms per dose.*

LIFESTYLE

Practise relaxation techniques such as yoga, meditation, t'ai chi, and walking in the fresh air and sunlight.

Exercise is helpful; aim for 30 minutes aerobic exercise five times a week.

Get enough sleep to aid relaxation and support immunity and recovery.

Wear organic underwear, or even avoid underwear in the summer months if you are wearing a dress.

OTHER THERAPIES

Massage, including shiatsu and reflexology, can help balance the body.

Homeopathy helps heal the whole body.

CONVALESCENCE

A period of time that allows recovery from illness used to be integral to treatment. Nowadays, an emphasis on getting up and about as soon as possible can lead to chronic immune problems such as post-viral fatigue.

HERBS

Tonic herbs stimulate and restore vitality, increase appetite, and boost digestion.

Oatstraw is nutritious and restorative for the nerves, and boosts strength. Avoid with gluten sensitivity.
➤*Infuse 1–2 tsp dried oatstraw in 175ml (6fl oz) boiling water. Drink 3–4 times daily.*

Horseradish root boosts circulation. See box, opposite.
➤*Add daily to sandwiches and meat and fish dishes.*

Angelica root is a digestive stimulant and rebuilding tonic. Avoid in pregnancy and therapeutic doses if diabetic.
➤*Take 2–5ml tincture in a little water 3 times daily.*

ESSENTIAL OILS

Certain oils act as tonics and offer adrenal support following a debilitating illness.

STAYING FRESH

To stop very soft varieties of dates, such as Medjool dates, drying out, store them in the fridge. Other dates will keep in a cool, dark cupboard for up to 4 weeks.

Pine is a tonic recommended for weakness and fatigue following illness.
➤*Add 3 drops to a diffuser and inhale.*

Ginger can help to stimulate the appetite.

Cardamom treats debility and nervous exhaustion, and stimulates appetite.
➤*Add 5 drops ginger or cardamom to 10ml jojoba oil and use in a massage to boost circulation and aid relaxation.*

FOOD

Nutritional needs post-illness can vary depending on the illness. As a general rule eat easily digestible, nutrient-dense foods and drink plenty of hydrating fluids. Water is ideal, but herbal teas and clear broths also help to maintain hydration.

Berries are rich in vitamin C and bioflavonoids, which help to support a healthy immune system.
➤*Eat fresh or add to a smoothie.*

Dates contain iron, fibre, and carbohydrates for energy.
➤*A handful will boost energy levels when you don't have the appetite for a complete meal.*

Oily fish, such as salmon, mackerel, sardines, and trout, provides essential fats as well as easily digested protein and vital minerals.
➤*Have 2–3 portions a week, lightly grilled or steamed.*

Herbs and spices such as cinnamon, nutmeg, rosemary, sage, and thyme add flavour as well as antiseptic and circulation-boosting compounds.
➤*Sprinkle cinnamon or nutmeg over warm milk before bed.*

WHAT TO AVOID
Refined carbohydrates, sugars, alcohol, high-bran foods, and red meat. Also stimulants such as coffee, which can deplete, rather than restore energy.

SUPPLEMENTS

These ensure essential nutrients when appetite is low and stocks depleted.

FOCUS ON

Horseradish root

PROFILE
Thought to originate from eastern Europe, horseradish was a popular remedy in the Middle Ages.

PROPERTIES
This nutritious herb is stimulating for the circulation and digestion. It also has clearing properties useful for respiratory conditions.

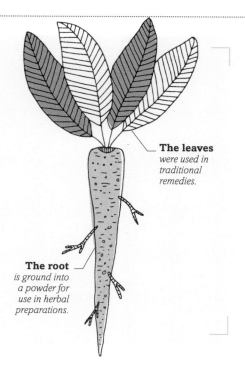

The leaves *were used in traditional remedies.*

The root *is ground into a powder for use in herbal preparations.*

Multi-vitamins ensure you get a broad spectrum of essential nutrients.
➤ *Take a daily supplement.*

Vitamin D levels can be low if bedridden and compromise immunity.
➤ *Take up to 1000iu vitamin D3 liquid supplement daily.*

Zinc supports wound healing.
➤ *Take 14mg daily.*

Vitamin C aids immunity and tissues.
➤ *Take 500mg to 1g daily. Look for a supplement with added bioflavonoids.*

Probiotic supplements help maintain a healthy gut flora if diet is disrupted.
➤ *Take a daily supplement with at least 10 billion live organisms per dose.*

LIFESTYLE

Fresh air and sunshine boosts recovery and vitamin D levels.

Gentle exercise such as yoga or t'ai chi can keep you supple.

Ask for help – support aids recovery.

OTHER THERAPIES

Homeopathy supports healing.

LUPUS

In auto-immune disorders such as lupus, the immune system mistakenly attacks and destroys healthy tissues, which causes pain and inflammation. Lupus commonly affects the skin, but areas such as the brain, kidneys, lungs, and other organs and tissues can also suffer. Systemic lupus erythematosus (SLE) is the most common type of the disorder, and this affects mainly women.

HERBS

Herbs can help to support deficient immunity and strengthen the liver, and antioxidant and antiviral herbs stabilize cells and tissues.

Siberian ginseng (Eleuthero) is a tonic antioxidant herb and strengthens immunity. Avoid with acute infections.
➤ *Take 3–5ml tincture in a little water 3 times daily.*

Astragalus acts as an immune tonic, strengthening and protecting the liver. Avoid with acute infections and immune-suppressant and blood-thinning drugs.
➤ *Take 2–4ml tincture in a little water 3 times daily.*

Turmeric is anti-inflammatory, antioxidant, boosts immunity, and helps detoxify the liver. It combines well with ginger and black pepper, which aid its absorption. Avoid therapeutic doses in pregnancy and with gallstones. May cause rashes.
➤ *See remedy, page 228.*

Ginkgo biloba, an antioxidant, promotes healthy cells and tissues. Avoid in pregnancy, if breastfeeding, or with anticoagulant or antiplatelet medicine.
➤ *Take a 66mg leaf extract tablet equal to 3300mg whole leaf, 1–3 times daily.*

WHAT TO AVOID

Immune-stimulating herbs such as panax ginseng and echinacea.

FOOD

A plant-based diet with fruits, vegetables, wholegrains, and only moderate amounts of lean meat and fish is ideal. Stay hydrated with 1.5–2 litres (2¾–3½ pints) fluid a day from water and herbal teas.

Oily fish, such as salmon, mackerel, tuna, and trout, have anti-inflammatory omega-3 fats.
➤ *Eat 2–3 portions a week.*

Dairy provides calcium and, if fortified, vitamin D for bone health – a particular concern because lupus medication can increase the risk of osteoporosis.
➤ *Have 2–3 portions daily.*

Nutrient-rich broth can reduce symptoms associated with lupus.
➤ *Have 240–500ml (8–16fl oz) daily.*

Coconut oil and olive oil nourish skin.
➤ *Use for cooking and dressings.*

WHAT TO AVOID

Alfalfa and soya can aggravate symptoms in some people.

➤ **CONTINUED...**

SUPPLEMENTS

Support the diet with key supplements.

Omega-3 fatty acids calm inflammation.
➥*Take 1–5g daily of a combined EPA and DHA supplement.*
Vitamin D can be low in lupus sufferers.
➥*Take 2000iu vitamin D3 daily.*
Spirulina, a naturally occurring algae, has amino acids and other nutrients.
➥*Take up to 3g a day in capsule form.*

LIFESTYLE

Yoga reduces stress to calm symptoms.
Regular sleep combats fatigue.
Avoid direct sunlight in peak hours as this may aggravate skin symptoms.

OTHER THERAPIES

Chiropractic and osteopathy relieve joint or back pain and headaches.
Acupuncture provides pain relief.
Meditation helps with depression and chronic tension or pain.

REMEDY

Liver detox

*Infuse 1–2 tsp **turmeric** (see p227) in 175ml (6fl oz) boiling water. Add a pinch of **ginger** and **black pepper** to aid absorption. Drink 3–4 times daily.*

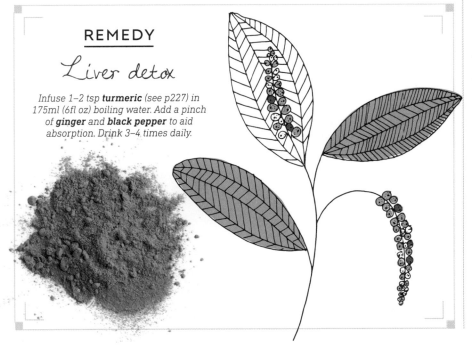

RHEUMATOID ARTHRITIS (RA)

This auto-immune disease is characterized by chronic joint inflammation, which causes the eventual destruction of cartilage and bone. Sufferers can be in constant pain and the disease can worsen over time, with a devastating impact on quality of life. Seek medical advice early on for preventative medications.

HERBS

Herbs help to regulate and strengthen the immune system, fight infections, and ease inflammation in the joints. Also, herbs help to remedy gut dysbiosis – a microbial gut imbalance – which can occur with RA.

Rehmannia can help to regulate immune function and control the inflammatory response.
➥*Take 2–6g daily in capsules.*

Devil's claw is anti-inflammatory and analgesic, so helpful for stiff joints.
➥*Take 2–8g daily in capsules.*
Ginger is anti-inflammatory, analgesic, and antioxidant to reduce damage to the joint tissues. Avoid with peptic ulcers and gallstones.
➥*Take the powdered dried root in capsules, 500mg to 1g, 3 times daily.*

WHAT TO AVOID

Immune-stimulating herbs such as panax ginseng and echinacea.

ESSENTIAL OILS

Anti-inflammatory oils can bring relief. If an inflamed joint is painful to touch, use essential oils in the bath or in a compress.

Clove is analgesic, helping relieve pain.
Ginger is stimulating and warming.
Nutmeg has warming properties, which can soothe inflamed joints.
➥*Add 2 drops of any of the above oils to 5ml unfragranced lotion and gently massage into the skin. If painful, use in a compress: add 3 drops oil to a bowl of warm water, soak a flannel in the water, wring it out, and apply to the joints; or dilute 5 drops in a bath dispersant and use in a warm bath.*

FOOD

Eat whole, unprocessed foods and a mainly plant-based diet.

Coconut oil and olive oil contain antioxidants that support joint health and immunity.
➥*Use both daily.*
Oily fish such as salmon have anti-inflammatory omega-3 fatty acids.
➥*Have 2–3 portions a week.*
Matcha, powdered green tea leaves, is high in the antioxidant polyphenol epigallocatechin-3-gallate (EGCG), which may reduce inflammation and slow the breakdown of cartilage.
➥*Drink daily as a hot or cold drink.*

" Anti-inflammatory essential oils can help to relieve inflamed and stiff joints."

WHAT TO AVOID

Red meat, sugar, fats, salt, caffeine, and the "nightshade" family of plants such as tomatoes, potatoes, aubergines, and peppers, which can worsen symptoms. Gluten and milk can also be triggers.

SUPPLEMENTS

Certain supplements can help to calm and control the body's inflammatory reactions.

Probiotic supplements help reduce inflammation and tenderness.
➡ *Take a daily supplement with at least 10 billion live organisms per dose.*
Omega-3 fatty acids can help reduce inflammation and ease joint pain.
➡ *Take 1–5g daily of a combined EPA and DHA supplement.*
Vitamin D may be deficient with autoimmune conditions. Food sources are scarce so a supplement is helpful.
➡ *Take 2000iu vitamin D3 daily.*
Borage oil contains a compound, gamma linolenic acid (GLA), which is converted into a hormone-like substance, prostaglandin E1 (PGE1), in the body. PGE1 is anti-inflammatory, so eases inflammation, stiffness, and swelling.
➡ *Take 1–2g daily.*

LIFESTYLE

Sunlight can be protective. Regular exposure to ultraviolet B (UVB) rays may reduce the risk of developing rheumatoid arthritis.
Yoga can help maintain a degree of flexibility, and also reduce stress.

FOOD INTOLERANCE

A food intolerance occurs when the body has difficulty digesting a food. Unlike an allergy, it is not triggered by the immune system and is rarely life-threatening. It can, though, upset digestion with symptoms such as discomfort, diarrhoea, and bloating.

HERBS

Antihistamine and immune-regulating herbs can help to manage responses to foods. Herbs to support digestion and restore the gut lining are also beneficial.

Aloe vera juice is anti-inflammatory, protective, and restores the gut lining. Avoid in pregnancy.
➡ *Take 15ml of juice twice daily.*
Nigella (black seeds) have antihistamine and anti-inflammatory properties.
➡ *Use the seeds in cooking, or take the black seed oil as directed.*
Thyme acts as an antihistamine, is anti-inflammatory, and improves digestive health. Avoid in pregnancy.
➡ *Infuse 1–2 tsp dried thyme in 175ml (6fl oz) boiling water. Drink 3 times daily.*

FOOD

If allergy testing is inconclusive, try removing suspect foods and reintroducing them to see if a reaction occurs. Foods that support digestive function are beneficial.

Apple cider vinegar can help to regulate the pH balance in the stomach.
➡ *Take 2 tbsp in 175ml (6fl oz) water between meals.*
Fermented foods such as sauerkraut, lacto-fermented pickles, and kimchi contain prebiotics and probiotics, which support efficient digestion.
➡ *Eat as side dishes and condiments several times a week.*

SUPPLEMENTS

Food intolerance may be a result of a poorly functioning gut, for example, if bacteria are out of balance or where stomach acid is low. Supplements can help to restore balance in the gut.

Probiotic supplements promote a healthy gut flora to support digestion.
➡ *Take a daily supplement with at least 10 billion live organisms per dose.*
Betaine HCl can support digestive acid production, helping digest foods more easily and cut the risk of a reaction.
➡ *Take daily as prescribed.*
Omega-3 fatty acids, derived from fish or marine plant sources, have an anti-inflammatory action that may help calm food intolerance.
➡ *Take 1g daily.*

LIFESTYLE

Find ways to de-stress. Stress can interfere with digestion, which can make symptoms worse.
Check other conditions. An intolerance may be linked to conditions such as chronic fatigue (ME), *Candida*, and digestive problems. Treating these may remove an intolerance.

OTHER THERAPIES

Homeopathy treats the whole body, which in turn can improve digestion.
Acupuncture can reduce inflammation.

COELIAC

This auto-immune disease is triggered by gluten, a type of protein found in wheat, rye, barley, and oats. Coeliac requires lifelong management as there is no cure. Symptoms include digestive upset, cramping, and fatigue. Other problems associated with coeliac include osteoporosis, fertility problems, and an increased risk of other auto-immune disorders.

HERBS

Herbs can improve gut health by soothing gut irritation and inflammation and easing spasms and bloating. Certain herbs work as immune system modulators to help balance the auto-immune response.

Marshmallow root is a mucilaginous herb so has soothing properties that help to calm, protect, and restore the gut lining. See box, right. Take separately from other medicines as it may impede their absorption.
➡*Make a decoction with ½–1 tsp dried marshmallow root in 250ml (9fl oz) cold water; leave overnight, and drink 130–250ml (4½–9fl oz) 3 times daily.*

Lemon balm soothes the mind and the digestive system. It eases spasms, is carminative, and promotes healthy digestion. Avoid with hypothyroidism.
➡*Infuse 1–2 tsp dried lemon balm in 175ml (6fl oz) boiling water. Drink 3 times daily.*

Liquorice, an anti-inflammatory, helps balance the immune response. Avoid with hypertension, in pregnancy, or large doses for prolonged periods.
➡*Add a pinch of the powder to a lemon balm infusion (see above).*

WHAT TO AVOID

Oats, tinctures made with grain alcohol, and herbs processed with barley wine, for example, rehmannia.

FOOD

A lifelong gluten-free diet is the main dietary treatment for coeliac disease. Regularly eating foods with certain key nutrients can help to manage symptoms.

A plant-based diet that includes plenty of fresh fruits and vegetables will provide a variety of nutrients and antioxidants that can help to heal and repair the gut.
➡*Aim to eat at least 3–5 portions of deeply coloured fresh fruits and vegetables daily.*

Nuts and seeds are a good source of fibre as well as containing beneficial and healing fats.
➡*Snack on a handful, or sprinkle on salads, soups, or yogurts.*

Clear broth is a good source of easily assimilated nutrients and amino acids that can help to heal the gut.
➡*Buy ready-made or make your own broth at home from organic bones and have a cup daily.*

SUPPLEMENTS

While diet is the main supportive treatment for coeliac, certain immune-supporting nutrients may also help.

Probiotic supplements can help to establish and maintain a healthy gut flora. Take extra care to check that supplements do not contain gluten.
➡*Take a daily supplement with at least 10 billion live organisms a dose.*

Vitamin D is a key nutrient for supporting immunity and can be deficient in those suffering with an auto-immune disorder. It is hard to obtain sufficient amounts of this vitamin from food alone so a supplement is beneficial.
➡*Take 400iu vitamin D3 daily.*

LIFESTYLE

Follow an organic diet if possible. There is a school of thought that pesticide residues found in non-organic produce can trigger immune diseases such as coeliac in sensitive individuals, so it's worth avoiding residues where you can.

Clean up your environment. Air fresheners, perfumes, and household cleaning products containing harsh chemicals and ingredients can all pollute the air in our homes and have been shown to depress immunity. Switch to products with natural ingredients.

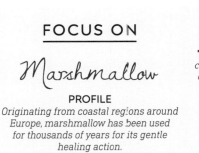

FOCUS ON

Marshmallow

PROFILE
Originating from coastal regions around Europe, marshmallow has been used for thousands of years for its gentle healing action.

PROPERTIES
This mucilaginous herb forms a protective layer with an anti-inflammatory effect, which is effective for calming gut and respiratory inflammation.

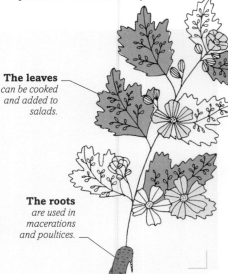

The leaves *can be cooked and added to salads.*

The roots *are used in macerations and poultices.*

MRSA

MRSA stands for methicillin-resistant *Staphylococcus aureus* and refers to one specific sub-species of harmful bacterium that have become resistant to antibiotic treatment. Natural alternatives help to boost immunity and in turn may be helpful in preventing infection taking hold in the first place.

HERBS

Herbs help boost immunity and many have complex antibacterial activity as they contain hundreds of active constituents that work together to fight bacterial infections, internally and externally.

Echinacea enhances the immune response and is antibacterial against *Staphylococcus aureas* and *Streptococcus*. Avoid with immunosuppressant medications.
➡ *Make a poultice with powdered roots and apply to infected wounds.*
Golden seal is active against a wide variety of bacterium including *Staphylococcus aureas*. Avoid in pregnancy, if breastfeeding, and with hypertension. Do not take internally for prolonged periods.
➡ *Take 2–4ml tincture in a little water 3 times daily.*

ESSENTIAL OILS

Many essential oils have powerful antibacterial, antifungal, and antiviral qualities. Because each plant has a unique chemical profile, different oils attack bacteria at different rates. Applying oils directly to the skin may be beneficial.

Thyme contains thymol, which is a powerful antiseptic.
Tea tree is strongly antibacterial.

Oregano contains a large amount of a substance called carvacrol, which has well-documented antimicrobial activity.
➡ *Add 3 drops of any of the above oils to the echinacea poultice (see left) to enhance healing to apply to the skin.*

FOOD

Foods with antibacterial properties and with gut-protecting nutrients can help to tackle infection. It's vital, too, to drink plenty of water daily – 1.5–2 litres (2¾–3½ pints) – because a dehydrated body is more vulnerable to infection.

Natural live yogurt contains a range of nutrients and beneficial bacteria to support immunity by building a healthy gut.
➡ *Use to dress vegetables, spoon onto a baked potato, or add to desserts.*
Asparagus contains natural prebiotics – substances that feed the friendly bacteria in your gut. Foods such as Jerusalem artichokes, onions, and garlic are also good sources.
➡ *Enjoy regularly when in season.*
Garlic is potently antibacterial when using freshly crushed cloves.
➡ *Try eating 1–3 cloves daily, starting with small amounts in frequent doses, crushed and blended into vegetable juices or in salad dressings.*

" Certain herbs have complex antibacterial activity, which helps to fight bacteria."

NATURAL PAIRING

Asparagus provides vitamin E. As this is a fat-soluble vitamin, pair asparagus with healthy fats, for example olive oil or nuts, to aid the vitamin's absorption.

Sweet potatoes contain beta-carotene, which is converted into immune-enhancing vitamin A in the body.
➡ *Try roasted or mashed, skin on.*

SUPPLEMENTS

Taking additional vitamins and antioxidants can help when fighting an active infection.

Multi-vitamins help support immunity.
➡ *Take a daily supplement.*
Vitamin C is an antioxidant and supports immunity and tissue healing.
➡ *Take 1.2g daily.*
Zinc works with vitamin C to support immunity.
➡ *Take 11mg daily.*
Probiotic supplements deliver good bacteria to the gut.
➡ *Take a daily supplement with at least 10 billion live organisms per dose.*
Propolis is rich in bioflavonoids, which help destroy disease-causing bacteria without harming friendly bacteria.
➡ *Take 500mg 1–2 times daily.*

LIFESTYLE

Avoid taking antibiotics for minor, self-limiting illnesses. Only take antibiotics for serious infections, as advised by a doctor.
Reduce stress. Stress can impede the immune system. Try techniques such as yoga, meditation, and visualization.

HOW TO MAKE

A BALM

Enriching balms, which contain butters, oils, and waxes, are extremely simple to make and are an effective way to nourish, heal, and soothe dry and damaged skin and nails. Aromatherapy essential oils can be added to provide additional therapeutic benefits. Tailor your choice of essential oils depending on their properties and the benefits you would like.

Makes about 85g (3oz)

YOU WILL NEED

15g (½oz) beeswax (or carnauba wax if vegan)

10g (¼oz) shea butter

2½ tbsp almond oil

2 tbsp jojoba oil

bain-marie (heat-proof bowl and saucepan)

17 drops of essential oils (a single oil or blend of oils)

lidded jars

thermometer

label

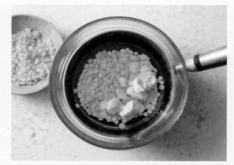

1 Sterilize the equipment: wash thoroughly then dry in an oven at 140°C (275°F) or in a microwave for 30–45 seconds. Gently heat all the ingredients, except the essential oils, in a bain-marie until melted.

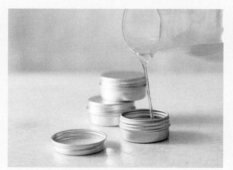

2 Once the ingredients are fully melted, pour them carefully into lidded jars.

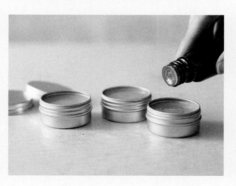

3 When the mixture is about 40°C (104°F), add up to 17 drops of your chosen essential oil or oil blend, dividing between the jars. (Essential oils should make up to 5 per cent of the ingredients for application to the body, and up to 1 per cent for the face.) Leave to cool with the lid off, then seal with an airtight lid. Label with the ingredients and the date.

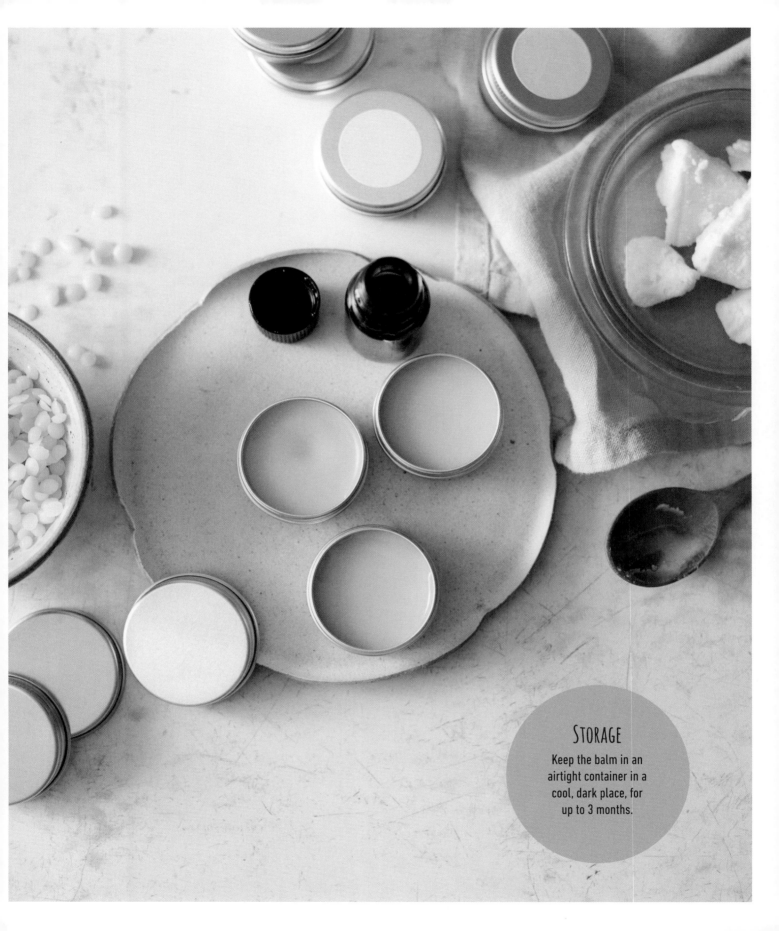

STORAGE

Keep the balm in an airtight container in a cool, dark place, for up to 3 months.

WOMEN'S HEALTH

Women's bodies face a unique set of challenges during menstruation, pregnancy, and the menopause, and normal hormonal changes can impact on how the body copes with a range of health concerns. In particular, loss of oestrogen after the menopause increases vulnerability to certain conditions. Discover how key nutrients and holistic healing can enhance fertility and boost health and vitality at all ages, as well as offer support for health concerns, easing symptoms and restoring balance.

STAYING WELL
WOMEN'S HEALTH

Throughout a woman's life, fluctuating or changing hormones can impact on many areas of health. Getting vital nutrients and using natural therapeutic remedies promotes vitality and enhances emotional and physical wellbeing, and in particular helps to boost fertility, support pregnancy, and enables the body and mind to cope during times of transition, such as the menopause.

FOOD

A balanced diet that supplies vital nutrients can boost vitality and fertility and help mitigate or even prevent many of the health problems that affect women.

WHOLEFOOD BENEFITS

A range of wholefoods helps boost fertility and optimize health during pregnancy and the menopause. Wholegrains such as wheat, barley, rice, and rye provide slow-release carbohydrates, which can help to prevent energy peaks and troughs linked to hormonal fluctuations, which can also inhibit ovulation.

MOOD-REGULATING PROBIOTICS

Probiotic live yogurt tops up good gut bacteria. As well as boosting immunity, there is increasing evidence of the role a healthy gut microbiome plays in regulating mood. Scientists believe that up to 95 per cent of the neurotransmitter serotonin, a mood stabilizer,

is produced in the gut. Live yogurt and other probiotic foods such as miso, kimchi, and sauerkraut, balance bacteria, helping to regulate emotions and avoid or limit mood swings.

Include foods such as pulses and beans in your diet, too. These act as prebiotics, feeding good bacteria already in the gut.

PHYTOESTROGENS

Dark green leafy vegetables, such as mustard greens, broccoli, cabbage, and kale, as well as being an important source of free radical-fighting antioxidants, also provide plant-based hormones known as phytoestrogens. These plant hormones work in a similar way to natural oestrogen produced by the body, so therefore help to make up for the loss of oestrogen that occurs around the time of the menopause.

FERTILITY BOOSTERS

Imbalances in hormone levels can affect fertility. Nuts and seeds (in particular flaxseeds) contain the omega-3 fatty acid, alpha-linolenic acid (ALA), which can help to balance hormones and

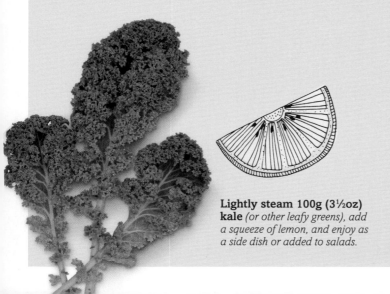

Lightly steam 100g (3½oz) kale *(or other leafy greens), add a squeeze of lemon, and enjoy as a side dish or added to salads.*

"Herbs that ease anxiety and reduce tension support strengthening tonic herbs."

boost fertility. Nuts and seeds also provide plant oestrogens to help regulate moods. Omega-3 fatty acids are found in oily fish, such as salmon and mackerel, too.

Full-fat dairy has fertility-boosting benefits. Cholesterol in full-fat dairy is thought to aid progesterone production, a key fertility hormone. Studies reveal that women who include full-fat dairy in their diet seem to have a higher pregnancy success rate.

BONE BUILDERS

Building and maintaining strong bones is essential for women's health. Pregnancy can deplete calcium stores and oestrogen loss in the menopause accelerates bone loss, putting women at risk of osteoporosis. Dairy products, leafy greens such as spinach and kale, and oily fish such as salmon and trout all provide calcium.

NATURAL IMMUNE BOOSTER

Garlic is antifungal and antibacterial. Sulphurous compounds in garlic support the liver, boosting immunity to guard against conditions such as thrush and possibly protect against cancer.

HERBS

Tonic herbs strengthen and enhance reproductive health and vitality. These are supported by herbs that ease anxiety and tension. Remedies should be halted immediately with conception and advice taken on which herbs are safe.

HERBS FOR WELLBEING AND BALANCE

Skullcap, a relaxing herb, enhances mental and emotional wellbeing and eases tension, for example in the premenstrual period. Chasteberry, a well-known tonic herb for women, tones tissues and balances hormones, so is helpful in the premenstrual period and can also help to lessen the impact of the menopause.

Antispasmodic herbs such as yarrow help to balance blood flow during menstruation, while lady's mantle acts as a tonic for uterine tissues to help promote a regular menstrual cycle. Both herbs also support liver health, helping to ensure that the body metabolizes and, where necessary, removes excess hormones.

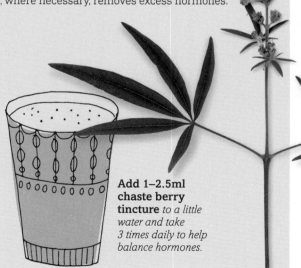

Add 1–2.5ml chaste berry tincture *to a little water and take 3 times daily to help balance hormones.*

Fertility-enhancing herbs

Schisandra berries, sometimes called the five-flavour-fruit because of the berries' complex flavour profile, have a strengthening tonic effect on the female reproductive system, enhancing reproductive function. Schisandra also has calming properties, helping to address feelings of anxiety and stress.

Shatavari, a member of the asparagus family commonly used to increase vitality, is also a nourishing tonic, which is thought to promote health in the female reproductive organs, and is often used specifically as an aid to fertility.

Herbs to support the menopause

Herbs that support the liver help to reduce and ease menopausal symptoms. The liver is vital to our overall health and wellbeing and its specific roles in functions such as balancing hormones, controlling blood sugar levels, and storing fuel for the body can all help to ease the transition that occurs during the menopause. Sage, yarrow, and lady's mantle all make effective liver tonics, supporting and strengthening liver function. Sage also has an oestrogenic effect that can help to control menopausal symptoms such as excessive sweating.

Essential oils

Essential oils are an effective and enjoyable way to balance moods and emotions and prevent chronic stress impacting on health. Many oils help to balance hormones to support the female reproductive system.

Regulating oils

Essential oils with balancing properties help to lessen the impact of hormonal fluctuations. Rose is both uplifting and relaxing, so helps to cope with hormonal changes, and it has a regulating and strengthening tonic effect on the uterus to limit premenstrual symptoms. Clary sage also helps to balance hormones, making it a useful oil for regulating menstruation. Geranium, as well as being cheering and reviving, is cooling and balancing and can be used to stabilize hormones, helping to regulate the menstrual cycle, and fennel helps to regulate menstruation and also has properties that help reduce fluid retention. Cypress is cleansing, toning, and deodorizing, so beneficial during the menopause to minimize or prevent symptoms such as hot flushes.

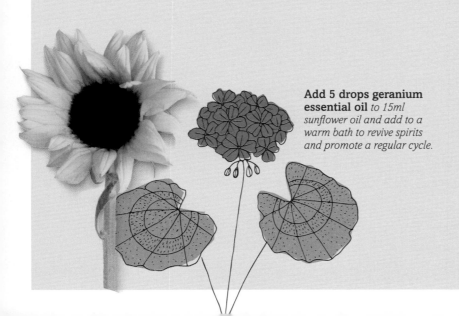

Add 5 drops geranium essential oil *to 15ml sunflower oil and add to a warm bath to revive spirits and promote a regular cycle.*

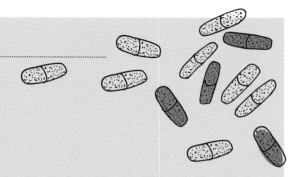

Reviving oils

Uplifting essential oils can be an effective tool for helping to cope with hormonal changes, enabling you to control emotions and keep mood swings in check. Neroli, derived from orange flowers, and patchouli, from a native Indian bush, both have a pronounced relaxing sedative quality as well as an uplifting effect, while ylang ylang, with its luxurious, intensely tropical floral scent, is also uplifting and an extremely beneficial oil for controlling mood swings.

SUPPLEMENTS

Certain nutrients play a significant role in boosting reproductive health, helping to balance hormones and support women's health at various stages. Supplementing the diet can be beneficial.

Vitamin boost

A daily multi-vitamin can help to support reproductive health, and increasing the levels of certain nutrients helps to fight inflammation to optimize health throughout the body.

Fertility essentials

Ensuring that your body is receiving sufficient amounts of certain nutrients gives a natural boost to fertility. Folic acid, zinc, and vitamin E all play an important role in regulating and balancing hormones. Women who have adequate levels of folic acid are less likely to experience problems with ovulation; a deficiency in zinc can lead to reduced fertility, hormone imbalances, and an increased risk of miscarriage; while vitamin E is also an important nutrient for balancing hormones.

Making sure you are getting sufficient vitamin D also boosts reproductive health. A lack of vitamin D is linked to low moods, reduced immunity, inflammation and cramping during periods, and a higher risk of fibroids. As this vitamin is mainly manufactured in response to sunlight, supplies often run low in the winter months and a supplement can help to restore levels.

Liver-supporting nutrients

Taking a B complex supplement can boost liver health if levels are low. The liver needs the entire B complex family to produce hormones and regulate hormone levels in the body, and B vitamins are also extremely important for maintaining energy levels and regulating moods.

"Essential oils with a balancing effect can help to lessen the impact of hormonal fluctuations."

TREATMENTS

WOMEN'S HEALTH

At certain times, hormonal fluctuations mean that women's bodies undergo significant, sometimes sudden, adjustments, for example, in pregnancy and in times of transition, such as the menopause. Infections can cause chronic conditions with repercussions on fertility and health. Holistic remedies help to balance hormones and ease symptoms. Pages 236–39 look at ways to support and maximize women's fertility.

PREMENSTRUAL SYNDROME (PMS)

PMS describes a collection of symptoms, both physical and emotional, that are linked to hormonal fluctuations during the menstrual cycle. Symptoms are most common in the week before menstruation, when oestrogen levels are high, and can be aggravated by environmental and dietary factors.

HERBS

Hormone-balancing herbs can be helpful, combined with relaxing herbs to ease anxiety and tension and improve mood, bitter herbs to boost liver function, and detoxifying and diuretic herbs to help reduce water retention.

Chaste berry acts on the pituitary gland to help balance sex hormones.
➡*Take 1–2.5ml tincture in a little water 3 times daily in the 2 weeks prior to menstruation.*

Vervain helps to balance hormones, lift mood, and relax mind and body. Excessive doses may cause vomiting.
➡*Take 2.5–5ml tincture in a little water 3 times daily.*

Skullcap is a nervous system tonic, easing agitation and anxiety and relaxing tension in the body.
➡*Infuse 1–2 tsp dried skullcap in 175ml (6fl oz) boiling water and drink 3 times daily.*

ESSENTIAL OILS

Oils can support the physical, behavioural, and psychological symptoms of PMS, such as fluid retention and irritability.

Fennel can help to treat fluid retention.
➡*Add 5 drops to 10ml almond oil and use in a massage.*
Rose helps relieve irritability and anxiety.
Clary sage can be very uplifting, helping with stress, anxiety, and depression.
➡*Add 5 drops of rose or clary sage to 10ml evening primrose oil for a massage. Or mix 5 drops of either oil to a bath dispersant and add to a daily bath.*

FOOD

Fresh wholefoods can boost wellbeing. Staying hydrated with water, herbal teas, and clear broths can help reduce bloating.

Oily fish, such as salmon and mackerel, are high in anti-inflammatory omega-3, shown to improve PMS symptoms.
➡*Eat 2–3 portions a week.*

Leafy green vegetables, such as kale, broccoli, and bok choy, are high in fibre, iron, and B vitamins, all of which can be helpful in reducing the symptoms of PMS.
➡*Add regularly to salads and stir-fries.*
Beans and lentils are healthy plant sources of protein, fibre, and iron.
➡*See recipe, opposite.*
WHAT TO AVOID
Highly salted foods can cause bloating and fluid retention. Excessive alcohol consumption and a high-fat diet can worsen PMS symptoms. Too many sweet treats and caffeinated drinks can lead to or exacerbate mood swings.

SUPPLEMENTS

A healthy diet and lifestyle can be supplemented with specific nutrients that are known to help relieve pain and discomfort and help to keep the emotions on an even keel.

Magnesium can ease headaches, sugar cravings, cramps, and anxiety.
➡*Take 400mg daily.*
Borage oil is rich in omega-6 gamma-linolenic acid (GLA), an anti-inflammatory essential fatty acid that can help to reduce breast tenderness and other PMS symptoms.
➡*Take 1–2g daily.*

LIFESTYLE

Relaxation techniques, such as yoga and meditation, help reduce stress, which, unchecked, can worsen the symptoms of PMS.

Exercise boosts energy levels and aerobic exercise in particular increases natural opioids (endorphins) in the brain to help improve mood.

Getting sufficient sleep is important. If you are not getting enough sleep, this can impact on your ability to cope with the symptoms of PMS, so it is essential to get the right amount of restful sleep.

OTHER THERAPIES

Homeopathy and acupuncture both help to balance hormones and manage the symptoms of PMS.

Flower remedies provide support, in particular helping to address the emotional causes of PMS.

RECIPE

Fibre-boosting dish

Make a 3-bean salad with **cannellini beans, kidney beans** and **green beans**. Add a squeeze of **lemon juice** to aid iron absorption.

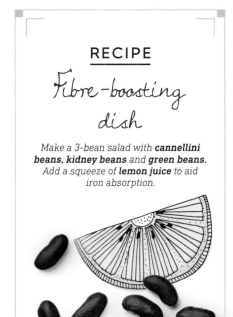

PERIOD PROBLEMS

Periods can be irregular, heavy, and painful. Painful pelvic cramps, known as primary dysmenorrhoea, occurring just before or during menstruation, are usually caused by inflammatory substances called prostaglandins produced in the uterine lining during menstruation.

HERBS

Antispasmodic herbs relax the uterus and ease pain, while circulation-boosting herbs and those that act as uterine tonics aid blood flow to help regulate menstruation.

Yarrow gently stimulates circulation in the abdomen to help regulate blood flow and improve both heavy and scant periods. Avoid with sensitivity to the *Asteraceae* plant family. Prolonged use can increase skin photosensitivity.
➡️*Juice the fresh flowering herb and take 3 tsp daily in water.*

Cramp bark is antispasmodic, helping to relax uterine muscles and ease cramping, and promotes healthy blood flow, which also helps reduce pain.
➡️*Take 4–8ml tincture in a little water 3 times daily.*

Lady's mantle helps regulate periods, reduces heavy flow, and acts as a strengthening tonic to uterine tissues.
➡️*Infuse 2 tsp dried lady's mantle in 175ml (6fl oz) boiling water and drink 3 times daily.*

Chamomile eases spasms to promote a healthier blood flow. Avoid if sensitive to the *Asteraceae* plant family.
➡️*Apply a warm chamomile poultice to the abdomen to relieve cramping.*

ESSENTIAL OILS

Essential oils help relieve pain, regulate hormones, and can be antispasmodic.

NOT QUITE RIPE?

Starch in bananas converts to simple sugars during the ripening process, so eat bananas before they are overripe to avoid a higher sugar hit.

Marjoram is antispasmodic and analgesic.
➡️*Add 5 drops to 10ml jojoba oil and massage into the abdomen and lower back, or add 5 drops to a hot compress.*

Fennel can help to regulate cycles where periods are light or scanty and painful.
➡️*Add 5 drops to 10ml grapeseed oil and massage into the abdomen and lower back, or add 5 drops to a hot compress.*

Lavender is calming and pain-relieving.
➡️*Add 5 drops to 10ml almond oil and use in a massage. Or add 8 drops to a bath dispersant and add to a warm bath.*

FOOD

Wholefoods and fresh vegetables and fruits help to maintain energy and curb cravings, as well as reduce bloating.

Apples have soluble fibre and slow-release sugars to beat cravings.
➡️*Eat daily as a snack.*

Leafy green vegetables, such as kale, broccoli, and bok choy have iron and B vitamins to help maintain energy.
➡️*Add to salads and stir-fries.*

Flaxseed has healthy fats and hormone-balancing phytoestrogens.
➡️*Add 1–2 tbsp ground flaxseed to cereal or porridge.*

Bananas contain potassium, vitamin B6, and slow-release carbohydrates to boost energy and avoid mood swings.
➡️*Use as a base for a smoothie.*

➤ CONTINUED...

SUPPLEMENTS

Certain supplements can help to regulate the menstrual cycle.

Multi-vitamins ensure adequate amounts of essential vitamins.
➤ *Take a daily dose.*

Bioflavonoids are antioxidant, anti-inflammatory, and have a hormone-balancing effect.
➤ *Take 500mg a day.*

Vitamin B6 deficiency can result in irregular cycles or absence of periods.
➤ *Take 50mg daily.*

Magnesium can help combat cravings and ease painful cramps.
➤ *Take 400mg daily.*

Vitamin D can interrupt the production of prostaglandins, and is also anti-inflammatory to help reduce cramping.
➤ *Take 600iu daily.*

Cinnamon is rich in antioxidants and has a mild analgesic effect, shown to relieve period pains as effectively as over-the-counter painkillers.
➤ *Take a 420mg capsule 3 times daily, or drink cinnamon tea, in the first 3 days of a period.*

LIFESTYLE

A regular exercise routine of at least 20 minutes a day can ease cramps. For severe cramps, try light stretching or yoga in the early part of a period. Yoga also enhances mood and reduces pain in women affected by the physical and psychological discomfort of periods.

A hot water pad or bottle brings relief and comfort from cramps.

Add a cup of Epsom salts to a warm bath to relax and give a light detox.

OTHER THERAPIES

Acupuncture is an effective form of pain relief for severe period pains.

Massage therapies, such as shiatsu and reflexology, are balancing and relaxing.

VAGINITIS AND VULVITIS

Inflammation of the vagina and/or vulva can cause itching, discomfort, and discharge. Causes include *Candida albicans*, bacterial infections, sexually transmitted infections, and chemical irritation from products.

HERBS

Antibacterial and antifungal herbs fight infections, supported by immune tonics. Anti-inflammatories soothe, heal, and restore health to the vaginal tract.

Echinacea acts as an immune tonic. Avoid with immunosuppressants.
➤ *Take 500mg to 1g daily as capsules.*

Golden seal is antimicrobial and healing. Avoid in pregnancy, if breastfeeding, and with hypertension. Do not take internally for prolonged periods.
➤ *Take 10–15 drops tincture in a little water 3 times daily, or add a few drops to a hip-height sitz bath.*

Calendula soothes inflammation, is antimicrobial, and promotes healing.

White dead-nettle cleanses and tones the vaginal tract. See box, below.
➤ *Infuse 1–2 tsp of either dried calendula or white dead-nettle in 175ml (6fl oz) boiling water, leave to cool, and add to a hip-height sitz bath.*

ESSENTIAL OILS

Some oils have antibacterial properties to fight bacterial infections.

Lavender is analgesic and antibacterial.
➤ *Add 5 drops to a warm, hip-height sitz bath and take a 15-minute soak.*

FOOD

Eat foods rich in antioxidant vitamins and immune-boosting nutrients. Dehydration increases vulnerability to infection so drink 1.5–2 litres (2¾–3½ pints) of water daily.

Coconut oil contains caprylic acid, which is a natural antifungal.
➤ *Use in cooking, add to smoothies and dressings, or eat 1–2 tbsp daily neat.*

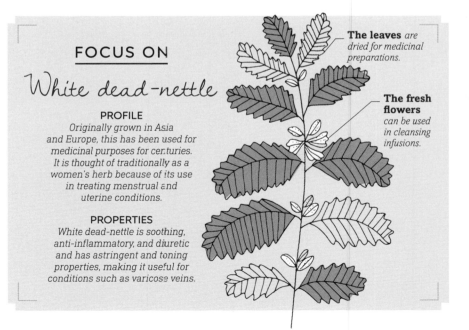

FOCUS ON

White dead-nettle

PROFILE
Originally grown in Asia and Europe, this has been used for medicinal purposes for centuries. It is thought of traditionally as a women's herb because of its use in treating menstrual and uterine conditions.

PROPERTIES
White dead-nettle is soothing, anti-inflammatory, and diuretic and has astringent and toning properties, making it useful for conditions such as varicose veins.

The leaves *are dried for medicinal preparations.*

The fresh flowers *can be used in cleansing infusions.*

Garlic, often called nature's antibiotic, can help to combat infection.
➡️ *Eat raw, for example in dressings, or use during cooking.*

Barley contains beta-glucan, a type of fibre with antimicrobial properties that boosts immunity, speeds healing, and may help antibiotics to work better.
➡️ *Eat on its own or as a rice substitute.*

Berries boost immunity with vitamin C, antioxidants, and bioflavonoids.
➡️ *Sprinkle over barley porridge.*

SUPPLEMENTS

A healthy diet can be supplemented with nutrients to help fight infections.

Multi-vitamins and minerals form the basis of a supplement regime.
➡️ *Take a daily dose.*

B vitamins, needed for cell replication, are often deficient with vaginal infections.
➡️ *Take a B complex with at least 25mg of each of the main B vitamins.*

Vitamin C promotes collagen formation, which is important during an infection.
➡️ *Take 1g daily.*

Vitamin E can strengthen resistance to chlamydia infections.
➡️ *Take 300iu daily. Or break open a capsule and rub the oil on the area.*

Zinc supports the immune system.
➡️ *Take 15mg daily.*

Probiotic supplements can help maintain immune health.
➡️ *Take one that delivers 5–10 billion live organisms per dose.*

LIFESTYLE

Use unperfumed soaps, and avoid washing the affected area if irritated; also avoid chemical irritants.

Avoid douching as this can wash away good bacteria.

OTHER THERAPIES

Homeopathy supports healing.

ENDOMETRIOSIS

This is where the uterus lining grows into other tissues, often causing pain and fertility issues. Linked to high oestrogen levels, it affects 7–15 per cent of women of reproductive age in the developed world.

HERBS

Uterine tonics help to tone the tissues. Herbs can also ease inflammation and spasms, lower excess oestrogen, and boost blood flow to the uterus.

Chinese angelica, a uterine tonic, stops blood stagnation. Avoid in pregnancy and therapeutic doses if diabetic.
➡️ *Take 3–5ml tincture in a little water 3 times daily.*

Lady's mantle, a strengthening tonic, helps reduce heavy bleeding and pain.
➡️ *Take 2–4ml tincture in a little water 3 times daily.*

White peony balances hormones and can ease spasms.
➡️ *Take 2–5ml tincture in a little water 3 times daily.*

Mugwort, a uterine stimulant, improves blood flow and cleanses tissues. Avoid therapeutic doses in pregnancy.
➡️ *Infuse 1–2 tsp dried mugwort in 175ml (6fl oz) boiling water. Drink 3 times daily.*

WHAT TO AVOID
Oestrogenic herbs such as black cohosh, hops, and alfalfa.

FOOD

A plant-based, organic diet can lower the risk of endometriosis and ease symptoms. Drinking plenty of water with high-fibre foods helps control oestrogen levels.

Brown rice and high-fibre grains boost digestion and can help lower oestrogen.
➡️ *Eat wholegrains such as rice daily.*

> "*A plant-based, organic diet is thought to lower the risk of endometriosis.*"

Dark green leafy vegetables such as broccoli and kale are antioxidant-rich and can help to modulate oestrogen.
➡️ *Eat 1–2 servings daily.*

Alliums, such as garlic and onions, have sulphur compounds that boost liver health to help remove excess oestrogen.
➡️ *Use liberally in cooking each day.*

WHAT TO AVOID
Sugar, caffeine, and alcohol are linked with higher oestrogen levels.

SUPPLEMENTS

Supplementing with anti-inflammatory nutrients may reduce symptoms.

Vitamins C and E are antioxidants that can help fight inflammation.
➡️ *Take 1g vitamin C and 1200iu vitamin E daily.*

Omega-3 fatty acids are anti-inflammatory to help ease pain.
➡️ *Look for a supplement with around 100mg EPA and 700mg DHA.*

Propolis can boost fertility in women with endometriosis.
➡️ *Take 500mg 2 times a day.*

LIFESTYLE

Detox your home. Hormone-disrupting chemicals such as parabens are found in household cleaners and cosmetics.

Stay active. Regular exercise is linked to a lower risk of endometriosis.

5

RECIPES FOR WELLNESS

DIPS

Ready in moments, these mouthwatering dips are an effortless way to top up your nutrients. Plant-based sources of protein and flavour-boosting herbs and spices make these healthy dips a must to stock in the fridge. Simply prepare all the ingredients, blitz to the desired consistency, then serve with crudités, oat cakes, or tortilla chips.

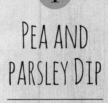

1

PEA AND PARSLEY DIP

Packed with protein, fibre, and micronutrients, peas are tiny nuggets of nutrition, while parsley has a natural diuretic action, boosting urine production and easing bloating.

SERVES 4 • **PREP TIME** 10 MINS

125g (4½oz) garden peas, cooked

1 avocado, peeled and pitted

1 clove of garlic

2 spring onions, chopped

2–3 tbsp parsley, chopped

½ tsp ground cumin

1 tsp tamari

2 tbsp lemon juice

1 tbsp olive oil (add towards the end of blitzing)

Nutritional info per serving:
Kcals 132 Fat 10.5g Saturated fat 2g Carbohydrates 4.5g Sugar 1.5g Sodium 72mg Fibre 3.5g Protein 3g Cholesterol 0mg

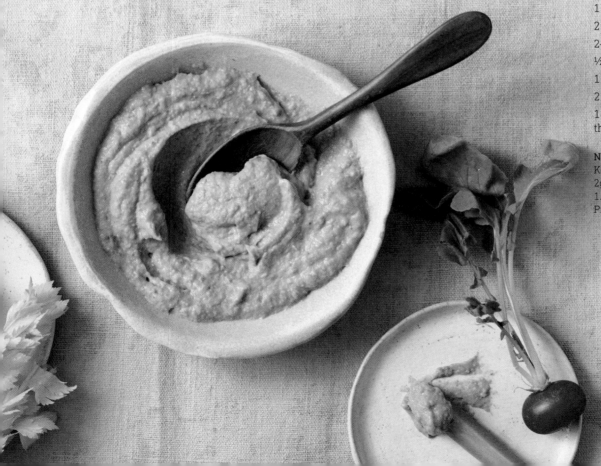

2

RED BEAN AND YOGURT DIP

Red kidney beans are high in cholesterol-lowering fibre, and natural yogurt provides probiotics for gut health as well as calcium, protein, potassium, and phosphorus for bones, helping to guard against conditions such as osteoporosis.

SERVES 4 • PREP TIME 5 MINS

125g (4½oz) red kidney beans, drained and rinsed

60g (2oz) red onion, diced

1 clove of garlic

1 tsp red chilli, deseeded

1 tsp ground cumin

1 tbsp tomato purée

1 tbsp olive oil

1 tbsp rice wine vinegar

150g (5½oz) natural yogurt

Nutritional info per serving:
Kcals 102 Fat 4.5g Saturated fat 1g Carbohydrates 9g Sugar 4.5g Sodium 83mg Fibre 3.5g Protein 5g Cholesterol 4mg

3

CANNELLINI BEAN DIP

High in protein and calcium for strong bones, cannellini beans also contain cholesterol-lowering soluble fibre for heart health.

SERVES 4 • PREP TIME 5 MINS

300g (10oz) cannellini beans, drained and rinsed

1 clove of garlic

1 tbsp lemon juice

1 tbsp tahini

1½ tbsp coriander leaves

Nutritional info per serving:
Kcals 110 Fat 3g Saturated fat 0.5g Carbohydrates 12.5g Sugar 0.5g Sodium 4mg Fibre 6g Protein 6.5g Cholesterol 0mg

4

PESTO DIP WITH COCONUT YOGURT

Home-made pesto sauce is packed with nutrients and provides unsaturated fats for heart health. Coconut yogurt is a tasty alternative to dairy and a great source of vitamin B12, which supports nerve health, and mood-boosting vitamin D.

SERVES 4 • PREP TIME 5 MINS

20g (¾oz) pine nuts

1½ tbsp basil leaves

1 clove of garlic

1½ tbsp olive oil

200g (7oz) coconut yogurt, to serve

Nutritional info per serving:
Kcals 168 Fat 13g Saturated fat 3g Carbohydrates 8g Sugar 6.5g Sodium 20mg Fibre 6.5g Protein 1g Cholesterol 0mg

5

CREAMY AVOCADO DIP

This creamy dip is full of anti-inflammatory essential fats from the avocado, while coriander provides fibre, vitamin C, and blood-boosting iron.

SERVES 4 • PREP TIME 5 MINS

1 avocado, peeled and pitted

85g (3oz) red onion, chopped into quarters

½ tbsp coriander

250g (9oz) coconut yogurt

Nutritional info per serving:
Kcals 115 Fat 9g Saturated fat 2g Carbohydrates 4g Sugar 3g Sodium 83mg Fibre 2g Protein 3.5g Cholesterol 0mg

PELVIC INFLAMMATORY DISEASE (PID)

PID is an infection of the female upper genital tract, including the uterus, fallopian tubes, and ovaries. Often it is linked to the bacteria that cause chlamydia and gonorrhoea. Symptoms include abdominal pain, painful urination, and bleeding between periods. Left untreated it can cause irreversible damage to the fallopian tubes, raising the risk of ectopic pregnancy and infertility. Medical attention is vital; natural remedies can support treatment.

HERBS

Herbs help to fight infection and boost immunity and pelvic circulation. Relaxing herbal baths can soothe abdominal tissues.

Echinacea strengthens the immune response to help fight infections. Avoid with immunosuppressants.
➡ *Take 1–2ml tincture in a little water hourly for acute infections, then 3–5ml tincture in a little water 3 times daily.*

Calendula is antibacterial and detoxifying, and stimulates the pelvic lymph nodes and blood circulation. Avoid internal use during pregnancy.
➡ *See remedy with lavender flowers, below.*

Cleavers stimulates and cleanses tissues via the lymphatic system. It is also diuretic, helping to eliminate waste.
➡ *Infuse 2 tsp dried cleavers in 175ml (6fl oz) boiling water. Drink 3 times daily, or enjoy the fresh juice in the spring.*

FOOD

A balanced, nutrient-dense diet will support other treatments. Being hydrated discourages infection so aim to drink 1.5–2 litres (2¾–3½ pints) of water daily.

Green tea is rich in antioxidant and anti-inflammatory compounds that support immunity.
➡ *Drink 2–3 cups a day, hot or cold.*

Brightly coloured, antioxidant-rich foods, such as blueberries, cherries, tomatoes, squash, and peppers have a protective effect.
➡ *Include in your daily diet.*

Olive oil and coconut oil are anti-inflammatory.
➡ *Use for cooking and dressings.*

> " *Being well-hydrated helps to discourage infection, so drink plenty of water.* "

SUPPLEMENTS

If you are taking antibiotics, supplements can help to rebuild the immune system.

Probiotic supplements repopulate the gut with beneficial bacteria, vital for a fully functioning immune system after a course of antibiotics.
➡ *Take a supplement with at least 10 billion live organisms per dose.*

Vitamin C is vital for healthy immunity and collagen formation, which supports the integrity of body tissues so they are less prone to infection and scarring.
➡ *Take 1–2g daily.*

Zinc boosts immunity, accelerates healing, and may ward off recurrent infections.
➡ *Take 15mg daily.*

Olive leaf has antibacterial and antifungal activity, boosting immunity. Avoid with low blood sugar or low blood pressure.
➡ *Take 250–500mg, 1 to 3 times daily.*

LIFESTYLE

Use condoms with a new sexual partner until they've had a sexual health check.

Avoid douches. These can remove beneficial organisms naturally present in the vagina that fight infection.

OTHER THERAPIES

Acupuncture may boost immune health.
Homeopathy can treat the whole body.

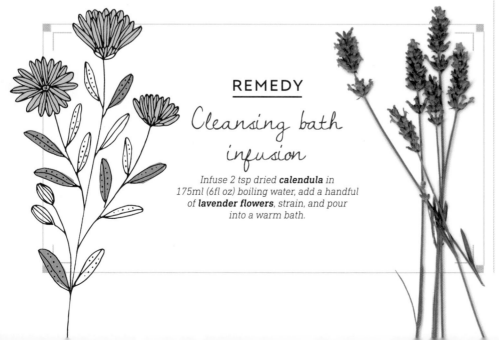

REMEDY

Cleansing bath infusion

Infuse 2 tsp dried **calendula** in 175ml (6fl oz) boiling water, add a handful of **lavender flowers**, strain, and pour into a warm bath.

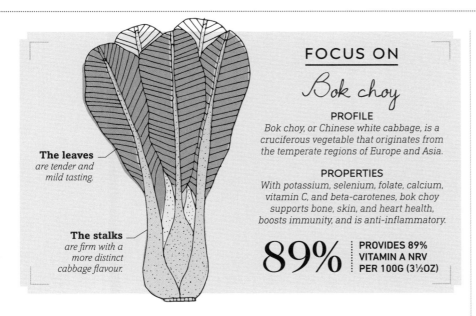

FOCUS ON

Bok choy

PROFILE
Bok choy, or Chinese white cabbage, is a cruciferous vegetable that originates from the temperate regions of Europe and Asia.

PROPERTIES
With potassium, selenium, folate, calcium, vitamin C, and beta-carotenes, bok choy supports bone, skin, and heart health, boosts immunity, and is anti-inflammatory.

The leaves *are tender and mild tasting.*

The stalks *are firm with a more distinct cabbage flavour.*

89% PROVIDES 89% VITAMIN A NRV PER 100G (3½OZ)

FIBROIDS

Uterine fibroids are benign tumors, which can be caused by genetics, environment, and/or hormonal factors. Although not life-threatening and often asymptomatic, they can lead to debilitating symptoms such as heavy bleeding, abdominal pain, constipation, and frequent urination. In some women, fibroids can cause miscarriage and affect fertility.

HERBS

Strengthening uterine tonic herbs help tone tissues and can reduce heavy bleeding; hormone-balancing and liver tonic herbs help to manage an excess of oestrogen; and antispasmodic herbs can ease pain.

Chaste berry helps balance hormones.
➡ *Take 2.5ml tincture in a little water 3 times daily.*
Lady's mantle tones the uterus to stem heavy flow and promote healthy tissue.
➡ *Infuse 1–2 tsp dried lady's mantle in 175ml (6fl oz) boiling water and drink 3 times daily.*

Yarrow eases abdominal congestion and heavy bleeding and supports the liver to help balance hormones. Avoid in pregnancy or with sensitivity to the *Asteraceae* plant family. Prolonged use can increase skin sensitivity.
➡ *Take 2–4ml tincture in a little water 3 times daily.*

FOOD

Switching to a plant-based diet can help to manage weight and hormone levels, both of which influence fibroid growth.

Lean protein, especially from oily fish, is anti-inflammatory.
➡ *Eat 2–3 portions each week.*
Cruciferous vegetables, such as broccoli, cabbage, kale, and bok choy (see box, above) contain a compound, indole-3-carbinol, which supports liver health and aids hormone balance.
➡ *Eat regularly. Try snacking on broccoli florets.*
Flaxseeds are a rich source of the omega-3 fatty acid alpha-linolenic acid (ALA) and polyphenols, both of which aid hormone balance and boost fertility.
➡ *Add 1–3 tbsp ground seeds daily to yogurts, fruit salads, or smoothies.*

WHAT TO AVOID
Fatty and processed meats can exacerbate inflammation. Refined carbohydrates and sugars cause spikes in hormone levels and these may be linked to fibroid growth.

SUPPLEMENTS

Certain supplements can help to reduce inflammation and support healthy hormonal balance.

Curcumin, found in turmeric, is an antioxidant and has anti-inflammatory compounds that research shows inhibit fibroid cell proliferation.
➡ *Take a 400mg capsule 2–3 times daily.*
B complex supplements supply the full family of B vitamins, which the liver needs to process hormones and regulate hormone levels.
➡ *Take a supplement that supplies 50mg of the main B vitamins.*
L-arginine is an amino acid that may slow or halt the growth of fibroids.
➡ *Take 500mg daily on an empty stomach.*
Vitamin D deficiency has been linked to a higher risk of fibroids.
➡ *Take 1500–2000iu daily.*

LIFESTYLE

Limit exposure to cadmium, found in enamelled pans, cigarette smoke, and very polluted environments, as it is linked to a higher risk of fibroids.
Exercise regularly. Being overweight combined with low levels of physical activity has been linked to fibroids.

OTHER THERAPIES

Homeopathy offers several remedies that can be supportive in treating fibroids.
Acupuncture is often recommended to help balance hormone levels and help to shrink fibroids.

POLYCYSTIC OVARIES

Polycystic ovarian syndrome (PCOS) affects 6–10 per cent of women of reproductive age. Insulin resistance is often a factor, which in turn leads to an increase in male sex hormones (androgens), such as testosterone, and can cause irregular menstruation, increased body hair, acne, fertility problems, and future diabetes.

HERBS

Herbs help to regulate hormones and menstruation, improving symptoms such as acne and hirsutism. If there is insulin resistance, herbs help control insulin levels.

Saw palmetto is an anti-androgenic (blocks the action of male hormones), to regulate hirsutism and menstruation.
➡️ *Take 1–2ml tincture in a little water 3 times daily.*

Liquorice helps lower testosterone levels. Avoid in pregnancy, with hypertension, or large doses over long periods.
➡️ *Take 1–3ml tincture in a little water 3 times daily.*

White peony helps reduce testosterone production. See box, above.
➡️ *Take 3–5ml tincture in a little water 3 times daily.*

Fenugreek seeds increase sensitivity to insulin and balance sugar levels. Avoid in pregnancy or with hypothyroidism. Take separately from other drugs as it may impede their absorption.
➡️ *Infuse 1 tsp dried fenugreek seeds in 175ml (6fl oz) boiling water and drink 3 times daily.*

FOOD

A low-carbohydrate diet helps to raise blood sugar levels slowly.

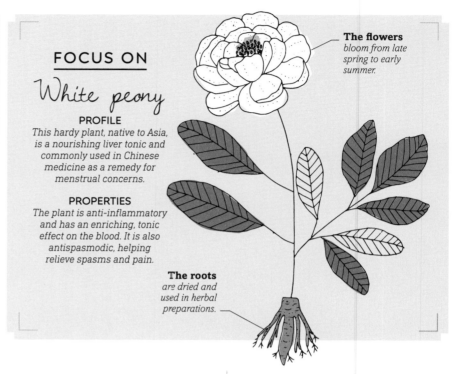

FOCUS ON

White peony

PROFILE
This hardy plant, native to Asia, is a nourishing liver tonic and commonly used in Chinese medicine as a remedy for menstrual concerns.

PROPERTIES
The plant is anti-inflammatory and has an enriching, tonic effect on the blood. It is also antispasmodic, helping relieve spasms and pain.

The flowers *bloom from late spring to early summer.*

The roots *are dried and used in herbal preparations.*

Kale and spinach provide B vitamins and potassium to help regulate hormones, sugar, and fat metabolism.
➡️ *Add to soups, stir-fries, and meals.*

Eggs are a complete protein source (with all the essential amino acids), with iron, folate, thiamine, and vitamins.
➡️ *Enjoy a daily egg if you wish.*

Barley releases energy slowly, has reproductive-supporting nutrients, and fibre to help process excess hormones.
➡️ *Use for risottos and porridge.*

SUPPLEMENTS

These can support a healthy diet to aid metabolism and balance hormones.

Multi-vitamins and minerals form the foundation of a supplement regime.
➡️ *Take a daily dose.*

Chromium helps to balance blood insulin levels.
➡️ *Take 200–400mcg daily with food.*

Zinc is helpful for balancing hormone and blood sugar levels.
➡️ *Take 10mg daily.*

B complex vitamins help the liver process hormones, and vitamins B2, B3, B5, and B6 support a healthy metabolism.
➡️ *Take a daily supplement with 25–50mg of the main B vitamins.*

Resveratrol, a compound in grapes and other plant foods, supports hormone balance and glucose control.
➡️ *Take 1500mg daily.*

LIFESTYLES

Lose weight. Obesity can contribute to polycystic ovaries.

Exercise daily to boost metabolism, aid weight loss, and control insulin levels.

Take time out to unwind as PCOS can lead to mood swings and depression.

OTHER THERAPIES

Acupuncture helps balance hormones and stimulates ovulation.

Homeopathy can help balance hormones.

Counselling and psychotherapy can be helpful for dealing with symptoms of depression.

PREGNANCY AND BREASTFEEDING CONCERNS

The symptoms women experience during pregnancy and breastfeeding are a testimony to how profoundly the body changes. Natural remedies can help with common concerns.

HERBS

Herbs can ease indigestion, nausea, anxiety, and insomnia, and some promote breast milk production. Generally herbs are avoided in the first trimester; the ones listed here are safe throughout pregnancy.

Ginger is helpful for nausea, indigestion, and is a strengthening tonic. Avoid with peptic ulcers and gallstones.
➡️*Take the powdered root in capsules, 250mg to 1gm, 3 times daily or as required.*
Lemon balm can ease indigestion and nausea and reduces depression and anxiety. Avoid with hypothyroidism.
➡️*Infuse 1–2 tsp dried lemon balm in 175ml (6fl oz) boiling water and drink as required.*
Fennel seeds soothe indigestion and can promote milk production.
➡️*Infuse 1–2 tsp fennel seeds in 175ml (6fl oz) boiling water. Drink as required.*

ESSENTIAL OILS

Aromatherapy can help to alleviate lower back ache and reduce stress and anxiety.

Lavender is analgesic and helps to relieve muscular pain.
Neroli can fight fatigue and aid sleep.
➡️*Add 2 drops of either oil to 10ml jojoba oil and use in a massage. Ensure the pregnant woman is supported and relaxed. Or mix 4 drops with a bath dispersant and use in the bath.*

FOOD

The body needs extra nutrients, vitamins, and minerals if pregnant or breastfeeding. It's vital to be hydrated, too – try to drink 1.5–2 litres (2¾–3½ pints) of water a day.

Dairy products provide extra calcium. Yogurt, especially live Greek yogurt, has both calcium and live cultures that are beneficial for the gut.
➡️*Include in the diet daily.*
Legumes, such as lentils, peas, beans, and chickpeas are good sources of fibre, protein, iron, folate, and calcium.
➡️*Add to soups and salads or whizz in the blender to make dips and spreads.*
Sweet potatoes are an excellent healthy source of beta-carotene, which converts to vitamin A in the body.
➡️*Roast in its skin or mash.*
Eggs are easily digested and a rich source of protein and vital nutrients.
➡️*Start your day with an egg or enjoy an omelette as a light meal.*

SUPPLEMENTS

These can be taken alongside a healthy diet to cover any nutritional shortfalls.

Multi-vitamins and minerals form the foundation of a supplement regime.
➡️*Take a daily dose.*

> " *Essential oils can be used to relieve lower back pain and reduce feelings of stress and anxiety.* "

FROZEN FRESH

An excess of fresh lemon balm can be frozen for later use. Try chopping the leaves, combining with water, and freezing in an ice-cube tray for up to nine months.

Vitamin C is essential for the immune system and is rarely included in multi-vitamins in adequate amounts.
➡️*Take 500mg to 1g daily as a "complex" that includes bioflavonoids and other synergistic compounds, such as rosehips.*
Vitamin D deficiency in pregnancy may be an issue in women with dark skin, particularly if they are city dwellers.
➡️*Take 400iu of vitamin D and 500mg to 1g of calcium daily.*
Omega-3 fatty acids from fish or algal sources such as spirulina support the heart and joints and are helpful for the baby's neural development.
➡️*Take 1g daily.*

LIFESTYLE

Switching to organic food where you can avoids taking in pesticide residues that could harm your baby.
Practise relaxation techniques. Stress depletes the body of essential nutrients – especially B vitamins – needed for babies to develop and grow. Yoga is ideal as usually classes include a period of meditation and relaxation. Yoga can also help you remain supple during pregnancy and get back into shape after the birth.
Quit smoking as this can affect circulation and breathing and introduces nicotine and the toxic metal cadmium into the body.

POSTNATAL DEPRESSION (PND)

A traumatic birth experience, lack of support, and stress can all lead to PND, a period of depression after giving birth. It is usually temporary and lifts with support from family, friends, and if needed, professionals.

HERBS

Antidepressant herbs and nervous system tonics can be supportive, helping increase confidence and strengthening both the mind and body.

St John's wort is an antidepressant and nerve tonic that lifts mood and restores vitality. Avoid in pregnancy and high doses in strong sunlight. When taken internally, interacts with many prescription medicines.
➡ *Take 2–5ml tincture in a little water 3 times daily.*
Damiana is a tonic and antidepressant.
➡ *Infuse 1–2 tsp dried damiana in 175ml (6fl oz) boiling water. Drink 3 times daily.*

Rosemary is stimulating and uplifting. Avoid therapeutic doses in pregnancy.
➡ *Take 1–2ml tincture in a little water 3 times daily.*

ESSENTIAL OILS

Therapeutic oils have an uplifting effect.

Neroli is an antidepressant and sedative.
Patchouli helps alleviate depression. See box, below.
➡ *Add 5 drops neroli or patchouli to 10ml jojoba oil and use in a massage, or mix 5 drops of either oil with a bath dispersant and add to a warm bath.*
Ylang ylang, a renowned antidepressant, helps to calm extreme mood swings.
➡ *Add 2–3 drops to a diffuser or add 5 drops to 10ml evening primrose oil and use in a massage.*

FOOD

A nutrient-dense, wholefood diet offers support during times of transition.

Oily fish, such as salmon and mackerel, are linked to lower rates of depression.
➡ *Eat 2–3 servings a week.*

Spinach, asparagus, and Brussels sprouts, as well as dried legumes such as chickpeas, beans, and lentils have the highest natural levels of folate, thought to help lift mood.
➡ *Eat regularly during the week.*
Yogurt with live cultures should be part of the daily diet to feed good bacteria in the gut, which helps regulate mood.
➡ *Add to cereals, dips, or meals.*
WHAT TO AVOID
Limit or cut out sweets, refined cereals, fried and fast foods, processed meats, alcohol, and sugary drinks.

SUPPLEMENTS

B vitamins, magnesium, potassium, and selenium can be low with depression. Vitamins C and D and amino acids lift mood.

B vitamins, especially B12 and folic acid, play a role in producing mood-affecting brain chemicals.
➡ *Take as part of a B complex.*
Vitamin D helps to lift mood.
➡ *Take 600–800iu vitamin D3 daily.*
Trace elements support the nerves.
➡ *Take in a daily multi-mineral.*
Vitamin C helps the body produce a mood-lifting chemical, norepinephrine.
➡ *Take 1g daily with food.*

LIFESTYLE

Spend time outside. Regular time in green environments has been shown to reduce depression. Also, sunshine helps the body make vitamin D.
Exercising 3–4 times a week can improve mood significantly.
Yoga promotes a sense of wellbeing.

OTHER THERAPIES

Psychotherapy and counselling can help when depression is hard to shift.
Massage provides relaxation as well as immune support.
Homeopathy supports emotional healing.

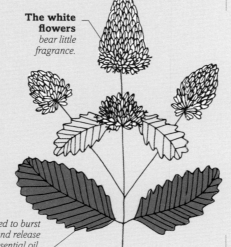

FOCUS ON
Patchouli

PROFILE
A native to India and Malaysia, patchouli's strongly scented essential oil is cultivated both for its therapeutic value and for using in perfumery.

PROPERTIES
Patchouli lifts the spirits, making an effective antidepressant. It is also antiseptic, antifungal, and toning, promoting skin-cell regeneration.

The white flowers *bear little fragrance.*

Leaves *are scalded to burst open the cell walls and release the musky essential oil.*

MENOPAUSE

Menopause is the gradual decline of oestrogen production as women age. Symptoms can include night sweats, hot flushes, insomnia, aches and pains, anxiety, and mood swings.

HERBS

Herbs can ease anxiety, liver tonics help balance hormones, and phytoestrogenic herbs help manage hormonal shifts.

Sage supports liver function. Avoid with epilepsy or a chance of pregnancy.
➡ *See remedy, right with lemon.*
Motherwort eases palpitations and anxiety. Avoid with heavy menstruation, if there is a chance of pregnancy, or with heart conditions.
➡ *Take 2–4ml tincture in a little water 3 times daily.*
St John's wort lifts depression, anxiety, and fatigue. Avoid if there is a chance of pregnancy and high doses in strong sunlight. If taken internally, interacts with many prescription medicines.
➡ *Infuse 1–2 tsp dried St John's wort in 175ml (6fl oz) boiling water and drink 3 times daily.*
Fenugreek seed is mildly oestrogenic to ease hot flushes, night sweats, mood swings, insomnia, and headache. Avoid with hypothyroidism or a chance of pregnancy. Take apart from other drugs as it may impede their absorption.
➡ *Take a daily 100mg capsule.*
WHAT TO AVOID
Warming herbs such as cinnamon, ginger, and cayenne, and also alcohol can exacerbate hot flushes.

ESSENTIAL OILS

Uplifting or calming oils in an aromatherapy massage are comforting and nurturing, helping to ease menopausal symptoms.

Rose helps to alleviate anxiety and helps regulate hormones.
Geranium can help to balance fluctuating hormones.
Clary sage helps regulate hormones.
➡ *Add 10 drops of any one of the above to 20ml (²⁄₃fl oz) base oil (jojoba for rose and geranium, almond oil for clary sage) and use in a full-body massage, or mix 5 drops with a bath dispersant and add to a warm bath.*
Cypress can be useful for hot flushes.
➡ *Add 4 drops to a bowl of cold water, soak a flannel, wring it out, and apply to the forehead or back of the neck.*

FOOD

A Mediterranean-style diet, with plenty of fresh produce and healthy fats, is the basis of good health during the menopause.

Nuts and seeds, especially flaxseeds, as well as tofu, pulses, and legumes have plant oestrogens to help regulate moods and combat vaginal dryness.
➡ *Snack on a handful each day.*
Celery, fennel, and dill have a compound anethole, which can calm hot flushes.
➡ *Drink a glass of fresh organic vegetable juice twice daily.*
Maca boosts libido, energy, and vitality.
➡ *Add 1–2 tsp powder to porridge or cereals each day.*

SUPPLEMENTS

Hormonal changes can affect how your body uses and absorbs certain nutrients. Supplements can remedy imbalances.

Omega-3 fatty acids, from fish or algal sources such as spirulina, help combat depression.
➡ *Take 1g daily.*
Vitamin E can relieve hot flushes.
➡ *Take 600–1200iu daily.*
Pine bark extract relieves hot flushes and night sweats and is energizing.
➡ *Take 120mg daily.*

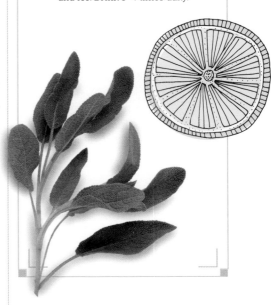

REMEDY

Liver-boosting tonic

*Infuse 1 tsp dried **sage** in 175ml (6fl oz) water, strain, cool, and add sliced **lemon** and ice. Drink 3–4 times daily.*

LIFESTYLE

Weight loss may reduce or eliminate hot flushes and night sweats.
A regular bedtime in a cool, dark room helps manage symptoms.
Yoga can reduce stress and improve sleep in menopausal women.

OTHER THERAPIES

Acupuncture can reduce hot flushes and night sweats.
Homeopathy supports the whole body during times of transition.
Hypnotherapy, psychotherapy, and counselling may be helpful.
Flower essences can encourage a positive attitude to this life transition.

MEN'S HEALTH

Men face their own particular health concerns, needing to pay attention to areas such as prostate health and testosterone levels, as well as be aware of emotional wellbeing, which can be neglected. Discover which nutrients are essential for reproductive and general health, and how herbs and essential oils provide valuable support, enhancing fertility and helping men to cope with everyday stress; and explore how diet and natural remedies can relieve problems and support healing.

STAYING WELL
MEN'S HEALTH

Optimal health for men involves a well-functioning cardiovascular system, strong bones and muscles to provide a sturdy structure, good prostate health and sexual function, and emotional wellbeing. The nutrients the body receives build the foundations for good health, and natural remedies can help to boost energy levels and manage stress, ensuring energy and vitality.

FOOD

A wholefood, largely plant-based diet with lean proteins, low in saturated fats from red meats, sugar, and alcohol promotes heart health, supports fertility, and maintains mental and physical vitality.

NUTRIENTS TO PROMOTE DIGESTION

Healthy digestion is a key component to health, helping to ensure the absorption of nutrients to fuel bodily functions, promoting heart and musculoskeletal health, and supporting fertility. Fermented foods such as live yogurt, kefir, sauerkraut, and miso contain probiotics to help populate the gut with beneficial bacteria, supporting digestion and ensuring the assimilation of nutrients.

Healthy gut bacteria is supported by prebiotics, which feed good bacteria already present in the gut and provide "resistant" starch – a type of dietary fibre that promotes regular bowel movements. Asparagus, chicory, globe and Jerusalem artichokes, radish, ginger, onions, garlic, and sweet potato are all nutrient-dense prebiotic foods that can form part of your daily diet.

NUTRIENTS FOR PROSTATE HEALTH

Looking after the health of the prostate – the walnut-sized gland in men located just below the bladder – is crucial for men's health as changes in prostate size can affect urinary and sexual function and increase the risk of cancer. Key nutrients support the prostate. For example, a carotenoid, lycopene, helps to slow the rate of prostate enlargement. Lycopene is most abundant in cooked tomatoes – heating increases its bioavailability; other sources include watermelon, pink grapefruit, guava, and papaya.

Green tea is rich in protective antioxidants and has a mild diuretic effect, which can improve urine flow and reduce inflammation in men where the prostate is enlarged. Leafy greens, such as broccoli, kale, cabbage, and sprouts, contain a compound, sulforaphane, which has cancer-fighting properties.

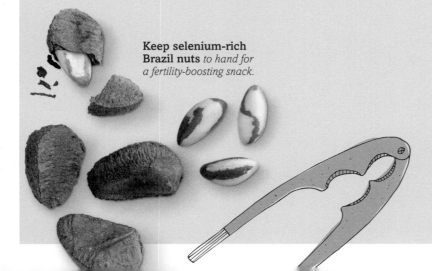

Keep selenium-rich Brazil nuts *to hand for a fertility-boosting snack.*

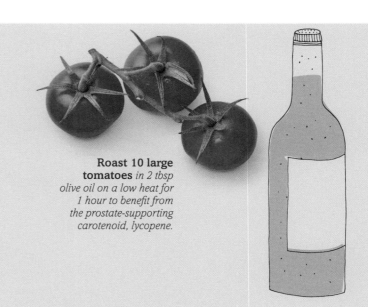

"Herbs that are restorative and energizing can be beneficial for men's health."

FERTILITY BOOSTERS

A varied, nutrient-dense diet with antioxidant-rich vegetables and fruit provides the nutritional foundation for good reproductive health. Lean proteins, including fish, eggs, and pulses such as beans and lentils are also a good source of vitamins and minerals. Some nutrients are especially supportive of men's fertility. Zinc, found in foods such as shellfish, dairy, and poultry, is thought to boost sperm count and improve motility – how well sperm move – while selenium, found in foods such as Brazil nuts, oily fish, brown rice, and eggs, promotes sperm count, shape, and motility. Iron, folate, and magnesium, found in foods such as dark green leafy vegetables, pulses, lean meat and fish, wholegrains, and nuts, are also vital for optimum reproductive health.

FOODS FOR BONE HEALTH

From the age of 30, men start to lose bone and muscle mass, so it is vital to get the right nutrients for musculoskeletal health. As well as calcium from dairy and leafy greens, nutrients such as zinc and manganese, found in macadamia nuts, are also beneficial. Sources of vitamin C, such as citrus, promote collagen formation for bone and muscle health, and healthy sources of protein, from lean meat and fish, pulses, and yogurt, support muscles with age.

HERBS

Tonic herbs and ones that support the nervous system and reproductive organs are beneficial for men's health. Restorative and energizing herbs are also beneficial.

RENEWING AND RESTORATIVE HERBS

Stress and busy lives can sap energy supplies, so herbs that stimulate and renew can be beneficial. Damiana, an uplifting herb with an antidepressant effect, also acts as an energy tonic for men, helping to renew vitality and vigour. Herbs can also have a restorative effect. Valerian is a powerful sedative herb that can aid sleep, allowing the body to rest and recuperate.

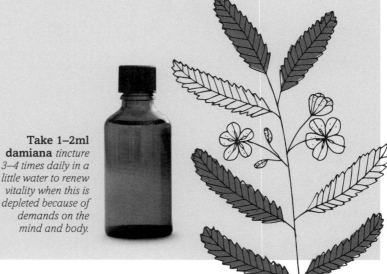

Herbs for fertility

Tonic herbs can be beneficial for male reproductive health. Saw palmetto is a strengthening tonic herb that is used to boost male reproductive health, and ashwagandha, a tonic herb that is used for overall health and vigour, is also used by Ayurvedic practitioners specifically to boost sperm count.

Polygonum (He shou wu) is a traditional Chinese herb that is thought to help boost the libido if this is waning as well as improve sperm count and poor sperm motility. Ginkgo biloba is used to stimulate peripheral circulation and has a direct effect on blood flow to the penile arteries and veins, which can help to overcome problems with erectile function.

Prostate health

An enlarged prostate is a common concern as men age. Certain herbs are used to help control the prostate and limit symptoms such as frequent urination. One of the effects of saw palmetto is that it helps to reduce elevated testosterone levels, which can contribute to an enlarged prostate, and it also has a diuretic effect to boost urine flow and ensure the removal of toxins. Nettle root also helps to regulate the prostate.

Essential oils

The inherent therapeutic benefits of oils can ease anxiety and help to avoid chronic stress impacting on health.

Calming and uplifting oils

Sandalwood's woody, spicy aroma revives and restores, relaxing jangled nerves and releasing tension and held-in emotions, while cedarwood's uplifting aroma eases tension and grounds emotions. Jasmine's warm, floral aroma is uplifting and aids awareness. Relaxing oils such as lavender promote restful, restorative sleep.

Sandalwood and cedarwood are also considered traditional aphrodisiacs with particular appeal for men, and ylang ylang's uplifting, arousing aroma helps to relax and dispel anxiety.

Oils for focus

Rosemary, black pepper, and lemon can enhance mental clarity and focus. If working life involves a lot of sedentary desk time, the mind can become distracted, so these oils can help to re-focus the mind and enhance motivation and concentration.

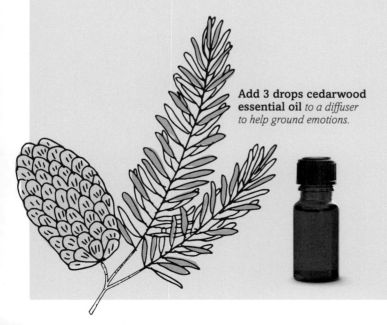

Add 3 drops cedarwood essential oil *to a diffuser to help ground emotions.*

"Therapeutic essential oils can help to avoid chronic stress impacting on health."

Oils to support the prostate

Frankincense, myrrh, and rosemary have anti-inflammatory and antiseptic properties that are thought to support prostate health.

Hair and skin benefits

Rosemary stimulates hair follicles to support healthy hair growth, while lavender soothes skin subjected to frequent shaving.

Supplements

Supplements can support a healthy diet by targeting specific areas of concern.

Circulation boosters

Cardiovascular health can come under strain from the effects of stress and lifestyle choices so targeted supplements can be helpful. L-arginine, an amino acid, acts as a precursor of nitrogen oxide, a molecule that helps maintain good circulation. Omega-3 fatty acids, derived from plant or marine sources, can also boost circulation, as well as support sperm production.

Promoting reproductive health

Supplements can maintain levels of nutrients that are key for male reproductive health. Selenium is vital for testosterone production and sperm formation; in particular, it is thought to protect against toxic heavy metals such as cadmium and lead, high levels of which can adversely affect sperm development. If the diet is low in selenium-rich foods, a supplement can be beneficial.

Zinc is needed for immunity and healthy sperm development, both prerequisites for optimum fertility. A healthy diet is the best way to get zinc, but a supplement can help if levels are low. Zinc deficiency is rare and too much can have side effects, so check levels before supplementing. Manganese boosts sperm function so a supplement is useful if levels need regulating.

Some supplements help to maintain or boost libido and sexual function. Antioxidant vitamin E supports blood vessels and muscles, including in the pelvic region, while maca powder, from a Peruvian root vegetable, boosts sexual performance in both sexes.

Supporting prostate health

Evening primrose oil, an omega-6 fatty acid, aids the production of prostaglandins, which may reduce the risk of prostate cancer.

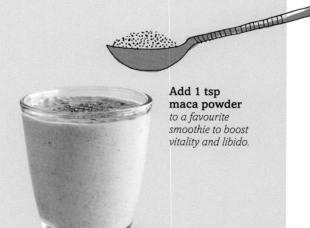

Add 1 tsp maca powder *to a favourite smoothie to boost vitality and libido.*

MEN'S HEALTH

Prostate health is a major concern for men as they age. Sexual health can also encounter problems, with factors such as stress, mental health, and certain conditions having an impact on function. Here, we explore how natural remedies can be beneficial for preventing and treating some common complaints and how lifestyle practices can support health. Pages 254–57 look at ways to support and maximize fertility in men.

BALANITIS

This skin condition results in inflammation, redness, irritation and soreness at the head of the penis, and can have a number of causes, including infection, skin irritation, and general skin conditions such as eczema and psoriasis. Treatment for the condition depends on the underlying cause.

HERBS

Herbs can help to reduce inflammation, as well as soothe and cleanse the tissues to promote healing and ease the discomfort. Applying anti-infective herbs to the skin will help to treat any infection.

Echinacea can be used internally to boost the immune response, and topically as a cleansing, healing wash. Avoid with immunosuppressants.
➡️*Make a decoction with 1–2 tsp dried echinacea root in 250ml (9fl oz) boiling water, cool, and use as a wash.*
Sarsaparilla is deeply cleansing and ideal for treating irritated and itchy skin conditions. See box, right.
➡️*Take 1–2ml tincture in a little water 3 times daily.*

Calendula is anti-inflammatory and antimicrobial to cleanse and heal.
➡️*Infuse 1–2 tsp dried calendula in 175ml (6fl oz) boiling water, cool, and apply. Or add to a base cream, 1:4 infusion to cream.*

LIFESTYLE

Hygiene is key to combating balanitis, so clean thoroughly under the foreskin.

Candida is a common cause of balanitis. If this has been diagnosed, follow the remedies for *Candida* on page 225.
Chemical irritation can cause inflammation. Avoid strong soaps, antibacterial washes, and highly perfumed bath products, and use non-biological laundry products if you think washing powders may be a cause. Some spermicides and lubricants can also cause irritation.

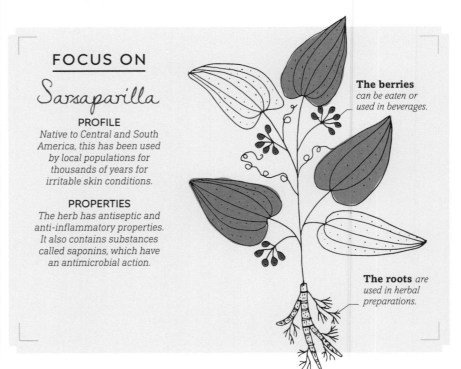

FOCUS ON
Sarsaparilla

PROFILE
Native to Central and South America, this has been used by local populations for thousands of years for irritable skin conditions.

PROPERTIES
The herb has antiseptic and anti-inflammatory properties. It also contains substances called saponins, which have an antimicrobial action.

The berries *can be eaten or used in beverages.*

The roots *are used in herbal preparations.*

"Herbs with an antispasmodic action can help to control muscles and so improve sexual function."

PREMATURE EJACULATION

Premature ejaculation is the most common sexual dysfunction in men under the age of 40. Long considered a psychological problem, research suggests that some men may have a chemical imbalance in the brain that makes ejaculation hard to control.

HERBS

Relaxing, calming herbs that support the nervous system are beneficial, as well as antispasmodic herbs to control muscles.

Schisandra acts as a strengthening tonic for hormones and calms anxiety without reducing alertness. Avoid with acute infection or if taking barbiturates.
➥ *Take 2–4ml tincture in a little water 3 times daily.*

Valerian is effective for relieving tension in the body and mind. Avoid with sleep-inducing medication.
➥ *Take 2.5–5ml tincture in a little water, 1–2 doses 2 hours apart, before sexual intercourse.*

Cramp bark is a muscle relaxant to help the body unwind and release tension.
➥ *Take 5ml tincture, 1–2 doses 2 hours apart, before sexual intercourse.*

WHAT TO AVOID
Circulatory stimulants in high doses such as ginkgo biloba, hawthorn, nettle, yarrow, prickly ash, feverfew, and rosemary.

SUPPLEMENTS

Alongside a healthy diet and exercise, supplements may help increase sexual stamina and performance.

A multi-vitamin ensures you are receiving essential nutrients.
➥ *Take a daily supplement.*
Vitamin E is an antioxidant, which helps support healthy blood vessels and muscles in the pelvic region.
➥ *Take up to 30iu daily.*
5-HTP can raise serotonin levels, which may help avoid premature ejaculation.
➥ *A daily low dose of 50mg may be sufficient.*
Folic acid is a B vitamin that can help regulate and stabilize moods, possibly helping to delay premature ejaculation.
➥ *Take 400mcg daily.*

LIFESTYLE

Stress, anxiety, and depression are linked to premature ejaculation so try to manage these conditions.
A strong pelvic floor helps to control ejaculation. Practise "Kegel" pelvic floor exercises to tone the muscles: draw up the muscles around the anus and urethra and hold for a few seconds. Repeat 3 times. Do this 10 times a day.
Condoms can decrease penis sensitivity, which may help delay ejaculation.

OTHER THERAPIES

Counselling can help deal with any emotional blocks that lead to premature ejaculation.

ERECTILE DYSFUNCTION (ED)

Sometimes referred to as impotence, erectile dysfunction describes the inability to develop or maintain an erection during sexual activity. The problem can strike at any age, although its incidence increases with advancing years. Erectile dysfunction was once thought to be purely psychological, but it is now known that physical conditions, such as atherosclerosis, diabetes, and hormone imbalances can play a part.

HERBS

Stimulating tonic herbs help raise vitality, mood, and improve overall wellbeing to enhance sexual function. Support these with strengthening heart and blood tonics to boost blood flow if circulation is sluggish.

Panax ginseng is a well-known strengthening tonic herb, which enhances vitality, stimulates the nerves, and boosts blood supply to improve function. Avoid with stimulants such as caffeine, asthma, nosebleeds, infections, or hypertension.
➥ *Take 1–2ml tincture in a little water 3 times daily.*

BITTER-SWEET
Dried schisandra berries are bitter-tasting, but can be rehydrated, strained, and sweetened with honey for a refreshing beverage.

➤ CONTINUED...

Damiana is a stimulating herb with an antidepressant action, which can help improve sexual response.
➡ *Take 1–2ml tincture in a little water 3 times daily.*

Ginkgo biloba stimulates circulation, improving blood flow to all the tissues to help re-energize. Avoid with anticoagulant medication.
➡ *Take a 66mg leaf extract tablet equal to 3300mg whole leaf, 1–3 times daily.*

WHAT TO AVOID
Hops, agnus castus, valerian, rehmannia, and skullcap can all dull your sexual responses.

ESSENTIAL OILS

Key aromatic essential oils work as natural aphrodisiacs, increasing the libido as well as improving the circulation. Oils can also help to relieve nervous anxiety and stress.

Sandalwood helps to relax nerves. It also has an antidepressant action, helping to revive spirits.

Jasmine has a warming, heady aroma that is powerfully uplifting, and is especially effective for nervous anxiety and emotional dilemmas.

Ylang ylang's exotic aroma makes this oil a well-known aphrodisiac. It also helps to reduce stress and anxiety.
➡ *Add 10 drops of any of the above essential oils to 20ml (²/₃fl oz) jojoba oil and use in a full-body massage. Or add 3 drops to a diffuser to inhale.*

SUPPLEMENTS

Try supplementing a healthy low-fat, wholefood diet with nutrients that help to maintain efficient circulation.

L-arginine, an amino acid, helps to synthesize nitrogen oxides in the body, which maintain healthy circulation. Low levels may contribute to ED.
➡ *Take up to 5g daily.*

Pine bark extract is a powerful antioxidant that has been shown to improve sexual function in men. It works well in combination with L-arginine.
➡ *Take 120mg daily.*

Maca is a Peruvian root vegetable, which is reputed to boost energy and improve sexual performance.
➡ *Take 1500mg daily as a capsule or powder; the powder can be blended into other foods if preferred.*

LIFESTYLE

Reduce stress. Taking measures to lower stress is important for dealing with ED. This is because the more stress your body experiences, the more adrenaline – the flight or fight hormone – it releases. This in turn has the effect of reducing blood flow to the extremities, including to the penis.

Stop smoking to improve your circulation. Smoking cigarettes damages blood vessels and nicotine makes them contract – both of which can restrict blood flow to the penis.

Losing weight brings several health benefits that can improve sexual response. Most notably, losing excess pounds improves heart health and circulation, which increases energy levels. It also boosts self-esteem, which can help with psychological factors.

Regular exercise such as swimming, running, and other forms of aerobic exercise that boost strength and heart health can help prevent erectile dysfunction. There is a strong link between leading a sedentary lifestyle and experiencing impotence.

OTHER THERAPIES

Psychotherapy and counselling can be beneficial if there are emotional or mental blocks to a fulfilling sexual life.

Acupuncture can be used to help improve sluggish circulation.

PROSTATE HEALTH

The prostate is a small gland in the male reproductive system. With advancing age, many men experience a decline in prostate health, which can range from an enlarged prostate to more serious conditions such as prostate cancer. Prevention, through attention to diet and lifestyle, is important to continued prostate health. Natural remedies can play an important role.

HERBS

Hormone-regulating herbs help to limit prostate enlargement, while herbs that tone tissues and reduce irritation and inflammation are soothing and reduce the frequency and urgency of urination. Antimicrobial herbs help fight infections.

Saw palmetto helps to balance hormones, controlling or inhibiting the release of ones that can lead to excessive growth of the prostate.
➡ *Take 1–2ml tincture in a little water 3 times daily.*

Nettle root relieves pain and helps limit prostate enlargement by reducing inflammatory chemicals in the body.
➡ *Take 2–5ml tincture in a little water 3 times daily.*

ANTIOXIDANT BOOST

Lightly steaming broccoli does reduce some of its vitamin content, but studies also show that it increase antioxidants such as beta-carotene and lutein.

Hydrangea is a traditional remedy for an inflamed or enlarged prostate and for painful inflammation of the urethra.
➡ *Make a decoction with 2 tsp dried hydrangea root in 250ml (9fl oz) boiling water and drink 3 times daily.*

Small-flowered willow-herb is toning, anti-inflammatory, and soothing, and is especially effective for the prostate gland.
➡ *Infuse 1–2 tsp dried small-flowered willow-herb in 175ml (6fl oz) boiling water and drink 3 times daily.*

FOOD

A wholefood and plant-based diet can help to reduce inflammation and maintain prostate health.

Tomatoes are rich in the nutrient lycopene, which has been shown to slow down prostate enlargement and prevent the condition benign prostatic hyperplasia (BPH), which leads to an enlarged prostate. Other lycopene-rich foods include watermelon, pink grapefruit, guava, and papaya.
➡ *Lycopene is released in greater quantities in cooked tomatoes so enjoy a rich tomato pasta sauce.*

Green tea has been shown to help improve urine flow and inflammation in men with enlarged prostate.
➡ *Have 2–3 cups daily.*

Broccoli, kale, cabbage, and Brussels sprouts have the compound sulforaphane, beneficial in preventing cancer, including prostate cancer.
➡ *Include in your diet daily.*

Pomegranate juice is high in protective antioxidants to support prostate health. It may also help slow the progression of prostate cancer. See box, right.
➡ *Have a 250ml (8fl oz) glass daily.*

WHAT TO AVOID
Excessive alcohol intake can damage prostate health. Sugar is linked to inflammation in the body, including the prostate. Red and very well done meat increases the risk of prostate cancer so limit your intake.

SUPPLEMENTS

Supplements can support a healthy diet to ensure you are receiving sufficient amounts of the key nutrients needed for prostate health.

Zinc inhibits the activity of an enzyme called 5-alpha-reductase, which is linked to prostate problems. Taking zinc supplements has been shown to reduce the size of the prostate and reduce symptoms of BPH.
➡ *Take 20–40mg daily.*

Amino acids, specifically a combination of L-alanine, L-glutamic acid, and L-glycine may help improve symptoms of BPH as well as urinary flow.
➡ *Take 300mg daily of each.*

Vitamin D is linked to a lower risk of prostate cancer.
➡ *Take 2000iu vitamin D3 daily.*

Evening primrose oil is an omega-6 fatty acid that helps the body produce prostaglandins, which in turn stops testosterone "binding" to the prostate and may help reduce the risk of prostate cancer.
➡ *Take 1g daily.*

LIFESTYLE

Exercise to improve fitness and lose weight to lower your risk of the prostate enlarging.

Reduce stress. This is thought to help improve symptoms such as urinary urgency, urinary frequency, and pain associated with an enlarged prostate.

Get some daily sun to improve vitamin D status, which has been shown to reduce the risk of prostate cancer.

Check your medications. Regular use of antihistamines, decongestants, and antidepressants can increase the risk of an obstructed prostate.

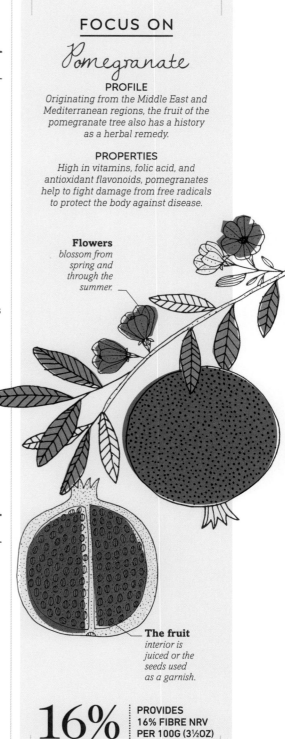

FOCUS ON
Pomegranate

PROFILE
Originating from the Middle East and Mediterranean regions, the fruit of the pomegranate tree also has a history as a herbal remedy.

PROPERTIES
High in vitamins, folic acid, and antioxidant flavonoids, pomegranates help to fight damage from free radicals to protect the body against disease.

Flowers
blossom from spring and through the summer.

The fruit
interior is juiced or the seeds used as a garnish.

16% PROVIDES 16% FIBRE NRV PER 100G (3½OZ)

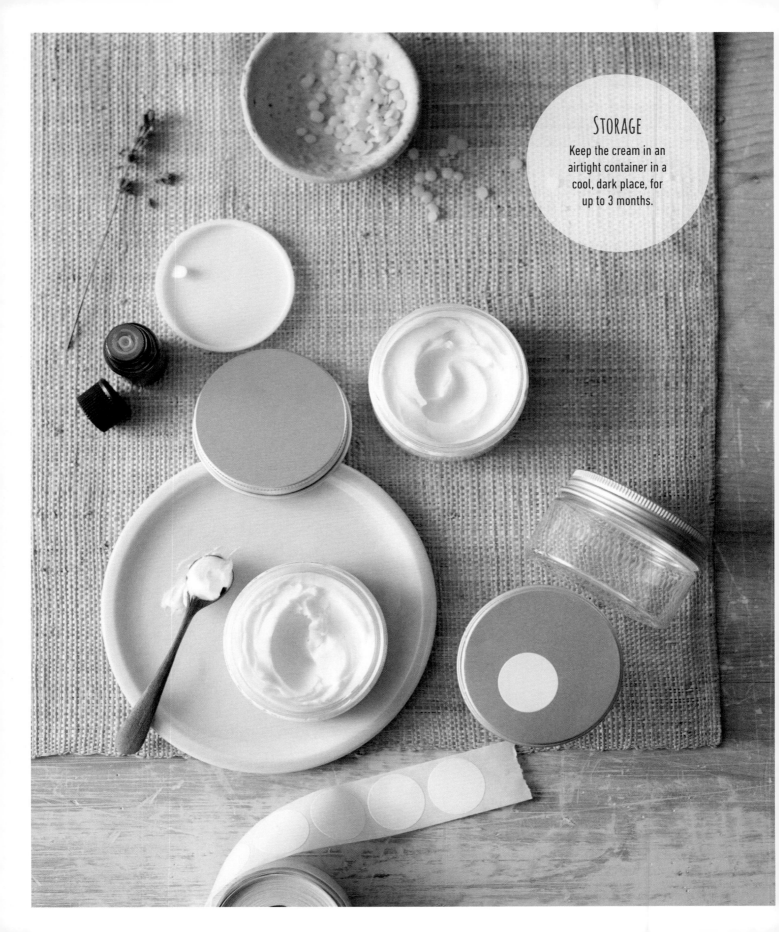

STORAGE

Keep the cream in an airtight container in a cool, dark place, for up to 3 months.

HOW TO MAKE
A CREAM

Creams use an emulsifying agent such as wax to combine oil-based and water-based ingredients – substances that don't usually mix – to make a stable product, or emulsion. Varying amounts of liquid are added to create the desired consistency. Choose oils and plant extracts that are particularly suited to your skin type, and do a patch test on a small area of skin first to check for a reaction.

Makes approx. 100g (3½oz)

YOU WILL NEED

1 tsp glycerine

4 tbsp mineral water

1 tbsp emulsifying wax

1 tbsp grapeseed oil

1 tsp beeswax (or carnauba wax if vegan)

20 drops of essential oils (a single oil or blend of oils)

1 small saucepan

1 bain marie

thermometer

small bowl

whisk, or electric hand-held mixer

lidded jars

label

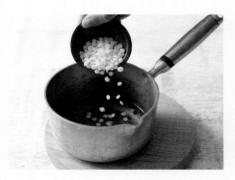

1 Sterilize the saucepan, bowl, and jars: wash thoroughly and dry in an oven at 140°C (275°F) or in a microwave for 30–45 seconds. In the saucepan, heat the glycerine and water to 70–75°C (158–167°F). Remove from the hob. Add the emulsifying wax and stir to dissolve, returning to the hob if necessary.

2 Place the oil-based ingredients – the grapeseed oil and beeswax – in a bain marie and heat to 70–75°C (158–167°F), until the ingredients are melted.

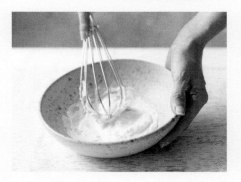

3 Combine the water and oil mixtures in a bowl, whisking to a smooth cream. Once below 40°C (104°F), add up to 20 drops of essential oils (these should make up to 5 per cent of the mixture if applying to the body, and up to 1 per cent for the face). Cool to room temperature. Pour into sterile jars and seal once fully cool. Label with ingredients and date.

CHILDREN'S HEALTH

Childhood is an exceptional time when the body undergoes a period of constant growth and areas such as the brain and immune system develop. Explore how the right nutrients now optimize growth and development, laying the foundations for health to allow children to reach their full potential, and how natural remedies can play a supportive role, helping to boost immunity. When inevitable illnesses occur, learn how diet can aid recovery and holistic remedies provide gentle healing solutions.

○ ○ ○ ○

STAYING WELL

CHILDREN'S HEALTH

During childhood, the body undergoes enormous developmental and physical changes and infections are common as the immune system matures. Getting the right nutrients in childhood has profound effects on growth and future health, and diet can be supported with natural remedies to help boost immunity and promote vitality.

FOOD

To support good health and optimum growth, your child needs a nutrient-dense wholefood diet.

PROTEIN

Protein is vital for growing children, helping to build, maintain, and repair cells and tissues in the body, while promoting strong muscles and healthy brain development. Many sources also supply micronutrients, such as iron, needed for growth and immunity. Dairy, eggs, lean meat, fish, and pulses provide healthy proteins.

FIBRE

Children need fibre to maintain a healthy gut and support regular bowel movements. Fresh fruits and vegetables make ideal fibre- and nutrient-rich snacks. Pulses such as lentils and beans, and wholegrains such as barley and brown rice also supply essential fibre – although avoid giving only wholegrain bread and pasta under the age of two as this can quickly fill up toddlers and risk them missing out on nutrients from other foods.

ESSENTIAL FATTY ACIDS

Crucial brain development occurs in childhood and the immune system also develops. Oily fish, such as salmon and mackerel, as well as providing protein, supply immune-boosting and brain-building anti-inflammatory omega-3 fatty acids. For older children, nuts and nut butters are another good omega-3 source.

BENEFITS OF DAIRY

Dairy products such as yogurt and milk provide a number of important benefits during childhood, when processes such as bone development and growth are ongoing. Bone is living tissue and childhood is an essential time for bone deposits to be made,

Lightly steam broccoli florets *and add regularly to meals or give as finger foods with a yogurt dip to provide calcium and immune-supporting vitamin C.*

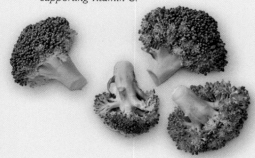

"Gentle herbal remedies can help to boost immunity during the childhood years."

ensuring healthy, strong bones by early adulthood, when bone density reaches a peak. Calcium is an essential component for healthy bone growth and for the development of teeth, and dairy is one of the main sources of calcium in childhood.

Dairy foods such as live yogurt also help to populate the gut with beneficial bacteria, which in turn play a role in developing a strong immune system. Healthy immunity may also reduce the chances of food allergies developing. Other sources of calcium include broccoli and fish such as sardines and mackerel.

STAYING HYDRATED

Often children don't recognize thirst, so encourage your child to drink healthy fluids, ideally water, to ensure adequate levels of hydration, to enhance growth and development, and support body systems. Offering water only from an early age helps your child to develop a preference for water over sugary drinks such as juice and squash, and to form a lifelong healthy habit.

PROTECTIVE FOODS

Manuka honey has strong antibacterial and anti-inflammatory properties that can help children to fight infection in the early years. Adding other antimicrobial foods such as garlic to meals gets your child used to stronger flavours.

HERBS

Herbs can be given in mild infusions, diffusers, or added to baths to support recovery and boost immunity.

CALMING ANTISEPTIC HERBS

Thyme has antiseptic properties to help fight viral infections and also helps to open airways and calm the coughing that can carry on after other cold symptoms have subsided. Wild cherry also calms irritated mucous membranes to relieve persistent coughs.

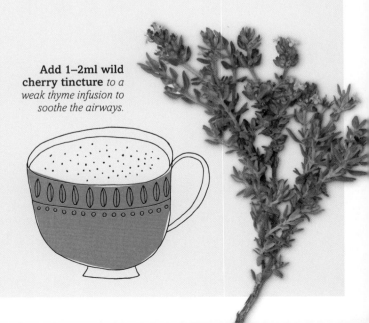

Add 1–2ml wild cherry tincture *to a weak thyme infusion to soothe the airways.*

Calming remedies

Anxiety in children, for example around changes to routines, can manifest in digestive upsets. Chamomile is a soothing herb that is well suited to children and can be used to help quell anxiety and calm digestion. Fennel is another gentle herb that can be used for babies and children to help soothe digestion.

Lemon balm has a cheerful aroma that is appealing to children, and the herb can be used to aid relaxation in both the mind and the body.

Older children may be happy to sip an infusion – perhaps sweetened with honey if this is helpful – and cooled infusions can also be added to baths for younger children and babies.

Skin soothers

Babies and young children have delicate skin that can be vulnerable to irritation and infection. Herbs that have an antimicrobial action can be useful for protecting young skin. Mullein flowers have established antibacterial properties that can help to ward off infection and are also non-irritant, so suitable for use on children's skin and scalps, for example, to prevent infection in cases of cradle cap. Mullein macerated oil can be rubbed into the scalp, or infused and used as a hair rinse.

Calendula is another gentle antimicrobial herb that is useful for soothing and controlling nappy rash. By helping to calm any redness and inflammation, calendula reduces the risk of infection and supports a healthy skin barrier.

Nit repellents

Head lice are extremely common in childhood with most children affected at some point. When head lice are circulating in a school or nursery, a rosemary infusion used in a hair rinse can be an effective preventative remedy. Strongly aromatic rosemary is thought to repel head lice and lower the risk of infestation.

Essential oils

A range of essential oils with appealing aromas can be used to promote health and wellbeing in your child.

Oils to ward off lice

Some essential oils are also useful for preventing head lice infestation. Tea tree and eucalyptus act as natural insecticides to help treat or prevent head lice infestation. In addition, neem oil

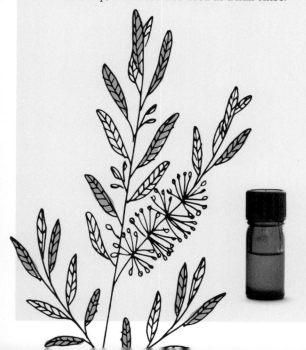

Add 3 drops tea tree essential oil *to 15ml mixed neem and sunflower oils, and massage into the scalp to ward off head lice during an outbreak.*

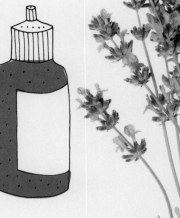
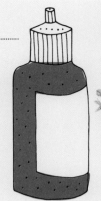

Add 8 drops lavender essential oil *to 15ml grapeseed oil, and add to a bedtime bath to promote restful sleep and support recovery after an infection.*

– a base oil used to dilute essential oils – is strongly antiseptic. Because neem is particularly potent it can be blended with other more neutral base oils such as sunflower or almond.

Skin-nourishing oils

Gentle essential oils with soothing actions can help to calm skin redness in children. Chamomile and lavender essential oils are popular with children. Chamomile has a soothing action that can calm inflammation and lavender has an anti-infective action that is useful if infection does take hold. Because of their sedative effects, both oils can also be used to promote sleep in children, giving the skin restorative time to rest and recover.

Base oils can also be useful for toning children's skin and scalp, especially where there is a tendency towards dryness. Coconut oil and olive oil can both help to maintain moisture.

Restorative oils

When a cough lingers after a viral infection, this can be tiring and prevent children from getting on with everyday activities. Frankincense essential oil can be used with children, in a diffusion or a supervised steam inhalation, to help deepen and calm breathing to restore vitality.

Supplements

A child on a healthy diet rarely needs supplements, and children should never take large doses of supplements. However, if your child is a picky eater you may worry about nutrient levels, so a supplement may be helpful.

Vital vitamins

A daily children's multi-vitamin and mineral supplement can ensure your child is getting vital nutrients if diet is a concern.

Vitamin C is important for immunity and tissue health; a child's supplement ensures an adequate intake if you think levels may be low. With indoor lifestyles, many children get insufficient vitamin D, synthesized from sunlight and vital for bone health, so vitamin D drops can top up stores, especially in winter.

Essential fatty acids

Omega-3 fatty acids promote both brain growth and emotional wellbeing, and also help to maintain a healthy skin barrier. If dietary sources are low, you may consider a supplement.

"Essential oils with appealing aromas promote wellbeing in children."

TREATMENTS
CHILDREN'S HEALTH

Babies and young children are susceptible to a range of conditions and infections as they grow and their immune systems develop. Most of these are not serious and often clear up of their own accord. Natural remedies can offer gentle treatments for children, supporting recovery and healing. As children can deteriorate rapidly, it is always important to keep a close eye and consult your doctor immediately with any concerns.

REMEDY
Tummy settler

*Add 2 drops **mandarin** essential oil to 10ml **almond oil** and gently massage into the abdomen in a clockwise direction to aid your baby's digestion.*

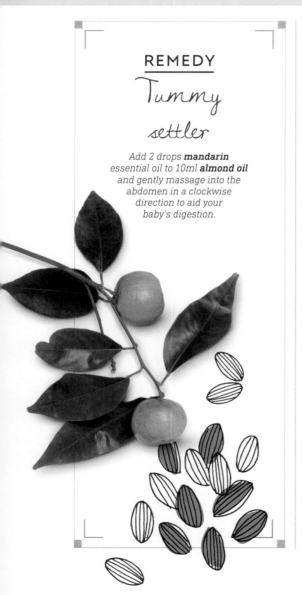

COLIC

Colic – inconsolable crying for hours – usually affects babies under three months old. The cause is unknown, but may be related to digestion.

HERBS

Carminative herbs can relax the gut wall as well as help to calm and promote rest.

Chamomile relaxes and calms digestion and eases tension and pain. Avoid with sensitivity to the *Asteraceae* family.
➡ *Make a warm poultice and place over the abdomen to relax and soothe.*
Lemon balm calms mind and body.
Fennel seed eases spasms, wind and bloating, and improves digestion.
➡ *Infuse ½ tsp dried lemon balm or fennel seed in 175ml (6fl oz) boiling water, cool, and add to a bath, or give 5ml to your baby in a dropper as needed.*

ESSENTIAL OILS

Gentle, antispasmodic oils can be helpful for soothing colic.

Roman chamomile is anti-spasmodic.
➡ *Add 2–3 drops to a diffuser to inhale.*

Mandarin is a digestive tonic.
➡ *Add 2–3 drops to a diffuser to inhale. Or see remedy with almond oil, left.*
Cardamom has antispasmodic activity.
➡ *Add 3 drops to a bowl of warm water, soak a flannel in the water, wring it out, and apply to the stomach.*

SUPPLEMENTS

Supplementing may help to improve your baby's digestion.

Probiotic drops have been shown to ease colic and other digestive problems.
➡ *Use as directed for babies.*

LIFESTYLE

Holding or rocking your baby during an episode can be calming and ease their distress, and swaddling them may be soothing.
During feeding, hold your baby upright to prevent them swallowing air.
If you're breastfeeding, avoiding tea, coffee, alcohol, and spicy foods can help.
Massaging your baby gently on the back or stomach may help.

OTHER THERAPIES

Osteopathy or chiropractic can help ease the distress of colicky babies.

NAPPY RASH

Red patches, sores, and/or blisters on your baby's bottom are a sign of nappy rash. Unless a rash is severe, most babies appear to be unbothered, but taking steps to clear up the rash can help prevent an infection setting in.

HERBS

Sore, irritated, and inflamed skin can be soothed with anti-inflammatory and emollient herbs, which can heal your baby's skin and keep it free from infection.

Calendula is anti-infective and soothes inflammation and redness to heal skin.
Chickweed is cooling and soothing, helping to calm red, irritated skin. See box, below.
➡️*Make a cream with a macerated oil or an infusion of either dried calendula or chickweed and apply to the skin.*

Witch hazel is cooling, soothing, and anti-inflammatory to promote healing.
➡️*Infuse 1 tsp dried witch hazel in 175ml (6fl oz) boiling water, cool, and use as a cleansing wash.*

LIFESTYLE

Apply a barrier cream to protect the skin from urine, its main irritant.
Get air to your baby's skin – let your baby go without a nappy when possible.
Apply breast milk. This has anti-infective substances to accelerate healing.
Avoid baby wipes. These can contain alcohol, fragrances, and preservatives, which can irritate the skin. Use plain water to clean your baby, applied with cotton wool for young babies and with a flannel for older babies.
Avoid talcum powder. Talcum powder is unnecessary and when mixed with cream can make your baby dirtier. It can become sticky and unpleasant if your baby is overheated and sweaty.
Change nappies often. Wash and pat dry thoroughly in between changes.

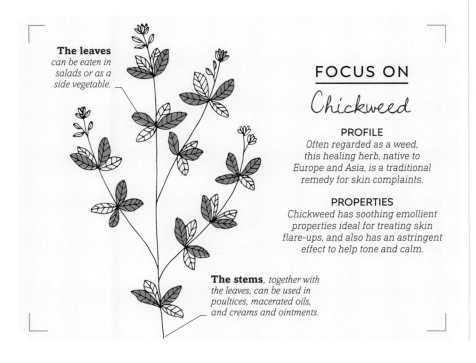

The leaves *can be eaten in salads or as a side vegetable.*

The stems, *together with the leaves, can be used in poultices, macerated oils, and creams and ointments.*

FOCUS ON

Chickweed

PROFILE
Often regarded as a weed, this healing herb, native to Europe and Asia, is a traditional remedy for skin complaints.

PROPERTIES
Chickweed has soothing emollient properties ideal for treating skin flare-ups, and also has an astringent effect to help tone and calm.

CRADLE CAP

Crusty, greasy, yellow patches on a baby's scalp are called cradle cap. Although this condition may be unsightly, it is not harmful, painful, or itchy for your baby and usually clears up of its own accord within a few months.

HERBS

Herbs that soothe inflammation and irritation can be beneficial when combined with gentle nourishing and moisturizing oils. Antibacterial herbs can also be used to help ward off any potential infection.

Mullein, a traditional remedy, is antibacterial and non-irritant.
Plantain is a soothing, toning, anti-inflammatory, and antibacterial herb.
➡️*Make a macerated oil with the leaves of either mullein flowers or plantain and apply twice daily.*
Heartsease is anti-inflammatory and cleansing, helping to cool and clear.
➡️*Infuse 1 tsp dried heartsease in 175ml (6fl oz) boiling water, cool, and use as a rinse after washing your baby's scalp.*

LIFESTYLE

Avoid harsh shampoos. Stick to those specially formulated for babies. Consider using non-foaming herbal-based shampoos that moisturize rather than strip natural oils from the scalp. After washing the hair, try massaging a couple of drops of olive or coconut oil into your baby's scalp.
Don't try to remove the flakes. Though tempting, this can break the skin or leave a sore area which is then vulnerable to infection. Instead, use a soft baby brush after washing to brush the scalp gently.

FEVER

A raised temperature is part of a healthy immune response to fight germs. In a child under five years old, a temperature above 37.5°C (99.5°F) is a fever. Most babies and young children recover after a few days, but young babies are less able to regulate their body temperature, so seek medical advice if your baby is under three months old and has a temperature above 37.5°C (99.5°F), or if your baby is three to six months old and has a temperature of 39°C (102.2°F) or more; if fever comes on rapidly; or if it is accompanied by symptoms such as lethargy.

HERBS

Herbs that promote perspiration help cool a high fever. Herbs also help to ease stress so the body can focus on fighting infection.

Limeflowers promote perspiration to control fever and calm and soothe.
➡ *Infuse ½ tsp dried limeflower in 175ml (6fl oz) boiling water and cool for your child to sip. For a baby over 3 months, add a stronger infusion to the bath or use in a compress.*

" Herbs that promote perspiration can help to cool the body and manage a fever."

Catmint induces perspiration to cool the skin and also calms and soothes.
➡ *Infuse ½ tsp dried catmint in 175ml (6fl oz) boiling water to sip during the day or use as a compress for a baby.*
Peppermint is cooling on the skin and it promotes sweating. Avoid with oesophageal reflux
➡ *Infuse 2–3 fresh leaves in 175ml (6fl oz) boiling water to sip throughout the day or use as a compress.*

ESSENTIAL OILS

These can provide a pleasant cooling sensation that can help to counter heat.

Lavender is cooling, making it beneficial for fever and the headaches associated with fever.
➡ *Add 4 drops to a bowl of cold water, soak a flannel or cloth in the water, wring it out, and apply to the forehead or the back of the neck.*

FOOD

Children with a fever may be listless, their appetites impaired, and they may be dehydrated. Offer comforting, nutrient-rich liquid foods that they can sip during the day. Continue to feed young babies breast or formula milk to hydrate them. Formula-fed babies may need additional cooled, boiled water to keep them well hydrated.

Clear broth is nourishing and hydrating as well as being an excellent source of electrolytes to help balance fluids.
➡ *Buy ready-made or make your own by stewing marrow or chicken bones and/or vegetables over a low heat for several hours. If your child has the appetite, add some chicken for protein.*
Water and other light beverages are important to keep your child hydrated.
➡ *Give plain water, or water with a squeeze of lemon, or try diluted fruit juices, coconut water, or birch water, which also provides extra sugars and*

HEALING BATHS

Herbal baths are a useful way to treat babies and infants. Add a cup of the herbal infusion to a bath to calm, soothe, and promote healing.

electrolytes. Traditional barley water is also a good hydrating drink: simmer 2 tbsp barley in 360ml (12fl oz) of water, covered, for an hour. Strain and then drink.
Honey is rich in antibacterial and antiviral compounds, which makes it especially beneficial if fever is accompanied by a sore throat.
➡ *Give your child a spoonful of Manuka honey as needed, or add 1 tsp honey to a soothing warm milk drink, weak black tea, or a herbal infusion such as chamomile or peppermint.*

LIFESTYLE

Dress your child in light layers and add or remove sheets or blankets as needed. Sponging your child with tepid water may improve his or her comfort.
"Watch and wait" is often the best approach when a child is ill. Given rest and care most fevers break on their own fairly quickly.
Consult your doctor or pharmacist about which medications can be given to help manage fever in babies and young children.

OTHER THERAPIES

Homeopathy aims to support the patient's innate ability to heal and children often respond well to individually chosen remedies.

TEETHING

A child's first teeth usually come through between the ages of three months and one year and they are often accompanied by painful, swollen gums, crying and irritability, difficulty sleeping, occasionally a slight fever, and possibly digestive distress. If your child has a high temperature or a severe digestive upset, these are more likely to be caused by a viral infection or other germ rather than be linked to teething and should be treated accordingly (see opposite).

HERBS

Herbs that help to calm your agitated baby, ease the pain of teething, and cool and soothe your baby's gums can be useful for managing teething pain and discomfort.

Catmint is a soothing and calming herb for your baby, which can help to ease pain and calm the restlessness that can accompany teething.

Chamomile is a mildly analgesic and anti-inflammatory herb, which can help to soothe the gums and also calm your baby. Avoid with sensitivity to the *Asteraceae* family.

Fennel seeds are refreshing and have anti-inflammatory properties that are soothing for teething gums.
➡ *Infuse ½ tsp of either dried catmint, chamomile, or fennel seeds in 175ml (6fl oz) boiling water, cool, and give a teaspoonful as required.*

ESSENTIAL OILS

These can be used in moderation to treat symptoms of teething. Essential oils that have an analgesic action can be used, diluted, on a baby's sore gums to bring some relief from the pain and discomfort.

Roman chamomile is a very gentle yet effective analgesic.
➡ *See remedy with coconut oil, below.*

FOOD

For a teething baby, chewing on harder foods helps to relieve the pressure of a new tooth pushing through the gums. During teething your baby's appetite may wane so choose foods that are nutrition-dense to ensure your baby is nourished. Also ensure your baby has plenty of hydrating milk and, if needed, water.

Apples, as well as being a healthy snack, also make an ideal comfort food during teething and are rich in vitamin C to support healthy gum tissues.
➡ *Give your baby cold slices of apple or even dried apples to suck and chew on while teething. You can also give cold stewed apple as a dessert or for breakfast to provide essential nutrients.*

Raw carrot sticks are the traditional hard food for teething babies to chew on. They are also rich in beta-carotene, converted to vitamin A in the body, which helps to support healthy tooth enamel in emerging teeth.
➡ *Give your baby a couple of peeled carrot sticks with a hummus dip as a healthy snack or as a finger food to go with a main meal.*

Cucumbers contain vitamin C, vitamin A, and magnesium, all of which are necessary for healthy teeth and gums. Cucumbers also have a high water content, making them super hydrating.
➡ *Cut cucumber into long sticks and serve cold from the fridge.*

Natural live yogurt contains good bacteria that can help to soothe the tummy upsets that may accompany teething. Yogurt also contains calcium to support healthy teeth.
➡ *Serve cold, straight from the fridge, to help soothe inflamed gums.*

LIFESTYLE

Many babies derive comfort from having something hard to chew on while they are teething. This can be a teething biscuit, apple, or carrot stick (see left), a baby toothbrush, or a cool teething ring.

A regular routine can ensure that your baby receives adequate rest to help him or her cope with the discomfort of teething. Even if your baby's sleep is likely to be broken, try to stick to regular bedtime and nap routines.

OTHER THERAPIES

Homeopathic remedies are a safe and gentle way to help ease the pain and distress of teething.

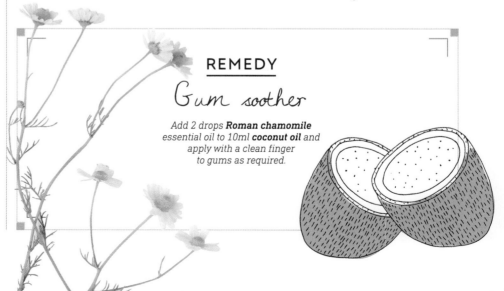

REMEDY

Gum soother

Add 2 drops **Roman chamomile** essential oil to 10ml **coconut oil** and apply with a clean finger to gums as required.

CROUP

This common childhood illness is characterized by a distinctive, bark-like cough caused by exposure to allergens or a viral infection. Although it can sound alarming, it is a fairly common condition in children and usually clears in a few days.

HERBS

Antiviral herbs can be used to fight any infection that is present. These can be supported by calming herbs, and anti-inflammatories and antispasmodics, which help to soothe and relax the larynx.

REMEDY

Throat-calming infusion

Add a few drops of **wild cherry** tincture to either dried **chamomile**, **thyme**, or **catmint** herbal infusion for your child to sip throughout the day as needed.

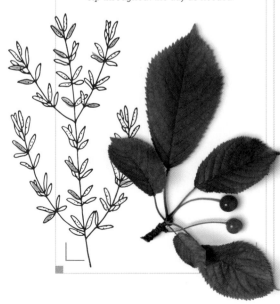

Thyme helps to calm spasms, opens the airways to ease breathing, and is also useful for fighting viral infection.
➡*Infuse ½ tsp dried thyme in 175ml (6fl oz) boiling water for your child to sip throughout the day as needed.*

Liquorice is antiviral, anti-inflammatory, and has calming properties for an irritated respiratory tract. Do not give large doses over prolonged periods.
➡*Add a pinch of the powder to herbal infusions such as chamomile, thyme, and catmint for your child to sip throughout the day as needed.*

Wild cherry relieves irritation of the mucous membranes to calm coughing and soothe. See box, opposite.
➡*This can be taken with either thyme, chamomile, or catmint; see remedy, left.*

ESSENTIAL OILS

Use antiseptic, expectorant, and calming essential oils diluted in a base oil to diffuse or to make a home-made chest rub.

Pine is antiseptic and expectorant.
➡*Add 3 drops to a diffuser for your child to inhale.*

Frankincense deepens the breathing and is a traditional remedy for treating respiratory conditions.
➡*Add 3 drops to 20ml (⅔fl oz) coconut oil and rub gently into your child's chest.*

Lavender is a deeply calming and soothing oil.
➡*Add 2–3 drops to a bowl of hot water. Ask your child to lean over the bowl, covering his or her head with a towel, and inhale the steam until it has cooled. Supervise to avoid your child getting too close and being scalded.*

FOOD

If your child is suffering with croup, he or she may not have a great appetite. Soft foods that are high in nutrients can help maintain energy and support immunity.

Dairy products such as natural yogurt or cottage cheese are easy to swallow and provide essential nutrients, protein, and energy.
➡*Top yogurt with fruit purées to add colour, flavour, and vitamins.*

Pulses are a good source of protein and when cooked are soft and easy to eat.
➡*Blitz cooked lentils or borlotti beans into a creamy, nourishing soup.*

Sweet potatoes contain beta-carotene, a vitamin A precursor, which can help support healthy lung function.
➡*Bake with their skins on and serve with a drizzle of honey.*

Water is essential to hydrate your child and help to lessen symptoms.
➡*Ensure your child sips water frequently. Or give diluted fruit juice, whose natural sugars help maintain energy levels, or fruity herbal teas.*

Clear broths provide nutrients, help hydrate your child, and are easy to eat.
➡*Buy ready-made or make your own by stewing marrow or chicken bones and/or vegetables over a low heat for several hours.*

LIFESTYLE

Keep your child calm. Anxiety and stress make croup worse so hold and comfort your child during an attack.

Investigate allergens in the home – dust, dander, mould, and synthetic fragrances are common triggers.

WATER FIRST

Your child may not always recognize thirst so keep a cup of water close by and encourage him or her to have some sips before a snack.

ROSEOLA

Roseola is a viral infection and is most common between six months and two years of age. It is caused by either the human herpes virus 6 or 7. In its early phase it mimics the symptoms of a cold, beginning with a sudden high temperature. As the fever subsides, a red rash appears on the chest and back and can spread to other areas. Your child may also have swollen lymph nodes around the neck, a sore throat, and a loss of appetite.

HERBS

Herbal remedies can help to make your child more comfortable. Choose herbs that promote gentle perspiration to help manage any fever, as well as calming herbs to ease feelings of anxiety, and antiviral herbs, which can be used to help contain the infection.

" Soothing, antimicrobial essential oils help to soothe skin rashes to promote healing and recovery. "

Catmint is calming and cooling, and its volatile oils help to fight the infection.
➡ *Infuse ½ tsp dried catmint in 175ml (6fl oz) boiling water for your child to sip throughout the day as needed.*

Elderflower gently promotes sweating, and is also soothing as well as having anti-infective properties.
➡ *Infuse 1–2 tsp dried elderflower in 175ml (6fl oz) boiling water, cool, and add to a warm bath.*

Chamomile is relaxing and can be used to soothe your child and help promote restful sleep. Avoid with sensitivity to the *Asteraceae* family.
➡ *Infuse ½ tsp dried chamomile in 175ml (6fl oz) boiling water for your child to sip before bedtime.*

ESSENTIAL OILS

Oils that are soothing and antimicrobial help to clear stuffy noses and soothe a rash, promoting the process of healing and recovery.

Roman chamomile is an extremely soothing essential oil.
➡ *Add 2 drops to 10ml base lotion and apply to areas of skin that have an irritable rash.*

Lavender is a deeply calming and healing oil.
➡ *Add 2 drops to 5–10ml bath dispersant and add to a warm bath.*

LIFESTYLE

Make sure that your child gets plenty of quiet rest in bed until the fever has abated to conserve energy and help speed recovery.

Ensure that your child drinks plenty of healthy fluids. Encourage your child to drink clear fluids – water is best, and cooled herbal teas can also be beneficial, or give an electrolyte rehydration solution to help prevent dehydration and promote recovery.

If your child has a fever, dress him or her in light layers and add or remove sheets or blankets as needed. Wearing light layers means that the body can cool down. If your child finds it comfortable and soothing, you can try sponging him or her with a tepid cloth.

Consult your doctor or pharmacist about which medications can be given to help manage fever in babies and young children.

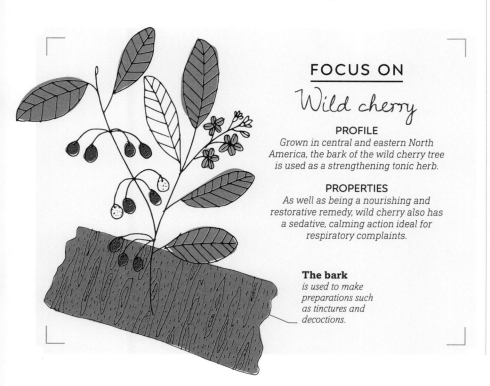

FOCUS ON

Wild cherry

PROFILE
Grown in central and eastern North America, the bark of the wild cherry tree is used as a strengthening tonic herb.

PROPERTIES
As well as being a nourishing and restorative remedy, wild cherry also has a sedative, calming action ideal for respiratory complaints.

The bark *is used to make preparations such as tinctures and decoctions.*

5

RECIPES FOR WELLNESS

ENERGY BITES

These moreish bites are nutrient-dense to help sustain energy as well as provide protective antioxidants. Blitz the dry ingredients, transfer to a bowl, then add the wet ingredients and combine. Roll into 3–4cm (1½–1¾ in) balls, cover in any topping, place on greaseproof paper, and chill in the fridge for an hour. Store in an airtight container in the fridge for up to 3 days.

1

COCONUT AND LIME BITES

With protein-filled nuts and carbohydrates from the dates, these light bites fuel the body. Dates are also high in fibre to aid digestion, while tangy lime provides vitamin C to support collagen synthesis for healthy skin and hair.

MAKES 8 BALLS • **PREP TIME** 15 MINS, PLUS CHILLING

Dry ingredients
45g (1½oz) almonds
45g (1½oz) cashew nuts
110g (3½oz) pitted dates
10g (¼oz) desiccated coconut

Wet ingredients
2 tbsp lime juice

For the topping
10g (¼oz) desiccated coconut

Nutritional info per serving:
Kcals 104 Fat 7.5g Saturated fat 2g Carbohydrates 6g Sugar 5g Sodium 3mg Fibre 1g Protein 3g Cholesterol 0mg

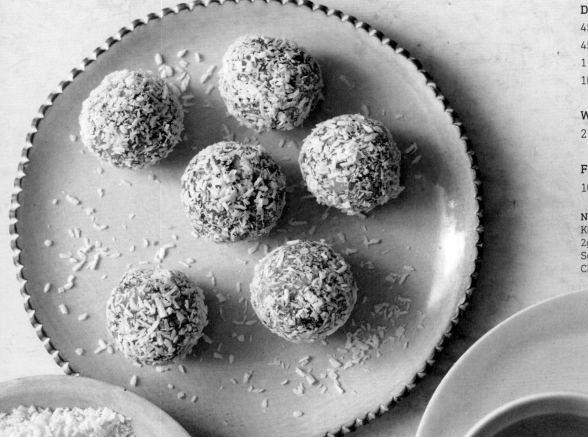

2

Nutty banana bites

Packed with essential nutrients, bananas are especially high in the electrolyte potassium, which helps to balance fluid levels and keep blood pressure in check.

MAKES 8 BALLS • **PREP TIME** 15 MINS, PLUS CHILLING

Dry ingredients

75g (2½oz) dried banana, chopped

60g (2oz) mixed nuts

1 tsp hemp powder

½ tsp chia seeds

Wet ingredients

2 tbsp smooth peanut butter

Nutritional info per serving:
Kcals 98 Fat 6g Saturated fat 1g
Carbohydrates 8g Sugar 6.5g
Sodium 33mg Fibre 0.5g
Protein 3.5g Cholesterol 0mg

3

Chocolate and goji berry bites

These high-protein snacks help to balance blood sugar levels. Also, goji berries, high in vitamin C and flavonoids, contain water-attracting polysaccharide sugars, which nourish and moisturize skin from the inside.

MAKES 8–10 BALLS • **PREP TIME** 15 MINS, PLUS CHILLING

Dry ingredients

100g (3½oz) mixed nuts

140g (5oz) pitted dates

1 tbsp cacao powder

1 tbsp goji berries

Wet ingredients

2 tbsp coconut oil

2 tbsp smooth peanut butter

For the topping

100g (3½oz) dark chocolate, at least 70 per cent cocoa content, melted

10g (¼oz) desiccated coconut

Nutritional info per serving:
Kcals 103 Fat 7g Saturated fat 3g
Carbohydrates 7.5g Sugar 6.5g
Sodium 12mg Fibre 0.8g
Protein 3g Cholesterol 0.3mg

4

Oatmeal and raisin bites

Oats are an excellent source of the soluble fibre beta-glucan. This binds to bad LDL cholesterol in the gut and prevents it from being absorbed into the bloodstream. Raisins add iron, B vitamins, and potassium to these energy-dense treats.

MAKES 8 BALLS • **PREP TIME** 15 MINS, PLUS CHILLING

Dry ingredients

45g (1½oz) oats

20g (¾oz) flaxseeds

85g (3oz) raisins

½ tsp cinnamon

Wet ingredients

60g (2oz) almond butter

1 tsp maple syrup

1 tsp vanilla extract

Nutritional info per serving:
Kcals 115 Fat 6g Saturated fat 0.5g Carbohydrates 11.5g
Sugar 8g Sodium 6mg Fibre 2g
Protein 3g Cholesterol 0mg

5

Raw fudge bites

Protein-rich nuts not only help to satisfy hunger pangs, but also contain omega-3 fatty acids and vitamin E to support skin and blood vessel health.

MAKES 8–10 BALLS • **PREP TIME** 15 MINS, PLUS CHILLING

Dry ingredients

100g (3½oz) mixed nuts

50g (1¾oz) desiccated coconut

Wet ingredients

100g (3½oz) smooth peanut butter

1 tbsp coconut oil

1 tbsp runny honey

½ tsp vanilla essence

For the topping

10g (¼oz) desiccated coconut

Nutritional info per serving:
Kcals 222 Fat 18.5g Saturated fat 8g Carbohydrates 5g Sugar 4g
Sodium 47mg Fibre 2g
Protein 7g Cholesterol 0mg

ADENOIDS AND TONSILS

The adenoids and tonsils work together as part of the lymphatic system, to help children build up immunity and fight infection. They are located at the back of the throat, and can become infected with bacteria or viruses, making breathing and swallowing difficult. There is also a link between large tonsils and adenoids and middle ear infection (see p83).

HERBS

Herbs that cleanse and support lymphatic tissues can be helpful for infections. Combine these with antimicrobial, soothing, and toning herbs, as well as herbs that help to boost immunity and manage fevers.

Cleavers is cleansing and stimulating, helping to support the lymph system and restore healthy tissue.
➡ *Infuse ½ tsp dried cleavers in 175ml (6fl oz) boiling water for your child to sip during the day as needed.*
Calendula is toning, with antimicrobial action. It helps to soothe inflammation.
➡ *Infuse ½ tsp dried calendula in 175ml (6fl oz) boiling water, cool, and give to your child to gargle and swallow.*
Wild indigo supports the immune system and helps to clear infection in the lymph tissues. Not suitable for children under 12 years old; do not take for a prolonged period.
➡ *Add 1ml tincture to infusions, or dilute in water and take 3–4 times a day.*

FOOD

With inflammation in the adenoids or tonsils, focus on high-nutrition, low-acid, soft foods that are easy to swallow.

Manuka honey

PROFILE
This healing honey is produced in New Zealand by bees that pollinate the native Manuka bush and has been used in remedies for thousands of years.

PROPERTIES
Manuka has a soothing effect, and has antiviral and antibacterial properties to help boost immunity.

The white or pink flowers *bloom for around six weeks in January, producing nectar for bees to gather.*

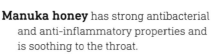

Manuka honey has strong antibacterial and anti-inflammatory properties and is soothing to the throat.
➡ *Give your child 1 tsp of Manuka honey as needed to soothe a sore throat and ease nasal congestion.*
Cruciferous vegetables such as broccoli, cabbage, and cauliflower have antimicrobial sulphur compounds.
➡ *Steam lightly to preserve flavour, or give your child a daily shot of broccoli sprout juice – one of the richest sources of sulphur compounds.*
Oily fish, such as salmon, mackerel, and sardines, are easy to swallow and provide anti-inflammatory fish oils.
➡ *Lightly steam or grill.*

LIFESTYLE

Gargling with warm salt water, for children aged 8 and over, can help reduce the swelling and pain of inflamed adenoids and tonsils.
Apply a cold pack or wrap some ice cubes in a towel and use as a cold compress on the throat. Or give your child an ice cube or ice lolly to suck.

Steam inhalations can be used to help relieve congestion in the chest and nasal passages. Always supervise young children during an inhalation to ensure that they don't get too close to the hot water and are scalded by the steam or the water. Similarly, a humidifier can be used to help to moisten the air in a room and soothe a sore throat.

OTHER THERAPIES

Homeopathy helps to support the whole body during times of illness.

" Herbs can cleanse and support the lymphatic tissues to help fight infection. "

IMPETIGO

This highly contagious, painful skin infection causes sores and blisters, usually on the mouth and face, and mainly affects children, although it can also affect adults. It is caused by one of two types of bacteria: *Streptococcus* or *Staphylococcus*, both of which are rapidly becoming resistant to antibiotics. If persistent, consult your doctor.

HERBS

Strong antibacterial herbs are needed to fight this infection. Herbs that help to boost your child's immunity are also important.

Calendula is antimicrobial and promotes rapid healing of skin lesions.
➥ *Apply the diluted tincture to the lesion or infuse ½ tsp dried calendula in 175ml (6fl oz) boiling water, cool, and give to your child to drink 3–4 times a day.*

Golden seal is an effective antimicrobial and anti-inflammatory herb to help combat infection and aid healing. Do not take internally over a long period.
➥ *Apply the diluted tincture to the affected area several times a day.*

Echinacea is effective when used topically to fight *Staphylococcus* infections, and, when taken internally, can also help to boost your child's natural immunity. Avoid with immunosuppressant medication.
➥ *Apply the diluted tincture to the affected area several times a day, or take internally, with your healthcare practitioner's advice.*

ESSENTIAL OILS

These have many skin-supporting properties. As well as being antimicrobial, oils can relieve the pain and itching of impetigo to promote rapid skin healing.

> *"Essential oils can help to remove the pain and itching of impetigo."*

Tea tree is a strong antiseptic and remedy of choice for many skin conditions.
➥ *Add 4 drops to 20ml (⅔fl oz) olive oil and apply to the affected area.*

Lavender is extremely soothing as well as pain-relieving.
➥ *Add 2 drops to 10ml unfragranced base lotion and apply to the affected area of skin.*

Patchouli is a deeply healing and soothing essential oil.
➥ *See remedy with jojoba oil, below.*

SUPPLEMENTS

For the best defence against infection, your child should eat a balanced, nutrient-dense diet with fresh fruits and vegetables and sources of protein. Supplements can help to support the diet during an infection.

Omega-3 fatty acids may help maintain the integrity of the skin and are also anti-inflammatory to support healing.
➥ *Give your child 250–500mg daily in liquid form.*

Probiotic supplements help to boost good bacteria in the gut. If your child is taking a course of antibiotics, probiotics are crucial to help restore balance in intestinal flora.
➥ *Give your child a daily supplement with up to 10 billion live organisms per dose.*

Zinc is necessary for the proper functioning of the immune system, enabling it to fight off infection.
➥ *Give your child 2–4mg daily.*

LIFESTYLE

Use a cotton pad, mild soap, and warm water to wash skin several times a day. Pat dry with a paper towel.

Keep the towels and clothes of the infected person separate from the rest of the family and wash daily.

Wear gloves when applying antibiotic ointment to your child's sores and wash your hands thoroughly afterwards.

Keep your child at home until the doctor is happy that he or she is no longer contagious.

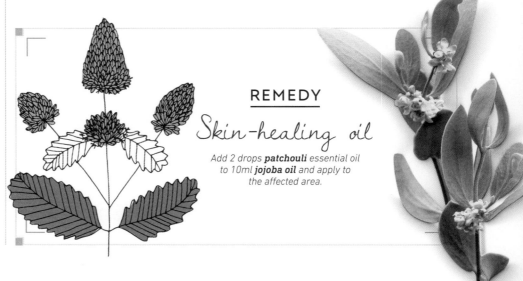

REMEDY

Skin-healing oil

Add 2 drops **patchouli** essential oil to 10ml **jojoba oil** and apply to the affected area.

HEAD LICE

Head lice (*Pediculus humanus capitis*) are human parasites, which live exclusively on the scalp, usually in young children. They feed on human blood and while the bites are not painful, they can be very itchy and cause allergic reactions. In severe cases, scratching and broken skin can lead to infections. Head lice are hard to remove, requiring time and patience. Also extra attention needs to be paid to hygiene while you deal with the infestation.

HERBS

Aromatic herbs can help repel head lice and prevent infection. Some herbs have antiparasitic properties, so can be used to help expel stubborn lice from the scalp.

Mugwort is antiparasitic and aromatic to deter head lice.
➡ *Infuse 2 tsp dried mugwort in 175ml (6fl oz) boiling water, cool, and use as a final hair rinse.*

Quassia chips have shown effectiveness in treating outbreaks of head lice.
➡ *Add a handful of chips to 1 litre (1¾ pints) boiling water and steep overnight, then strain the liquid. Apply to your child's scalp as a final rinse after washing and leave to dry, or spray into the hair after daily combing.*

Rosemary is strongly aromatic and anti-infective, helping to prevent head lice infestation.
➡ *Infuse 2 tsp dried rosemary in 175ml (6fl oz) boiling water and use as a final hair rinse.*

ESSENTIAL OILS

Using essential oils to treat head lice offers a natural alternative to chemical treatments. The nits lose traction in the oil and can be combed out with a fine-toothed nit comb. Some oils are also insecticides.

Tea tree is an extremely effective insecticide.
➡ *Add 5 drops to 10ml neem oil and massage into the hair and scalp, then wet comb the hair using a fine-toothed comb to try to remove nits.*

DELICATE SKIN

Essential oils are concentrated so if your child is under the age of four you may prefer to use a normal conditioner to help loosen and remove nits.

Eucalyptus has antiseptic properties that can help to soothe bites and also helps to tone and cleanse the skin.
➡ *Add 5 drops to 10ml conditioner and massage into the hair and scalp, then wet comb hair with a fine-toothed comb to try to remove the nits. Or make a tea tree, eucalyptus, and lime spritz with a bottle and spray atomizer (see remedy, below).*

LIFESTYLE

Use a fine-toothed nit comb to remove head lice. It may require several comb throughs to remove all of the nits and you may have to repeat this process every day, or every other day, over a period of several days to ensure that all the eggs are removed, so be patient.

Thoroughly check all family members at the same time as treating your child and treat any family member who is infected with headlice.

Vacuum all surfaces where children lie or play daily and wash stuffed toys during an infestation of head lice. Empty the bag or cylinder immediately.

Keep clothes, bedding, and towels of infected children and family members separate from other members of the family. Wash these items daily on the hottest possible setting and dry thoroughly, ideally in a tumble dryer.

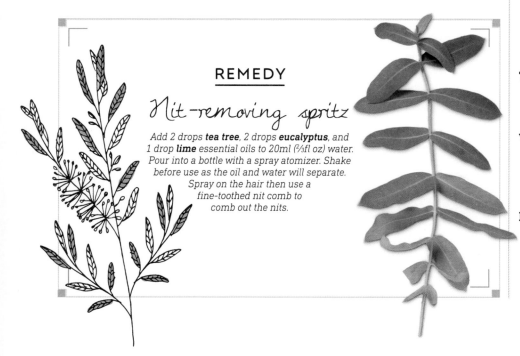

REMEDY

Nit-removing spritz

Add 2 drops **tea tree**, 2 drops **eucalyptus**, and 1 drop **lime** essential oils to 20ml (⅔fl oz) water. Pour into a bottle with a spray atomizer. Shake before use as the oil and water will separate. Spray on the hair then use a fine-toothed nit comb to comb out the nits.

BEDWETTING

Also known as nocturnal enuresis, bedwetting is common in children up to the age of six. Most children grow out of this over time as the bladder develops to a normal size and they become better at recognizing body signals. If your child starts wetting the bed again after a period of being dry you could ask your doctor for advice. Occasionally constipation or social problems such as bullying can be a factor in bedwetting, so these may need investigating.

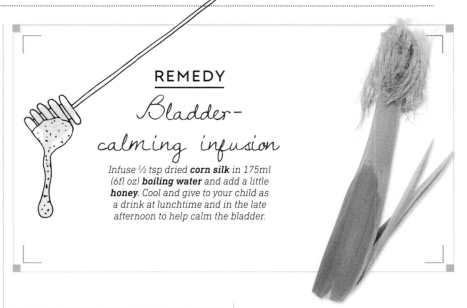

REMEDY

Bladder-calming infusion

Infuse ½ tsp dried **corn silk** in 175ml (6fl oz) **boiling water** and add a little **honey**. Cool and give to your child as a drink at lunchtime and in the late afternoon to help calm the bladder.

HERBS

Soothing and toning herbs and those that act as strengthening nerve tonics will help to calm and control an agitated bladder. These herbs can be combined with relaxing herbs that will help to ease the feelings of anxiety and stress that can accompany bedwetting.

Corn silk is a soothing and calming herb for the bladder, helping to reduce the risk of uncontrolled urination during the night-time.
➡️ *See remedy with honey, above.*
St John's wort eases anxiety around the issue of bedwetting and is also a soothing tonic for nerve tissue in the bladder. Avoid in strong sunlight. Taken internally, interacts with many prescription medicines.
➡️ *Make a macerated oil, adding a few drops of lavender essential oil, and use to massage your child's abdomen and spine before bed.*
Agrimony is toning and helps to calm anxious states. Avoid taking if suffering with constipation.
➡️ *Infuse ½ tsp dried agrimony in 175ml (6fl oz) boiling water and add a little honey. Give to your child to drink at lunchtime and in the late afternoon.*

FOOD

A wholefood diet will improve your child's health and wellbeing and ensure the proper growth and development of organs such as the bladder.

Fibre-rich foods, such as fresh fruits and vegetables, support regular bowel movements, which are especially important if constipation is a factor in bedwetting.
➡️ *Give your child 4–5 portions a day.*
Almonds are rich in magnesium, low levels of which have been associated with bedwetting.
➡️ *Try substituting almond milk for regular milk or alternate the two to ensure your child still gets enough calcium in his or her diet.*
Spinach is also a good source of magnesium.
➡️ *Try lightly sautéing with some garlic as an appealing side dish for your child.*

LIFESTYLE

Stress and changes such as family breakups, a new school, or a new baby can trigger bedwetting. Try to get to the root of the problem.

Constipation can restrict your child's bladder capacity, so ensure your child's diet is varied and that he or she is sufficiently hydrated throughout the day.
Get into a nightly regimen. Encourage your child to urinate at the start of the bedtime routine and again just before going to sleep.

OTHER THERAPIES

Homeopathy may help with the physical and emotional aspects of bedwetting.
Osteopathy and chiropractic can sometimes be beneficial.

" *A healthy, wholefood diet will ensure the proper growth and development of the bladder.* "

FIRST AID

Effective and timely first aid for minor complaints can minimize damage and accelerate healing. The inherent healing and protective properties in many plants make them a natural choice for first aid situations and nature provides a range of simple, often highly effective, remedies that work alongside the body's own immune response and traditional treatments to enhance healing. Discover the top herbs and plants for providing on-the-spot treatments and create an all-natural first aid kit.

TREATMENTS

FIRST AID

The body's immune responses and processes make it well-equipped to deal with many first-aid situations. While major injuries usually require professional treatment, natural remedies can also provide effective support, whether to help reduce swelling, stem bleeding, or generally revive. Build up your own holistic first-aid kit, with remedies, such as macerates, prepared in advance to have to hand when accidents occur.

BRUISES

The skin discolouration of a bruise is caused by blood seeping out from damaged vessels under an injury. As they heal, bruises turn from purple to pink, blue, or green—yellow, due to the breakdown of haemoglobin as it is reabsorbed into surrounding tissues.

HERBS

Herbs that help heal capillaries to limit internal bleeding are supported by herbs to reduce inflammation to speed healing.

Sage is toning, promoting rapid healing. Avoid therapeutic doses internally in pregnancy or with epilepsy and avoid taking for prolonged periods of time.
➡*Infuse 2 tsp dried sage in 175ml (6fl oz) boiling water, chill and apply as a compress.*

Daisy, or bruisewort, is a well-known remedy for bruises. It is anti-inflammatory and also helps to reduce the pain that can accompany bruises from the damaged tissues.
➡*Infuse the fresh flowers in 175ml (6fl oz) boiling water, cool, and apply to unbroken skin as a cold compress.*

Yarrow tones tissues, helps to stem the blood flow internally, and also has anti-inflammatory properties. Avoid internally during pregnancy or with sensitivity to the *Asteraceae* plant family. Prolonged use can increase skin sensitivity.
➡*Dilute 2–3ml tincture in a cup of cold water and apply to the affected area as a compress.*

ESSENTIAL OILS

Analgesic and anti-inflammatory essential oils can help to relieve the pain and swelling that can be caused when tissues under the skin are damaged.

Rosemary has pain-relieving properties that can help to manage the discomfort of bruises. Avoid with epilepsy.
➡*Add 4 drops to a bowl of ice-cold water, soak a flannel or cloth in the water, wring this out, and apply to the affected area.*

Lavender works as an analgesic oil to provide effective pain relief.

Helichrysum has anti-inflammatory properties that can help to accelerate tissue healing.

Black pepper has anti-inflammatory properties that make it a recommended treatment for bruises.
➡*Add 10 drops of either lavender, helichrysum, or black pepper essential oil to 20ml (⅔fl oz) arnica macerated oil and gently apply to the area. Or add 4 drops of either lavender, helichrysum, or black pepper essential oil to a bowl of ice-cold water, soak a flannel or cloth in the water, wring this out, and apply to the affected area.*

OTHER THERAPIES

Flower remedies, such as Five Flower or Rescue Remedy, can support treatment of symptoms of shock that may accompany significant bruising.

Homeopathy offers several remedies to help accelerate the healing of bruises.

" Herbs can support the healing of broken capillaries to limit bleeding and also help reduce inflammation."

CUTS

Cuts, grazes, and lacerations are common, usually minor, complaints. Our bodies are well-equipped to heal minor cuts themselves, but natural remedies can give a helping hand.

HERBS

Certain herbs have constituents that can speed up cell regeneration and wound-healing processes to help repair cuts rapidly. Combine these with antibacterial, antifungal, and anti-inflammatory herbs.

Yarrow is "styptic", meaning it can stem bleeding, and antibacterial to help keep cuts free from infection. Avoid internally in pregnancy or with sensitivity to the *Asteraceae* family. Prolonged use can increase skin sensitivity.
➡*Add a few drops of tincture to warm water to wash the wound.*

Self-heal is soothing and toning to tighten and heal cuts, stem bleeding, and prevent infection.
➡*Infuse the freshly crushed herbs in 175ml (6fl oz) boiling water, cool, and use to wash the cut.*

Calendula is antibacterial and speeds up the wound-healing process to prevent or limit scarring.
➡*Make a macerated oil with the fresh or dried flowers to use for a healing salve on cuts and wounds.*

ESSENTIAL OILS

Certain essential oils have wound healing and antiseptic properties; they are also able to promote the formation of scar tissue, making them ideal for first aid.

Myrrh has healing properties that are beneficial for slow-healing wounds.
➡*Add 5 drops to 10ml base oil and apply to the affected area.*

Helichrysum speeds up the wound-healing process.
➡*Add 4 drops to a bowl of cold water, soak a flannel or cloth in the water, wring this out, and apply to the area. Or add 2–3 drops to 10ml aloe vera gel and apply to the skin.*

Tea tree helps to promote the formation of scar tissue.
➡*Add 4 drops to a bowl of cold water, soak a flannel or cloth in the water, wring this out, and apply to the wound.*

LIFESTYLE

Clean the cut and apply pressure. It is important to remove grime from a cut by rinsing under water or wiping with wet cotton wool, from the centre outwards. Apply firm, even pressure to stem the bleeding. Don't keep checking to see if the blood has stopped as this can disturb the clotting process.

Use a hydrocolloidal bandage, available at most chemists, which helps keep the skin moist to promote faster healing and reduce pain.

OTHER THERAPIES

Homeopathic remedies can help speed the healing of cuts and wounds.

BURNS AND SCALDS

Minor burns and scalds and, without protection, sunburn are all common. While severe burns need immediate medical treatment, minor burns can be treated safely and effectively at home with natural remedies.

HERBS

Anti-inflammatory, cooling, and pain-relieving herbs can be applied directly to minor burns and scalds, including sunburn. They can reduce the redness and also help to soothe and heal the damaged tissues.

St John's wort reduces redness and inflammation to promote rapid healing and reduce pain. Avoid internally in pregnancy and high doses in strong sunlight. Taken internally, it interacts with many prescription medicines.
➡*Make a macerated oil with the fresh flowers to apply directly to burns.*

Calendula is anti-inflammatory and anti-infective to help heal skin. It works well with St John's wort.
➡*See remedy, below.*

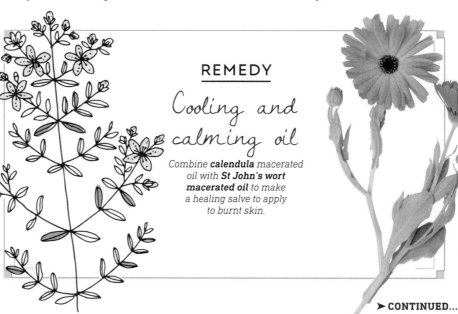

REMEDY

Cooling and calming oil

Combine **calendula** macerated oil with **St John's wort** macerated oil to make a healing salve to apply to burnt skin.

➤ CONTINUED…

Aloe vera gel is antiseptic, cooling, and anti-inflammatory to protect, soothe, and heal. Avoid taking internally during pregnancy.
➸*Cut the leaf and apply the fresh gel inside the leaf directly to unbroken skin.*

ESSENTIAL OILS

Look for essential oils that have pain-relieving properties and which promote healing of the skin.

Roman chamomile is analgesic and anti-inflammatory, speeding up the healing of the damaged skin. German chamomile helps to reduce redness.
➸*Add 4 drops to a bowl of cold water, soak a flannel or cloth in the water, wring this out, and apply to the area.*
Lavender is cooling, analgesic, and also promotes rapid healing, which in turn helps to reduce scarring.
Frankincense encourages the growth of new cells.
➸*Add 4 drops of either lavender or frankincense essential oils to a bowl of cold water, soak a flannel or cloth in the water, wring this out, and apply to the affected area. Or add 2–3 drops essential oil to 10ml aloe vera gel and apply to the burn.*

LIFESTYLE

Immerse burns in cold running water for at least 5 minutes, then keep skin cool for up to 3 hours with an ice pack or a cotton cloth soaked in cold water.
Take preventative steps to avoid sunburn. Apply a high-quality, at least factor 30, sunscreen with minerals such as zinc oxide, and cover exposed areas.

OTHER THERAPIES

Homeopathy offers support for the shock that can accompany burns, and also provides treatment for the physical damage of burns and scalds.

INSECT BITES AND STINGS

Most insect bites are simply annoying, causing some itching and red welts on the skin that disappear after a few days. For some, however, a single bite can produce an allergic-like reaction, or the area can take longer to heal than normal. Natural remedies can help support the healing process.

HERBS

Anti-inflammatory and cooling herbs can be used to soothe the affected area and help to relieve the itching and pain that accompany bites and stings.

Plantain is a soothing anti-inflammatory herb that has both toning and antibacterial properties.
➸*Crush or chew the fresh leaves and rub onto the bite, leaving the leaves in place as a poultice.*
Witch hazel has a toning and cooling effect on the skin and helps to reduce discomfort and itchiness.
➸*Soak a cotton wool pad in witch hazel water and use as a compress.*
Onion is anti-inflammatory and antibacterial to help cleanse and soothe insect stings.
➸*Slice a raw onion and rub this onto the sting.*

ESSENTIAL OILS

Essential oils not only have effective insect-repellent properties, they can also help to relieve the pain and itching caused by bites and stings.

Peppermint can relieve skin irritation and itching.
➸*Mix 2 drops with 10ml coconut oil and apply to the affected area.*

HIDDEN EXTRAS
Some lavender essential oils on the market have synthetic compounds added. Look for the botanical name *Lavandula angustifolia* to indicate a pure, authentic oil.

Lavender can help to prevent itching and scratching.
➸*Mix 2 drops with 10ml base lotion and apply to affected area, or use a cotton bud to apply the oil directly onto the centre of the bite or sting.*
German chamomile is both analgesic and anti-inflammatory, helping relieve the symptoms of bites and stings.
➸*Mix 2 drops with 10ml base lotion and apply to the affected area.*

LIFESTYLE

Go fragrance-free. There is evidence to suggest that mosquitoes are attracted to sweet, flowery smells so avoid perfumes and using highly fragranced sunscreens and body lotions.
Cover up. When there are mosquitoes wear long-sleeved shirts and trousers and cover the ankles and feet. There is evidence that mosquitoes are attracted to dark clothing, so light-coloured clothing may be preventative. Also, sleep under an insecticide-treated bednet in areas with malaria.
Burning citronella candles and incense can help to keep the immediate area clear of bugs.

OTHER THERAPIES

Homeopathic remedies can help reduce inflammation and calm allergic-like reactions.

NOSEBLEEDS

Nosebleeds are often caused by injury to the delicate blood vessels in the nose, often during or after a cold when there has been frequent nose blowing. Occasionally, nosebleeds are caused by a rise in blood pressure, so can be a concern for hypertension sufferers. Nosebleeds can also be more common in pregnancy due to hormonal changes.

HERBS

"Haemostatic", or styptic, herbs are herbs that contain substances to help stem bleeding. The herbs tighten and tone the tissues, which helps blood to coagulate more speedily and bleeding to cease. Styptic herbs can be used alongside any conventional treatments for the underlying causes of nosebleeds.

> " *Healing herbs can be used to tighten and tone tissues, which in turn helps the blood to coagulate and stems bleeding.* "

Yarrow is effective at stalling nosebleeds that occur often over a short period of time. See box, below. Avoid in pregnancy or with sensitivity to the *Asteraceae* plant family. Prolonged use can increase skin sensitivity.
➡ *Take 2–4ml tincture in a little water 3 times daily.*

Lady's mantle is "styptic" – able to stem bleeding. It does this by drying and toning tissues to halt the bleeding.
➡ *Infuse 2 tsp dried lady's mantle in 175ml (6fl oz) boiling water and apply to the nostril on a cotton wool plug.*

Herb Robert has a tightening and toning action that makes it a popular remedy for nosebleeds.
➡ *Infuse 2 tsp dried Herb Robert in 175ml (6fl oz) boiling water, gargle, and drink 90ml (3fl oz) when required. Or soak a cotton wool plug in the infusion and apply to the nostril.*

ESSENTIAL OILS

Therapeutic oils can be used to support the blood-clotting process.

Lemon is toning and antiseptic. It can help to speed up blood coagulation, in turn slowing down bleeding.
➡ *Make an ice-cold compress by adding 3 drops to a bowl of iced water, soak a flannel in the water, wring this out, and apply to the nose.*

LIFESTYLE

Dry rooms, for example where there is air conditioning or heating, can dry out the nasal membranes so they are more likely to bleed. Avoid over-heated rooms or too much air conditioning and try using a humidifier in dry rooms.

Chemicals in certain household products, as well as those in some nasal sprays, can make you more likely to experience nosebleeds.

Tip your head forward and pinch the fleshy tip of the nose continuously for 10–15 minutes to stem the bleeding. Seek urgent medical help if bleeding continues after 20 minutes.

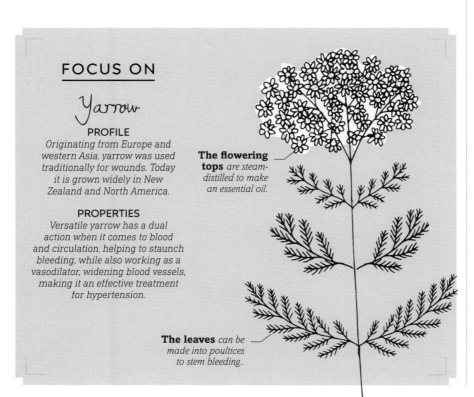

FOCUS ON

Yarrow

PROFILE
Originating from Europe and western Asia, yarrow was used traditionally for wounds. Today it is grown widely in New Zealand and North America.

PROPERTIES
Versatile yarrow has a dual action when it comes to blood and circulation, helping to staunch bleeding, while also working as a vasodilator, widening blood vessels, making it an effective treatment for hypertension.

The flowering tops *are steam-distilled to make an essential oil.*

The leaves *can be made into poultices to stem bleeding..*

SPLINTERS

A splinter trapped under the skin is an extremely common injury. However, although the damage is usually minor, a small splinter can cause a surprising amount of pain, and if it is not removed promptly and completely there is a risk of it becoming infected.

HERBS

Making a healing poultice with herbs can help to draw out the splinter, while anti-infective herbs can be used to help keep the wound clear of infection. Anti-inflammatory and healing herbs may also be beneficial to help the area recover once the splinter is removed.

Slippery elm powder has healing and soothing properties and can be used in a drawing paste to help draw out and remove splinters.

" Anti-infective herbs help to keep wounds free from infection, while anti-inflammatory herbs speed healing."

Marshmallow root powder heals internally and externally. It can be used as a drawing paste to remove splinters and to soothe the wound and promote healing. Take separately from other drugs as it may impede their absorption.

Plantain is toning, soothing, and antibacterial. See box, below.

➡ *Mix slippery elm or marshmallow root powder or plantain fresh leaves with boiled warm water, allow to cool, and apply as a poultice, or paste, to the affected area. Cover with a plaster or wound dressing, then leave the poultice in place for 24 hours to draw out the splinter.*

LIFESTYLE

Clean the area. Before you apply a healing poultice, wash your hands and the affected area with soap and water and gently pat the skin dry.

Use tweezers to remove the splinter once the herbs have drawn it out. Don't be tempted to squeeze out a splinter, as this may break it into smaller pieces that are harder to remove. Ideally use tweezers with a fine point, sterilizing them in boiling water or alcohol first.

Protect the damaged area. Aftercare of the affected site is important to avoid infection. Once the splinter has been removed, clean the area and apply a soothing ointment or salve such as hypercal or arnica, or an anti-infective such as myrrh. Keep the area covered with a bandage until it heals.

OTHER THERAPIES

Homeopathic remedies can help draw out stubborn splinters.

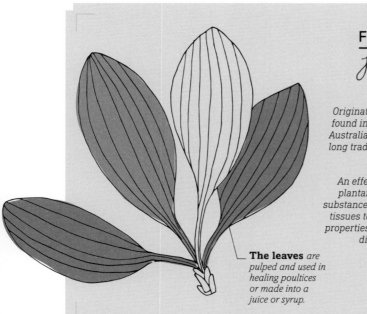

FOCUS ON
Plantain

PROFILE
Originating from Europe, but also found in Asia, North America, and Australia, this common weed has a long tradition as a first-aid remedy.

PROPERTIES
An effective anti-inflammatory, plantain also contains tannins, substances that help to knit damaged tissues together. Its antispasmodic properties can be useful for soothing digestive complaints.

The leaves *are pulped and used in healing poultices or made into a juice or syrup.*

GOOD ENOUGH TO EAT

As well as being an effective herbal remedy, the leaves of the marshmallow plant can be added to salads or cooked as a side vegetable.

REMEDY

Tissue-healing salve

Add **eucalyptus** and **peppermint**
essential oils to a combination of
elder leaf macerated oil and
St John's wort macerated oil
to create a healing salve.

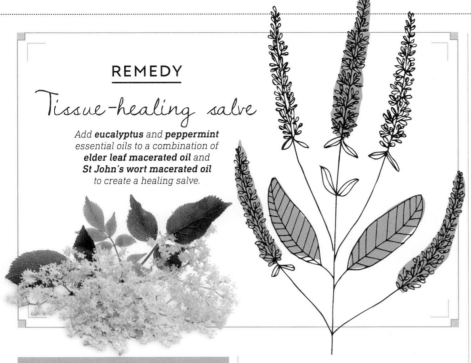

SPRAINS AND STRAINS

Injuries to muscles and ligaments
can occur during exercise, or result
from a fall or a knock. Sprains are
the result of torn, twisted, or
stretched ligaments, while strains
occur when muscles are torn or
stretched. Injuries can result in pain
and swelling and there may be
an inability to use or put weight
on the affected joint.

HERBS

Anti-inflammatory and toning herbs help
to reduce swelling, while analgesic herbs
and nerve tonics help to ease pain and
restore movement. Herbs can also be used
to promote the healing of damaged tissues.

Witch hazel is toning and cooling,
helping to reduce swelling.
➡*Infuse 2 tsp dried witch hazel in
175ml (6fl oz) boiling water. Use in a
cool compress.*

Elder leaf reduces swelling of sprains,
strains, and bruises. Use with St John's
wort, eucalyptus, and peppermint.
➡*See remedy, above.*
Comfrey is soothing and speeds up cell
regeneration and healing. Avoid on
infected or deep skin lesions. Seek
professional advice before internal use.
➡*Make a poultice with the crushed
leaves and apply regularly.*

ESSENTIAL OILS

These can be used to help reduce pain,
tenderness, and inflammation.

Peppermint is very cooling and can
help to reduce inflammation.
Marjoram is analgesic, helping to
reduce discomfort and pain.
Lavender has analgesic and anti-
inflammatory properties.
➡*Make a compress by adding 3 drops
of any of the above oils to a bowl of
ice-cold water, soak a flannel, then
wring it out and apply to the injury. Or
add 10 drops of any of the above oils
to 10ml arnica macerated oil and
gently massage into the injury.*

DEHYDRATION

The body is dehydrated if it loses
more fluid than it takes in, for example,
during strenuous exercise or on hot
days. Symptoms include thirst, dry
mouth, feeling lightheaded, tiredness,
and dark, strong-smelling urine.
Dehydration is also a common cause
of low blood pressure (see p148).

HERBS

Weak, refreshing infusions rehydrate and
soothing mucilaginous herbs restore.

Fennel seed is gently refreshing,
helping to clear, cleanse, and rehydrate.
Marshmallow leaf is rehydrating and
helps protect the mucous membranes.
Take separately from other medicines
as it may impede their absorption.
➡*Infuse 1 tsp of either of the above
dried herbs in 175ml (6fl oz) boiling
water and sip throughout the day.*
Ginger calms, soothes, and restores,
promoting healthy digestion and the
absorption of nutrients and water.
Avoid with peptic ulcers or gallstones.
➡*Infuse fresh slices in 175ml (6fl oz)
boiling water and sip during the day.*

WHAT TO AVOID

Psyllium husks while rehydrating, and
astringent herbs that contain tannins,
such as yarrow and agrimony, because
these can inhibit water absorption.

LIFESTYLE

Drink water throughout the day. If
exercising hard, have fluids on hand.
Sports drinks or rehydration solutions
can help to replace lost electrolytes
quickly in an emergency.
Use a spray bottle with tepid water
to prevent overheating.

FAINTING

Fainting is a sudden temporary loss of consciousness. It usually results in a fall, often preceded by weakness or unsteadiness. It can occur if blood pressure drops quickly or blood flow to the brain is reduced, or it can be linked to extreme stress or pain.

HERBS

Circulatory stimulants stabilize blood flow. Some herbs boost circulation to the head in particular to help reduce faintness.

Rosemary, a strengthening tonic, boosts circulation, especially to the head. Avoid therapeutic doses in pregnancy.
➽*Take 1–2ml tincture in a little water 3–4 times daily.*

Ginkgo biloba dilates blood vessels to boost circulation. Avoid in pregnancy, if breastfeeding, and with anticoagulant and antiplatelet medicines.
➽*Take a 66mg leaf extract tablet, equal to 3300mg whole leaf, 1–3 times daily.*

Ginger boosts circulation to peripheral areas. This warming herb works well with cinnamon. Avoid with peptic ulcers and gallstones.
➽*See remedy, below.*

ESSENTIAL OILS

Therapeutic oils can help to manage stress, fear, pain, or emotional shock.

Peppermint can stimulate the circulation and calm the nerves.

Neroli has a sedative action and calms states of anxiety.
➽*Add 2 drops of either of the above essential oils to a tissue or hankie to inhale, or dilute 2 drops of either oil in 10ml sunflower oil and apply to pulse points as required.*

LIFESTYLE

If you are standing in a crowded space, cross your legs and tighten the tummy muscles to avoid fainting. If you feel faint, lie down, or sit down with your head between your knees to restore blood flow to the brain. Rest for 20 to 30 minutes after fainting.

Stay hydrated to help normalize blood pressure and avoid fainting.

OTHER THERAPIES

Flower remedies. Keep some Rescue Remedy or Five Flower Remedy on hand to restore and revive.

Homeopathy offers a number of remedies to restore balance.

REMEDY

Strengthening infusion

*Infuse some freshly sliced **ginger root** in 175ml (6fl oz) boiling water, add a pinch of stimulating **cinnamon** to boost circulation and sip as needed.*

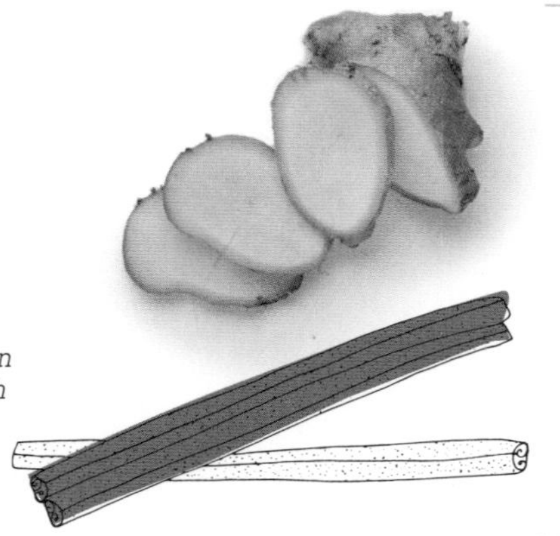

SUNSTROKE

If the body is severely overheated, its natural cooling mechanisms may become overwhelmed and fail, leading to sunstroke. Body temperature can rise dangerously, resulting in symptoms such as dizziness, nausea, exhaustion, and severe headache. The condition requires immediate treatment.

HERBS

Cooling, rehydrating, and sustaining herbs can be applied to stabilize the body once the acute symptoms of sunstroke have been treated. Herbs that regulate sweating, calm the heart rate, and help to relax the body may also be beneficial.

Lemon balm is cooling as it promotes perspiration and it is also calming for your body and mind. Avoid with hypothyroidism.
➽*Infuse 1–2 tsp dried lemon balm in 175ml (6fl oz) boiling water and drink as required.*

Aloe vera is cooling, soothing, and rehydrating. Avoid internal use during pregnancy.
➽*Drink 15ml juice twice daily, or dilute the gel or juice in water to use as a compress on your brow and neck.*

Peppermint helps to cool skin when applied topically. Avoid with oesophageal reflux.
➽*Infuse 1–2 tsp fresh or dried herb in 175ml (6fl oz) boiling water and use as a wash, or add to your bath.*

WHAT TO AVOID

Warming herbs such as cayenne, ginger, and cinnamon. Tinctures containing alcohol, which would not be suitable for dehydrated, overheated conditions.

ESSENTIAL OILS

Therapeutic oils can be used to help relieve headaches and nausea and lift exhaustion after excessive exposure to heat and sun.

Ginger can help to reduce any feelings of nausea.
➡ *Add 2 drops to a tissue and inhale, or add to a diffuser.*

Lavender relaxes, soothes, and cools.
➡ *Add 2 drops to 10ml aloe vera gel, mix well, and apply to any areas of over-exposed skin.*

LIFESTYLE

Rest is essential for recovery. Make yourself comfortable in a dark, cool room and allow time to recover.

Rehydration is important. Add ½ tsp of salt to a glass of water and sip frequently to rehydrate and equalize the balance of body fluids.

Have a tepid, but not cold, bath to help the body cool down. If the skin is also burned, add a generous handful of baking soda to soothe the pain.

OTHER THERAPIES

Homeopathic remedies can be used to treat feelings of weakness and exhaustion, helping to revive both the body and mind.

SHOCK

Physical shock, caused by factors such as severe fluid or blood loss, has a profound effect on the body, reducing blood flow, which can cause faintness, nausea, shaking, and pale, cold, clammy skin. Immediate action is needed to keep the person warm, and emergency treatment sought. Physical shock should not be confused with emotional shock (see p37), which can follow a traumatic event. Herbal remedies help to restore strength once physical symptoms are stabilized, and essential oils revive emotions after physical trauma.

HERBS

Following acute treatment for physical shock, blood-building herbs, circulatory stimulants, and tonic herbs help to restore circulation and blood levels to aid recovery.

Panax ginseng boosts circulation and eases symptoms such as a weak pulse or cold sweats. Avoid with nosebleeds, asthma, acute infections, hypertension, or stimulants such as caffeine.
➡ *Take a 500mg powdered herb capsule 4–6 times a day.*

Hawthorn is a heart tonic that is used to help strengthen heart contractions and boost circulation. Avoid with heart medications.
➡ *Take 3–5ml tincture in a little water 3 times daily.*

Nettle is a strengthening blood tonic, which helps to promote red blood cells and revitalize the body.
➡ *See remedy, below.*

ESSENTIAL OILS

Essential oils have properties that help to reduce the impact of physical shock on the mind and emotions. The therapeutic oils calm and rebalance, supporting a return to strength after physical shock.

Neroli is the "Rescue Remedy" of essential oils. It has a powerful sedative action and is therefore extremely relaxing.

Cedarwood is an extremely grounding oil and promotes feelings of courage and strength.

Cistus helps to balance emotions and is stimulating for the senses, helping you to reconnect with your body.
➡ *Add 2–3 drops of any of the above essential oils to a diffuser to inhale. Or mix 5 drops of any of the above oils into a bath dispersant and add to a warm, reviving bath.*

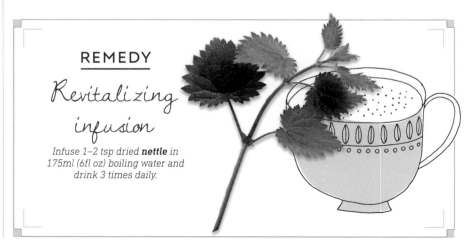

REMEDY

Revitalizing infusion

*Infuse 1–2 tsp dried **nettle** in 175ml (6fl oz) boiling water and drink 3 times daily.*

HOW TO MAKE
AN ESSENTIAL OIL COMPRESS

A compress infused with therapeutic oils can provide targeted local relief. Warm compresses can loosen tissues, relieving muscle tightness and stiffness, while cold compresses help reduce swelling and inflammation, soothe pain, and limit bruising.

Makes 1 compress

YOU WILL NEED

hot or cold water, enough
to fill a bowl

6 drops essential oil
– a single oil or a blend

large bowl

flannel

towel or cling film

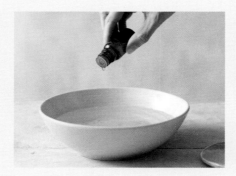

1 Fill a large bowl with either hot or cold water, depending on the instruction and the benefits required. Add the essential oil or blend of oils.

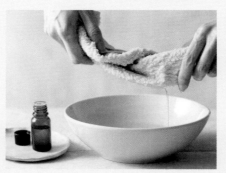

2 Place a flannel in the water and make sure it is soaked through. Remove the flannel and squeeze out the excess water.

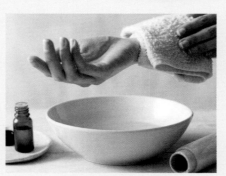

3 Apply the flannel to the affected area, then wrap the flannel with a towel or some cling film to insulate it. Leave the compress in place until the flannel has reached body temperature, then repeat the process 3 times.

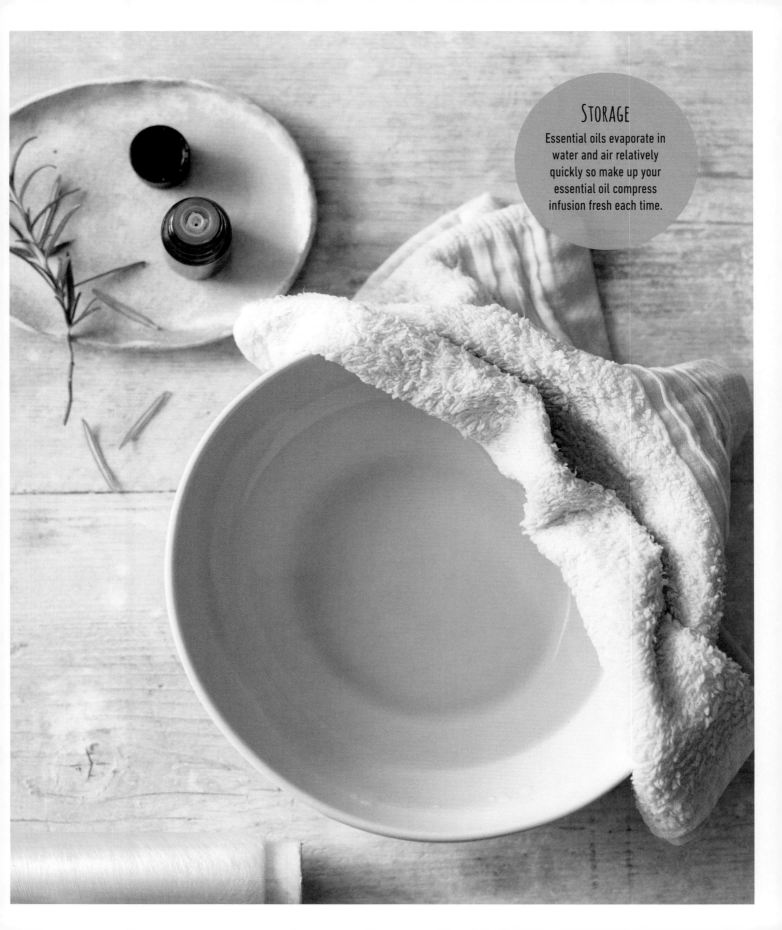

Storage

Essential oils evaporate in
water and air relatively
quickly so make up your
essential oil compress
infusion fresh each time.

CHARTS AND SAFETY GUIDELINES

Throughout the book, supplement doses are recommended and cautions given for individual herbs and essential oils. Here we explain why supplement doses can vary from official nutrient guidelines and give general safety advice on herbs and oils.

SUPPLEMENT DOSAGE CHART

Nutrient Reference Values (NRVs) express the minimum amounts that most healthy people need each day from food and supplements to avoid nutrient deficiencies. Where an NRV cannot be determined, regulators use Adequate Intake (AI) to make their recommendations. NRVs are adjusted for gender, age, and pregnancy. Values can also vary slightly in different countries. The table (right) provides a general guide only for healthy adults.

There are also Tolerable Upper Intake Levels (ULs) for some nutrients, which represent a recommended maximum daily intake generally considered safe. However, for various reasons, nutritionists may advise an ever higher dose in a supplemental range (SR). For example, a person may have problems absorbing a certain vitamin or mineral, or may have a chronic illness or dietary deficiency that has depleted levels of a nutrient. Some ailments respond well to short-term supplementation with higher levels of nutrients, which helps to restore balance. If in doubt about which nutrient or which amount is right for you, consult a nutritionist and/or doctor.

VITAMINS	NUTRIENT REFERENCE VALUE (NRV)	TOLERABLE UPPER INTAKE LEVEL (UL)	SUPPLEMENTAL RANGE (SR)
Vitamin A (retinol) and Beta-carotene	Vitamin A: 2664iu Beta-carotene*: 5-8mg	10,000iu Beta-carotene: ND	Vitamin A – 10,000iu+ Beta-carotene 10–40mg
Vitamin B1 – thiamine	1.1mg	ND	5–150mg
Vitamin B2 – riboflavin	1.4mg	ND	10–200mg
Vitamin B3 – niacin	16mg	35mg	100–1800mg as nicotinamide
Vitamin B5 – pantothenic acid	6mg	ND	20–500mg
Vitamin B6 – pyridoxine, pyridoxal-5-phosphate	1.4mg	100mg	10–200mg
Vitamin B7 - biotin	30mcg	ND	100–1000mcg
Vitamin B12 – cobalamin	2.5mcg	ND	300–5000mcg
Folic acid	200mcg	ND	500–5000mcg
Vitamin C – ascorbic acid	80mg	2000mg	250–2000mg
Vitamin D3 – cholecalciferol	200iu	4000iu	5000iu+
Vitamin E - alpha-tocopherol	17.9iu	1500iu	150–1200iu
Vitamin K – phylloquinone	75mcg	ND	70–150mcg
Bioflavonoids – citrin, hesperidin, rutin, quercetin, etc.	ND	ND	500–3000mg

Key for chart
ND = not determined
mg = milligrammes
mcg - microgrammes
iu = international unit (used for fat-soluble vitamins A, D, and E)
* There is no NRV for beta-carotene. Adequate intake is based on how much vitamin A equivalent is supplied.

MINERALS	NUTRIENT REFERENCE VALUE (NRV)	TOLERABLE UPPER INTAKE LEVEL (UL)	SUPPLEMENTAL RANGE (SR)
Calcium	800mg	2500mg	1000–2500mg
Chromium	40mcg	ND	100–600mcg
Copper	1mg	10mg	2–10mg (metabolism of copper is highly individual)
Iodine	150mcg	1100mcg	100–1000mcg
Iron	14mg	45mg	15–50mg+
Magnesium	375mg	350mg	300–800mg
Manganese	2mg	11mg	2–20mg
Molybdenum	50mcg	2000mcg	100–1000mcg
Phosphorus	800mg	4000mg	400–3000mg
Potassium	2g	ND	3–8g
Selenium	55mcg	400mcg	200–800mcg
Zinc	10mg	40mg	10–70mg

CONVERSIONS

A range of measures are used in the book for herbal preparations and essential oils. You can use the conversions below if preferred.

CONVERTING ML TO DROPS FOR TINCTURES AND OILS
1ml = 20 drops
2ml = 40 drops
3ml = 60 drops
4ml = 80 drops

CONVERTING ML TO TSP/TBSP FOR BASE OILS
10ml = 2 tsp
15ml = 1 tbsp
30ml = 2 tbsp
100ml = 3½fl oz

USING HERBS SAFELY

Most herbs can be used safely, but there are times when certain herbs should be avoided. To use herbs safely, follow the guidelines and dosage instructions; if in doubt, consult a qualified herbalist and/or doctor. Cautions on individual herbs are given in the book.

DURING PREGNANCY AND WHEN BREASTFEEDING
Medicinal herbs should be avoided in the first three months unless advised by a qualified herbal practitioner and agreed by a doctor. When pregnant or breastfeeding, some herbs should not be ingested, as advised in the book.

FOR BABIES AND CHILDREN
Some restrictions apply under the age of 12. The Children's section has safe herbs for babies and young children, with age limits where needed. Consult a qualifed herbalist before giving herbs to babies and children.

CONTRAINDICATIONS
Herbal remedies can be helpful for many chronic conditions, including asthma, cardiovascular disease, and diabetes, and help to counter the side effects of drugs. By restoring balance they can help to reduce high doses of medication. But certain herbs are contraindicated with some medications. If taking prescribed or over-the counter medicine for a condition, consult your doctor and/or a qualified medical herbalist before taking herbs.

USING ESSENTIAL OILS SAFELY

Essential oils are concentrated so need diluting in a base oil or other dispersant to avoid irritation. Extra care is needed around the eyes and mouth, and oils should not be ingested. Some restrictions apply, as outlined below. Cautions on individual oils are given in the book.

DURING PREGNANCY
Avoid using sage, hyssop, basil, and camphor during pregnancy. In the second and third trimesters, oils especially recommended are bergamot, Roman chamomile, eucalyptus, geranium, ginger, grapefruit, lavender, lemon, lemongrass, lime, mandarin, neroli, patchouli, petitgrain, rose otto, rosewood, sandalwood, sweet orange, tea tree, and ylang ylang.

WITH EPILEPSY
Rosemary, sage, hyssop, and camphor are not recommended with epilepsy because they may trigger seizures. Other oils can indirectly improve epilepsy by removing triggers such as stress. Reactions to oils can vary so consult a qualified aromatherapist and your doctor before using oils with epilepsy.

FOR BABIES AND CHILDREN
Caution should be taken using essential oils on babies and children to avoid irritating their senstive skin. Gentle oils such as lavender, Roman chamomile, and mandarin are best, used well diluted, or in a diffuser or inhalation.

INDEX

RESOURCES

Neal's Yard Remedies
www.nealsyardremedies.com
Supplier of essential oils and herbs. For courses in herbal medicine and aromatherapy, call 020 3119 5904, or email: courses@nealsyardremedies.com

G. Baldwin & Co
www.baldwins.co.uk
Supplier of herbs and essential oils.

The National Institute of Medical Herbalists
www.nimh.org.uk

Aromatherapy Trade Council
www.a-t-c.org.uk
Provides information and news on essential oils.

International Federation of Professional Aromatherapists
www.ifparoma.org
Provides a register of qualified aromatherapists.

British Association for Applied Nutrition & Nutritional Therapy
www.bant.org.uk

British Acupuncture Council
www.acupuncture.org.uk

British Homeopathic Association
www.britishhomeopathic.org

British Association for Counselling and Psychotherapy
www.bacp.co.uk

Society of Homeopaths
www.homeopathy-soh.org

The Dispensary
www.thedispensary.org.uk

Natural Health News
www.naturalhealthnews.uk

ACKNOWLEDGMENTS

The authors at Neal's Yard Remedies would like to thank: our great editor, Claire Cross from DK, who continues to be a delight to work with. All of our teachers who have helped to pass on their passion and expertise for natural health. Romy Fraser, founder of Neal's Yard Remedies, and Peter Kindersley who took up the baton of ownership helping to keep herbal remedies and natural health alive and thriving and available to all.

DK would like to thank: the great team at Neal's Yard Remedies for their expertise and guidance throughout.

Photography Tara Fisher
Food styling Maude Eden and Shambala Fisher
Photoshoot prop styling Linda Berlin
Illustration Ryn Frank
Proofreading Claire Wedderburn-Maxwell
Indexing Hilary Bird